D1109800

SOCIAL ASPECTS OF OBESITY

Culture and Ecology of Food and Nutrition

A series edited by *Harriet V. Kuhnlein*, McGill University, Quebec, Canada; *Peter L. Pellet*, University of Massachusetts; and *Christine S. Wilson*, Annapolis, Maryland

---

Volume 1
Social Aspects of Obesity
Edited by Igor de Garine and Nancy J. Pollock

This book is part of a series. The publisher will accept continuation orders which may be cancelled at any time and which provide for automatic billing and shipping of each title in the series upon publication. Please write for details.

SOCIAL ASPECTS OF OBESITY

Edited by

Igor de Garine
*Centre National
de la Recherche Scientifique
Lasseube, France*

and

Nancy J. Pollock
*Victoria University
Wellington, New Zealand*

Gordon and Breach Publishers

Australia   Austria   China   France   Germany   India   Japan
Luxembourg   Malaysia   Netherlands   Russia   Singapore   Switzerland
Thailand   United Kingdom   United States

3 Boulevard Royal
L–2449 Luxembourg

British Library Cataloguing in Publication Data

Social Aspects of Obesity. – (Culture &
Ecology of Food & Nutrition, ISSN 1024–5316; Vol.1)
  I. Garine, I. De   II. Pollock, Nancy J.
  III. Series
  616.398

    ISBN 2–88449–185–6 (hardcover)
          2–88449–186–4 (softcover)

Cover photograph courtesy of James R. Bindon.

CONTENTS

Contents

INTRODUCTION TO THE SERIES

Volumes in this series will reflect the interests of professional nutritional anthropologists, social nutritionists and other food, health and behavioral scientists, together with agricultural specialists, economists and program and planning officers, matching the breadth and range of subjects in the parent journal, *Ecology of Food and Nutrition*. Book topics may include quantitative and qualitative assessments of diets; resource utilization; ethnographies of diet in their cultural and ecologic settings, together with their health and policy implications; food behaviors and behavioral effects of eating; cultural, ecologic, economic or political constraints on diet and nutrition and local techniques to counter them; uses and nutrient composition of indigenous foods; statistical and other methods of study, for example, of health status, diet practices, food production, use and adequacy. Geographic distributions of foods and non-nutritive ingestants and their health consequences are of interest, as are traditional diets and changes in them. Other desirable themes for publication are nutritionally valuable indigenous foods and economically viable preparation practices for specific groups such as infant feeding and weaning, pregnant and lactating women and the elderly; growth; food storage practices, losses and waste; comparative diet and lifestyle studies of different groups within the same environment. Interactions among diet, environmental stress such as disease, parasitic infections and health are suitable subjects, as are diet and clinical disease. We encourage manuscripts with holistic, cross-disciplinary and cross-cultural study approaches to food and nutrition as they affect human beings.

PREFACE

Observing overweight and its pathological consequences has been a focus for western scientists over several decades. The diagnosis is clearly negative. In 1977, Garrow and Warwick reflected the general consensus when they wrote: "Obesity is common enough to constitute one of the most important medical and public health problems of our time, whether we judge its importance by shorter expectation of life, increased morbidity or costs to the community in terms of both money and anxiety."

Food and body shape are highly symbolic objects for which emotional as well as scientific factors have to be taken into account. Only recently has "moderate fatness" been granted some positive values, such as those demonstrated in an article "The good body: When big is better" (Cassidy, 1991). This new value is probably due to intellectual fashion, but is also the result of looking outside western urban civilization and discarding some of its sociocentrism. In a context of food uncertainty, storing energy in the form of fat has indisputable adaptive consequences including successful reproduction.

There are levels at which overweight has proven negative, especially when assessed in terms of biological consequences according to a variable hierarchy of criteria. In western culture it also has psychopathological consequences. It is likely that the general attitudes towards fatness and obesity by a human group have some psychological and, possibly, biological implications.

The human being is a seasonal animal. Nutritional status is linked to variations in food supply, which still operate in rural areas and developing countries. In the rather egalitarian socioeconomic framework of traditional societies, overweight—usually mild—is easily gotten rid of. It is not necessarily linked to class privileges, nor is it the result of a series of material and psychological events in a life story leading, in urban industrialized countries, to a culturally stigmatized pathological state which is very difficult to overcome.

Today it is possible for anyone who has the financial means to consume any type of food in any quantity, at any time of the year, escaping ecological constraints and social rules. As Stini (1981) remarks, man's ability to store fat as a nutrient reserve had an interest for a species periodically submitted to nutritional stress. One wonders if this feature is still adaptative when considering the overfed, sedentary western urbanite. Fischler (1979) speaks of "gastro-anomie" and of the anxiety linked to it. In line with the human tendency to play with biological adaptation in order to satisfy cultural wants, which are not totally attuned to optimal physical needs, western civilization has developed an ideal of body shape which is almost impossible to achieve according to the material and psychosocial conditions of modern urban life. Seeking the sinewy silhouette of hunter-gatherers in western societies is as paradoxical as attempting to make women obese—and untransportable—among the nomads of the Sahara.

As Cassidy (1991) remarked, going beyond the message of fat: "Look how much abundance I have. . . " to a more etheric model. . . "I'm so safe I can afford to ignore abundance. . . " is a very sophisticated and strong way of demonstrating "distinction" in Bourdieu's sense (1979), that results in a rather psychopathological attitude towards overweight. As Aimez (1979) wrote, ". . . our society is displaying a feeling of acute guilt in relation to eating. . . bulimia, anorexia, and toxicomania flourish. . . ." Far from being genuine in the human population, as it appears from historical records and observation of non-western societies, this attitude may be linked to historical factors in the leading cultures of northern Europe. Puritanism and its inhibiting attitudes towards sex and food, expressed by a fat, permissive body, are likely to underlie the view that thin is beautiful. This concern is at stake when demonstrating spirituality, efficiency and high socioeconomic status in a thin, ascetic body. Then overweight is regarded in a disapproving manner.

Fear of body fat is a feature of industrialized urban modern civilization. It reaches obsessional levels in northern hemisphere Protestant cultures, though it is milder in southern European Catholic countries. This fear has been spread worldwide by the dominant style of life of the west, backed by its media monopoly. Better information on overweight—treating it as a complex biological, psychological and social phenomenon, and considering it as a "total social fact" (Mauss, 1900 [1923]) that involves biological, psychological and socio-cultural aspects—may help to develop rational attitudes toward it and diminish the heavy psychological stress that it incurs in western societies. Such a strategy might be universally beneficial.

Hopefully, since it looks at overweight in a pluridisciplinary manner across a range of cultures, this book will make a contribution to that end.

Igor de Garine

REFERENCES

Aimez, P. 1979. Psychopathologie de l'alimentation quotidienne. *Communications. Paris. Editions du Seuil* **31**, 93–107.

Bourdieu, P. 1979. *La distinction—critique sociale du jugement.* Paris. Editions de Minuit.

✗Cassidy, C. 1991. The good body. When big is better. *Medical Anthropology* **13**, 181–213.

Fischler, C. 1979. Gastro-nomie et gastro-anomie. *Communications. Paris. Editions du Seuil* **31**, 189–210.

Garrow, J.S., and P. Warwick 1977. Diet and obesity. In J. Yudkin (ed.), *Diet of Man—Needs and Wants.* Applied Sciences Publication, London, pp. 127–144.

Mauss, M. 1900 [1923]. *Essai sur le don—forme et raison de l'échange dans les sociétés archaiques. Sociologie et Anthropologie,* Presses Universitaires de France, Paris, pp. 144–273. [First published in *Année sociologique* 1, 1923–1924].

Stini, W.A. 1981. Evolutionary aspects of human body composition. *Karger Gazette* **42, 43**, 1–4.

INTRODUCTION

An Overview of Obesity Issues
Across Several Cultures

A variety of issues associated with the social aspects of fatness and obesity are presented in the following articles. The aim is to broaden the viewpoint on obesity to include a number of social and cultural features, including rituals of fattening. Case studies such as those on the Sumo wrestlers of Japan (Hattori, chapter 2) or the Annang of Nigeria (Brink, chapter 4) show that a large body size is not only acceptable among some populations, but fattening practices are socially supported to ensure the development of large bodies. More specifically, large body size may bring prestige. Furthermore, the credit accrues to the whole group supporting the fattening practice, rather than to an individual.

Body size is considered here within a wider concept of body image. Both cultural factors and biological factors are included. A fundamental premise of the papers presented here is that the body is part of a society's cultural order. Local tenets of social and cultural order incorporate aspects of body image. The shape of particular bodies and the messages they convey are part of a larger value system that is a distinctive feature of each society. The cultural value system may include enlarging the body, or reducing its size. The means by which a particular body shape is attained and maintained are also culturally specified.

The body may have been lost to sociology in the latter's rejection of biological arguments, but Turner's (1984) reexamination of the relationship between the body and the mind has turned around the idea put forward by Hobbes that considered the mind to have greater significance than the flesh. Turner considers the body both as symbol and a physical entity. He places the body at the centre of the environment and of political struggles, where the socially interpreted body becomes a means of self-identification. Restraints, whether of the interior body through discipline or by representation of the exterior body in social space, are a key feature of his argument.

When we look at the body as shaped according to cultural norms, rather than according to some external criteria, we must consider how the delimitations of large body size—and small body size—fit within the concept of obesity as designated by western life statistics and medical criteria. Obesity as a concept is a dimension of body image that is formulated around a particular society's considerations of acceptable body size. It is thus an anthropological and sociological topic as well as a psychological one, though much of the written material on obesity in western societies stems from psychological and medical concerns rather than sociological ones (see Beller, 1977; Mann, 1974 for overviews of the broader social and medical approaches). As Turner argues in his plea for reinstatement of the body in the sociology of knowledge, "dietary management has emerged out of a theology of the flesh through a moralistic medicine, and has established itself as a science of the efficient body" (1984:3). This focus by western societies on control of the body as a demonstration of the superiority of the intellect, mind over matter, has caused us to lose sight of the place of body image in our value systems.

The word "obesity" in English has come to have strong negative overtones through the development of philosophical tenets that support the idea that the flesh must be controlled by the spirit, so regulation of diet is a means of demonstrating control by the mind over the body. Where such control is not exercised, a person is labelled as obese, or out of control. "Obesity is the effect of language and ideas on our bodies" (Turner, 1984:174).

The western idea of obesity reflects the conflict between desires and control, where the latter is expected to predominate over the former. The dilemma lies in a natural propensity to eat to fuel the system, and an unnaturally imposed system of control to reach a target body image established in a particular cultural and social context. The body is shaped according to culturally accepted principles that are enacted in attempts to make it fit societal norms or bear the brunt of negative comments. A contradiction thus arises between the body as a natural entity and the body as a cultural entity; as Turner reminds us, "our bodies are a natural environment while also being socially constituted" (1984:7).

In other societies such dichotomies as mind/body, desire/control and nature/culture are not as clearcut. The body may be at once both a substantive and symbolic entity, and a natural entity subject to cultural prescriptions. In particular the body is a social rather than an individual entity, where the collective consciousness is the prevailing factor.

The chapters that follow draw attention to aspects of obesity that are not very apparent in the literature. They draw on case material from societies in all five continents and thus afford opportunity for cross-cultural comparisons. Much of the previous work has centered on British and American research findings. Case studies in this book that come from non-western societies clearly illustrate that western biological and medical criteria for obesity are inappropriate if they are used without reference to their cultural contexts. Other case studies, such as those from Japan and Europe, pose the dilemma faced by some subsets of societies that choose vegetarianism (Ossipow, chapter 7) or Sumo wrestling as their life-style, or find the wider cultural norm too limiting (van Otterloo, chapter 6; Charzewska, chapter 10; Leonetti et al., chapter 11).

Societies undergoing a rapid introduction to consumer goods, such as Malaya, Nauru and Samoa (Wilson, chapter 12; Pollock, chapter 5; Bindon, chapter 13; Greksa, chapter 14) are caught between traditional values that support a particular body shape and modern medical concerns about diseases associated with so-called overweight. It is abundantly clear in Teti's article on Calabrian rituals (chapter 1) that some of these concerns, which have become obsessive in parts of the western world, are overridden by local customs and celebrations. In Italy, as in Nauru, Samoa and Nigeria, ecological factors such as natural disasters have been a contributory factor to fattening procedures in the past, if not as much so today.

The place of body size within concepts of body image is dealt with by the authors of these chapters at various levels. Some address the difficulties of applying the generalized concepts of obesity and overweight or body fatness to particular societies, while others attempt to place their case studies first within a broader cultural framework for that society, and then into the general framework of obesity and body image. Measurement against norms of ideal body size, health risks associated with deviation from those norms, and genetic proscriptions are three significant areas that loom large in the literature and are addressed here. The papers on fattening practices serve to demonstrate how we need a broader social image than that extant in western thinking if we are to appreciate fully the cultural significance of such rituals. All the chapters pick up the medical versus the social concerns in the process of examining food intake and socioeconomic factors that contribute to body image and social order.

Let us examine some of the main topics associated with obesity in the literature in order to highlight the contribution this volume makes to this growing area of debate.

Fattening Processes

Social and cultural processes that ensure certain sectors of a population become large-bodied are underreported in the literature. Where such events are described, they have been included within coming-of-age rituals or as part of the social process of setting apart certain sectors of the community such as the upper hierarchy. Chiefs and chiefly children may be fed the bounty of the land as a symbol of the health and well-being of the community. For example, throughout Polynesia and in Fiji and parts of Micronesia high-ranking people received the best food and the greatest abundance. Captain Cook's journals describe the scene of a chief being fed many taros and fish and puddings, as well as receiving turtle and the best fish caught (Beaglehole, 1962). Cook was amazed by this procedure, but others, notably missionaries, viewed it in a more derogatory light, labelling it profligatory or the height of debauchery (Ellis, 1831). Not only did they view food in a different light from Polynesians, but they carried this difference through into their own values of body size. Such attitudes encompass the difference in values between the British view of the body and food, and those held elsewhere in the world even in the late eighteenth century.

De Garine (chapter 3), Pollock (chapter 5), and Brink (chapter 4) have underlined that such fattening processes were an ecological mechanism to ensure the survival of the chiefly sector through times of food scarcity. In that sense fattening had both a biological and a cultural purpose. We can analyse it as providing nourishment which can be drawn upon during times of drought and famine, and thus it not only enabled the fattened women and men to survive to reproduce, but supported the whole group's continuity, as Brink (chapter 4) has argued for the Mbobo.

Whether that biological outcome was the most important for those practicing such fattening processes is hard to assess. Most of the accounts also stress the attribute of beauty associated with a large, well covered body. As Ishige (chapter 16) has illustrated, in Japanese society a plump body shape was adulated in the literature and painting; this changed only in 1953 with the arrival of American influence, including a new body image.

Thus, fattened individuals became the show-pieces of their society. Their body size was a notable asset, and gave them high status, as Prinz (chapter 15) noted for the Azande men. In the Pacific it is hard to unravel the fattening process from that of lightening the skin, both of which contributed to the local view of beauty (Pollock, chapter 5). Thus, a number of people of large girth in any society may have conveyed messages other than those of direct survival. They were fed with whatever food was available to enhance their high status, and that status also required that they take on large body size. They represented a picture of strength and beauty, as well as an achieved status denied to other sectors of the population (Teti, chapter 1). So, the fattening process should be included as part of the adornment process as well as part of biological survival.

This picture of fattened bodies as beautiful conflicts directly with the western body image that lauds a slim body. Attempts to slim and thus to reach the ideal body image in Holland, as documented by van Otterloo (chapter 6), represent the counterside, the alternative view of beauty that is widespread in western cultures. Dutch women, particularly those in the middle class, made stringent efforts to attain a slim body for themselves and their children. They were more successful, according to van Otterloo, than their working-class counterparts because the latter had less time to devote to caring for their body size; therefore, they became fatter than they wanted to be.

A third dimension of these fattening processes was the ritual events that ensured the feeding of selected individuals by others either in public or in extreme secrecy. Van Gennep's (1960) three stages of separation, seclusion, and reintegration may be applied to these rituals. The participants emerge in full beauty and strength to be admired by the larger public. Brink's analysis of the Fattening Room for the Annang (chapter 4) stresses the importance of learning during the seclusion phase, so that the participants in that culture emerged as ritual specialists.

Thus, the fattening process has a strong symbolic dimension. Its significance may be designated for women—as in the case of Nauru and the Annang—for men—as in the case of the Massa and the Japanese Sumo wrestler—or for both sexes—as in the case of Tahiti. In all these instances selected persons, or a designated group, undergo the fattening process in order to achieve a given body image. These bodies then become the means by which a series of messages are conveyed to other people of that society and beyond. That a well-rounded body is a sign of strength or beauty is in the eye of the beholder. Such fattened bodies are as much art objects as they are reproductive members of society. Beauty and health are two reasons given for holding a particular body image. The body is a means of conveying aspects of group identity.

Measures of Obesity

A number of different measures to define obesity have been proposed in the literature. These enable a numerical value to be assigned against which it is possible to assess whether a particular body is over- or undersized. Body mass index (BMI) has been the value most widely used in the United States and Britain; this correlates weight in kg with height in cm squared to yield a figure somewhere between 20 and 30 as a desirable weight/height ratio for western adults. The Quetelet and skinfold thickness measures have been used similarly to indicate the amount of fat on a body. More recently waist-to-hip ratio has been proposed as a better measure of body size, with different standards for men and women (Bray, 1979). Lean body mass is also considered a better measure of the health risks associated with fatness. Ashwell, Cole and Dixon's summary of all these measures (1985) concludes that intra-abdominal fat can be correlated with waist-to-hip circumference to yield a measure with the greatest reliability.

Many workers are beginning to question these measures. Some are concerned about methodological issues such as the replicability of measurements from person to person or about the scale, while others question the end uses for which these measures are devised. One of the major concerns is whether they are meant to establish an average or an ideal body size. Since they are derived from select groups of participants, not from a random selection of any given population—if that were possible—they can be labelled an average only of those sampled.

Keys et al. (1972) have argued that average values are not appropriate for all populations because body size changes over a lifespan. In a later paper, Keys (1980) warned that we cannot assume relative body weight is a reliable measure of fatness and obesity, as many other factors need to be taken into account.

Beller (1977) preferred to use relative rather than absolute measures in her discussion of the concepts of Fat and Thin, mainly pertaining to western societies. She and others have used Sheldon's somatotypes, endomorph, ectomorph and mesomorph, in their discussions of how western society has viewed fat and thin bodies over time, and correlations of these body types with personality types. Whichever measure a specific researcher espouses, it can be relative only to a particular population, since a large number of environmental and genetic variables must also be considered, as discussed below. As Beller (1977) has noted, environmental factors raised by Roberts (1953), such as heat and sunlight, along with genetic factors, have long been considered to influence body shape.

Parizkova's paper in this volume (chapter 9) challenges the issue of whether American measures can be applied to the Czech population. She suggests that even using a number of the measures combined only serves to complicate rather than clarify the picture. Her concern is to show how body fat patterns change during a person's lifetime, differentiating between men and women. But the measures developed in western societies are not adequate to assess a person at these different age levels. They are too culturally restrictive.

Health Risks

Measures of obesity have been derived and used as indicators of the risks of certain diseases or of mortality. Such studies have sought to establish a correlation between a particular BMI or Quetelet index and the risks of that person suffering coronary heart disease, hypertension and associated diseases such as diabetes mellitus. Keen focus on such associations has led to collaborative work between medical researchers, physical anthropologists and actuaries. Their focus has been mainly on western populations.

Large body size was identified as a risk to survival in 1911 when the first life insurance data were being compiled. These studies established the baseline for acceptable versus nonacceptable standards of body size in both the United States and Great Britain (Bray, 1979). As a result, standard average tables have become established that correlate height with weight.

Bray (1979) lists height/weight or BMI (W/H squared), subscapular skinfold, or circumference at waist as preferred measures of obesity. He suggests a BMI of 30 is a significant measure of excessive mortality. Bray's measures are favoured as absolute statements of risk for noninfectious diseases.

With increased concern about anorexia nervosa in western societies, a disease associated with body image, Beere (1990) has compiled a handbook of tests and measures of self-perception of body size "to provide the respondent with an opportunity to report their perceptions of their body size." One such study analysed responses to a questionnaire to assess attitudes toward weight, appearance, eating and fitness in families of persons with anorexia nervosa in New Zealand (Hall, Liebrich and Walkey, 1983). Such attitudinal measures are used as indicators for both patient and doctor to assess how far outside the accepted norm a person's particular body image is. The very existence of such overall measures may be as much the cause as it is part of the treatment of such psycho-medical illnesses associated with body image.

These average values of association between body size and health risk have been found to be flawed (Keys et al., 1972). Life insurance statistics are overstated, according to Keys (1980) and Cahnman (1968), since no significant correlation between death and high body weight has been found. So we cannot conclude that obesity is a cause of increased mortality. Nor is there a correlation between coronary heart disease and overweight. Keys and Cahnman see the arguments against obesity stemming from upper- and middle-class values which have led to discrimination against obese girls, in whom obesity is seen as a defect. To emphasize this alternative view, Keys argues that "the best prospect for avoiding early death is to be somewhat above the average in relative weight" (1980:304).

Obesity has even become a disease itself, not just a precursor of one. As the literature has burgeoned and western society becomes more phobic about controls over body size, so medical researchers have identified a number of different types of risk which they use to admonish individuals to lose weight (Trowell and Burkitt, 1981). A number of western or noninfectious diseases are cited as likely to befall overweight individuals.

Obesity and overweight are most frequently associated with coronary heart disease, hypertension, and diabetes (Bray, 1979). Scrimshaw and Dietz have also supported this argument (see chapter 8). Van Itallie (1986) has shown that obesity has adverse effects on health and longevity for some populations in the United States. Gober and Stemmermann (1981) have argued that Hawaiians have a higher rate of coronary heart disease than Japanese living in Hawaii because of their sporadic heavy feeding and low physical activity, both of which contribute to their being overweight. Prior (1976) made a similar argument for New Zealand Maori and Cook Islands populations, and Zimmet and Whitehouse (1981) have pinpointed obesity as a disease factor that is particularly associated with diabetes and cardiovascular disease in Pacific Island populations.

However, a number of authors have contested this association between obesity and western diseases. Andres (1980) suggests that the risks of mortality associated with obesity have been overemphasized; rather we need clarification, particularly by increasing our understanding of mild to moderate obesity (1980:385). Vague (1956), too, has identified more specific issues, namely gender and physiology, in his argument that obesity in males is more likely to lead to metabolic disturbance than obesity in females. Hallstrom and Noppa (1981) have concluded from their studies that there is no significant difference between the obese and the non-obese with regard to susceptibility to disease.

In this volume Parizkova (chapter 9) considers overweight a problem for Polish children, who are then encouraged to attend "fat camps." Van Otterloo recognizes that her Dutch women are trapped by these medical correlates of large body size, but have neither the means to eat better nor to exercise more and thus attain the slim image upheld by the wider society.

So it appears that there is no clear evidence that obesity is the single direct cause of death, even in U.S. populations where much of this work has been carried out. Rather, a number of related factors must be isolated that may be indicative of some relationship between body size and health risk. Physiological factors, growth patterns, genetic predispositions and a familial base to obesity may all predispose an individual to suffer one or more of these diseases. And food intake and exercise or energy output are strongly implicated. Some of the arguments are based on contemporary features, while others are rationalized in terms of adaptation and modernization arguments.

Certain *physiological* factors have been identified as associated with obesity. In some populations obesity lessens the response to diet-induced thermogenesis (Jaquiers, 1987), while fat patterning in the Papua New Guinea population has been found to change most in young people, with females being fatter than males (Norgan, 1987). Björntop and Zimmet (1979) found that fat cell enlargement occurred in their Tuvalu sample, a Polynesian population.

A number of studies, such as that by Rolland-Cachera and Bellisle

(1986) have concluded that there is no correlation between adiposity and food intake.

In this volume Leonetti et al. (chapter 11) have examined the association between levels of adrenaline and adipose tissue regulation and levels of educational achievement in Japanese-American students. They concluded that higher levels of adrenaline may represent an adaptive condition expressed in adipose tissue regulation; therefore, high adrenaline is associated with educational success, while low adrenaline may be associated with obesity and lower educational achievement.

Studies of *growth patterns* in particular populations have shown that in western societies upper class children tend to be fatter but become leaner as they become adults, while children from lower socioeconomic classes are thinner as children but tend to become fatter in later life (Baecke et al., 1983; Bray, 1979; Cockington, 1980; Stunkard et al., 1972). Bindon and Pelletier (1986) and other researchers have recorded the rapid growth of Samoan babies in their first year, particularly those who were bottlefed. These infants deposited fat cells which might be hard to lose later in life. Huenemann et al. (1966) found in their study of U.S. teenagers that food practices were only one factor associated with obesity.

Parizkova (chapter 9) has noted the importance of the amount of fat in the Czech population over stages of growth from childhood to adulthood. She concludes that obesity in industrial countries is a problem at all ages, not only for health, but for social and cultural reasons. In an earlier paper (1986) she had noted that malnutrition in the early years can lead to later obesity if the nutritional status of the population improves. Thus, growth patterns need to be monitored within a range of social factors affecting obesity.

Associations between obesity and *reduced fertility* have been documented by Frisch and MaArthur (1974). They observed that since the menstrual cycle decreases with rapid weight loss and emotional stress, critical body weight is necessary for maintenance of menstruation. Any abnormal increase or decrease in body fat can reduce the menstrual flow. Even though this argument is controversial, it needs to be taken into account, along with genetic arguments, when attempting to reassess the reproductive rates of populations for which a good supply of body fat has been considered adaptive both to irregular supplies of food and to climatic conditions. This holds true particularly in the tropics, in Pacific societies such as Nauru and Samoa (Pollock, chapter 5; Bindon, chapter 13).

Genetic arguments have been used to account for differences in body size between populations. Neel (1962) proposed a much-cited argument that some populations have a particular genotype for diabetes mellitus which was particularly efficient in the release of insulin in times of an abundant food supply. Large body size made this propensity even more efficient. This hypothesis has become known as the thrifty gene theory, as the gene was believed to allow these populations to maintain a store of fat over times of food scarcity to draw on when needed. But with population increase, decline in the standard of living and food types available, and a more regular supermarket-type food supply, Neel argued that a so-called thrifty genotype is no longer useful. Rather, some populations have a high rate of obesity because of this particular diabetes mellitus genotype. Thus, for Neel obesity is the result of a genetic predisposition to diabetes, and not the cause of diabetes, as others have argued.

Bindon (chapter 13) uses the thrifty genotype argument to account for obesity in the Samoan population. He suggests that there were good reasons for a genetic predisposition for obesity in the past when the food supply was irregular; therefore, thrifty genes may have served this population well, enabling them to survive periods of food shortage and to reproduce. But now that the food supply has become regular, that genetic predisposition is proving a detriment to health. His detailed study of physiological factors associated with diet in four Samoan communities has shown that females are more at risk of developing obesity than males. Thus, he considers the genetic factor to be stronger for women than for men.

Cassidy's (1992) adaptation argument includes tallness, boniness, muscularity and fattiness within her concept of "bigness." She also opposes obese to fat in order to show why bigness can be idealized and preferred, acting as symbols of power. She relies heavily on literature from the United States and the western world to support her argument that "fat is associated with the trappings of social power" (1992:201). The power message overrides biological adaptation because it allows those immersed in abundance to ignore survival issues (1992:203). But underlying that power is a strong adaptation which is both biological and cultural.

The key factor in these arguments for a genetic case for obesity is the association between this thrifty gene and modern life-style. An intensive study of human biological factors in four Samoan communities has relied on the argument that modernization has rendered the thrifty gene deleterious (Baker, Hanna and Baker, 1986). Bindon's study, which was part of that larger project (and Pelletier, 1986; chapter 13, this volume), suggests changes to wage labour and purchased food contribute to a marked degree of obesity in Samoans. Greksa's work (see chapter 14), which was part of the same study, focuses on energy use. He found that Samoans decreased their occupational energy expenditure with modernisation, while they increased their energy intake. This was particularly notable for modern American Samoans. Input is exceeding energy output now that a supermarket array of foods and fast foods are available. The genetic factor that was once a life-saver has become deleterious, leading to obesity.

A *familial base* of obesity, that may be in part genetic, has been identified by Knowler et al. (1983) as a strong risk factor for diabetes. In their study of the Pima Indian population in the southwestern United States, they have argued that today's abundant food supply together with the "thrifty genotype" may be cause for concern about that population's high levels of obesity. They suggest that "Neel's 'thrifty genotype' may mediate differences in sensitivity to insulin in various metabolic pathways" (1983:112).

While Garn and Clark's (1976) examination of family patterns of obesity found similarities between the weights of parents and children, Withers (1964) noted that human obesity tends to be familial but not specifically associated with diabetes. Studies of anorexia nervosa have found it to occur particularly in families where parents have a history of being overweight. It is very difficult to establish whether obesity occurs in families because of hereditary factors or because of household customs pertaining to the type and amount of food eaten.

Gender has been a common correlate when examining populations in which obesity and so-called overweight are being questioned. Such questions are as much political as they are medical. Beller (1977) discusses the history of the gendered basis of obesity, arguing that it has developed with patriarchal control of western societies. Male power extends to wanting to see their wives/women "in control" also. The ultimate result of this is great psychological pressure to conform, leading to anorexia and bulimia. Brumberg (1988) argues that for anorexics appetite is seen as a sign of sexuality and indicates lack of self-restraint. However, Hallstrom and Noppa (1981) found very small relationship between obesity and the likelihood of mental illness in their study.

The social stigma of a fat body pertains to both genders (Czajka and Parham, 1990), but Garn and Clark's (1976) study of cultural pressures on women to be thin found that western adolescent females report more positive attitudes toward a small body size. Wooley and Wooley (1979) noted no distinctive features of eating styles of obese persons in their study; nevertheless, excess body fat was the most stigmatized physical feature that "only the most extraordinary behaviour will enable them [overweight people] to become and remain thin" (1979:69).

The gender variable has most frequently been pulled out by those examining obesity and socioeconomic status. Sobal and Stunkard (1989) have listed some 24 studies that show that women of lower socioeconomic status in the United States are more likely to be obese than women of upper socioeconomic status. Goldblatt, Moore and Stunkard's (1965) longitudinal British study showed no difference in overweight and obesity according to socioeconomic status (SES) in boys, and trivial differences in girls, but the differences between the genders became clearer in adults. In developing societies, however, Sobal and Stunkard (1989:263) found that SES is directly associated with obesity.

These gender studies, particularly those correlating income and body size, need a lot more work. The socioeconomic factors are hard to correlate cross culturally, where often a good subsistence diet may mask a low level of cash income. In the Pacific, women may be confined to the home for cultural reasons, and thus lack exercise as well as cash income and indulge their love of food. Any visitor must be invited to share food, and feasting is a regular invitation for overindulgence. Drinking *kava*, a locally made narcotic beverage, which is mainly a male pastime, is said to maintain a slim body. So there are many factors in the life-style that cannot be compressed into a SES measure to compare with western life-styles.

Food intake has been cited frequently as the main cause of obesity, with the indication that if that person could only control what he ate he would become a slimmer and more acceptable social being. Both total calories and specifically "bad" calories, such as those from high fat, high sugar, and low fibre content have been blamed for the frequency of obese persons (Trowell and Burkitt, 1981). These three factors have been cited as particularly significant for Polynesian populations (Bindon, 1981; Prior and Tasman Jones, 1981), as they have been introduced to a society that previously had a high fibre, low fat, low sugar diet of root and tree starches and fish (Pollock, 1992).

The recommended daily caloric intake has been reviewed by nutritionists several times in the last twenty years, thus changing the target goal for those who aim to keep their intake close to that recommended norm. That has stabilized recently at 2,700 kcalories for men in light to medium work, and 2,200 kcalories for women. But others have argued that it is not so much the total calories as the origins of those calories, whether in fat, or refined flour and sugar, that contribute to the unhealthy diet of obese people (Mann, 1974).

Cautions about linking food practices too closely with obesity have been raised by several authors. Huenemann et al. (1966) have warned that food intake is only one factor, while Sobal and Stunkard (1989) have argued that there is a loose linkage between food intake and body weight; rather they argue for a wider genetic-environmental interaction. Similarly, Mayer (1953) has preferred to consider the multiple etiology of obesity in man as based on both genetic and environmental factors. He concludes that obesity is more than just overeating.

The attitudes of vegetarians to food throw some light on why some people select nonmeat foods in order to feel healthy and avoid obesity. Ossipow (chapter 7) has documented a number of aspects of the attitudes to the body held by Swiss vegetarians. They tend not to get fat, and hold a strong moral position that fat omnivores represent a body poisoned by meats and denatured products. A "light" body, based on a vegetarian diet is clean and preferably thin. In another study (Stern et al., 1982) comparing the attitudes to food of Mexican Americans and Anglos in Texas, the Mexican Americans had a strong sense of fatalism about their own obesity, and they were skeptical of Anglos' desires to be lean. Cultural including of moral issues rather than material concerns permeates these viewpoints.

Marked *changes in food intake over time* have been cited as one explanation for the prevalence of obesity today. Brown and Konner (1987) have shown how body size is an adaptation to food shortages in the past. Among others, Fischler (1981) has argued that contemporary nutrition disorders are a consequence of archaic traits being reactivated by recent developments disturbing natural biological wisdoms (1981:68). He proposes what he calls the omnivore's paradox that new food offers potential dangers, yet there is a drive to sample new food. He concludes we are in a state of what he calls "Gastro-anomy" with no cultural clues as to the correct choice of food, as the choices are now based on individual, not social, decisions.

Beller's (1977) history of obesity focuses on another version of that paradox, namely the urge to produce good food for the family and yet at the same time not to overfeed them. This is a particular dilemma for the woman as cook. She documents the changes in attitudes to body image over time, showing how western populations have held fatness in high regard until the recent past. It is only in recent times that "thin" has become the ideal. It is a patriarchal ideal that became established in the upper classes in Victorian times, and has been further refined over the last hundred years in both British and American societies.

Addressing specific changes in the diet, Eaton and Konner (1985) have argued that meat has come to predominate over vegetables. In paleolithic times the diet was predominantly vegetable-based, with less total fat, more essential fatty acids and a much higher ratio of polyunsaturated to saturated fats than the present diet centered around meat in the western hemisphere.

This change to a modern diet high in fat, refined sugar and flour and low in fibre is cited as the main feature of obesity as a disease of modernization or westernization (Coyne, Badcock and Taylor, 1984, for the Pacific; Birkbeck, 1981, for New Zealand; Prior and Tasman Jones, 1981, for Maori and Polynesians). More specifically Zimmet and Whitehouse (1981) have emphasized both genetic and dietary factors as the major contributing cause of diabetes, the focus of their work in several Pacific populations.

Socioeconomic Factors

A number of studies in the United States and Britain have indicated that certain sectors of those populations are at greater risk from obesity than others (see Zimmet and Baba, 1990; Silverstone, Gordon and Stunkard, 1969). These risk factors become clearer when studies take into account social, cultural and economic variables. Stunkard's studies (for example, 1977; Sobal and Stunkard, 1989) have documented socioeconomic status and educational level in a number of studies of different sectors of American society.

Goldblatt, Moore and Stunkard (1965) have made a strong case for the decrease in the prevalence of obesity with increase in socioeconomic status. Rolland-Cachera and Bellisle (1986) have posed the question why U.S. working-class children are fatter than upper-class children. Focusing particularly on women, Silverstone, Gordon and Stunkard (1969) found that obesity is markedly more prevalent in lower-class women than upper-class women, though social class is not as strong an indicator of obesity in men (1969). Hallstrom and Noppa (1981) came to the same conclusion, adding that obese women had low performance in school in the United States Moore. Stunkard and Stole's Manhattan study (1962) showed that 30 percent of women in the lowest socioeconomic class were obese while there was less discrepancy for men. They were not sure whether obesity was the cause or the result.

The study by Leonetti et al. (chapter 11) of Japanese-American students in Washington state looked particularly at the association between levels of adrenaline and adipose tissue regulation and the level of educational achievement. They found that low adrenaline may be associated with obesity and lower educational achievement in this population.

Body Image

Certainly body image is an important variable that has not been considered enough in studies of obesity. Cahnman (1968) and DeJong (1980) have both warned us of the severe stigma of obesity, and its consequences for setting the obese apart and labelling them as physical deviants. The issue is also picked up by Beller (1977) in her depiction of the cultural characteristics demarcating the fat from the thin. As Stern et al. (1982) have shown in their San Antonio heart study, Mexican Americans demonstrated a high level of fatalism about their own potential for obesity, even though suburban Mexican Americans were leaner than low income Mexican Americans. The Mexican Americans felt the Anglos were too concerned about losing weight, and were skeptical of their desire to be lean. The authors conclude that cultural factors rather than social factors distinguish the attitudes and behaviour related to obesity of the Mexican Americans and Anglos in their study.

Even though many studies have noted women's rather than men's greater propensity to become obese, Drenowski and Yee (1987) have shown that for men in the United States, certainly for those in the upper middle class, thinness is valued as a body image, tending to be valued as an end in itself as well as a means of prolonging life and avoiding ill health.

The burden of guilt and anxiety about excess baggage of fat (Beller, 1977) and the negative associations the obese draw between their body image and not being able to get access to a job, enter college or reach salary levels they desire all point to the strong negative image in the United States of the obese. Czajka and Parham (1990) pinpoint social prejudice and discrimination as significant factors associated with the pressure to be thin. Such messages are particularly influential when they come from health professionals, the media and colleagues.

Conclusions

When obesity or large body size is considered within the wider concept of body image, as argued here, a number of issues are raised. Previously, obesity had been considered mainly as a medical or health concern, or a psychological problem, with individuals seen as deviating from an established norm. A few authors have demonstrated that socioeconomic and ethnic factors also are pertinent to the understanding of obesity as a health issue. But the articles in this volume stress the social aspects with a focus on the place of large body size within a society's total value system.

Contrary to the western view of obesity as due to lack of self-control, whether by overeating, lack of exercise, or genetic factors, we will see that particular fattening practices are subject to rigorous social controls that are often carried out within ritual celebrations. Such a view of fattening raises new issues not only about the applicability of narrowly defined concepts to other cultural situations, but also about the parameters within which obesity has been dealt with so far. After all, smoking too was a ritual activity which spread to become a health concern.

Thus, cross-cultural concerns with body image require that we look deeper into the concept of obesity and its synonyms. We need further ethnographic descriptions of body size within the overall value systems of particular societies, so that we can develop a more systematic approach to body image and the variety of meanings of body size whether small or large.

Nancy J. Pollock

REFERENCES

Andres, R. 1980. Effects of obesity on total mortality. *Annals of Internal Medicine* **103**, 1003–1005.

Ashwell, M., T.J. Cole and A.K. Dixon. 1985. Obesity: New insight into the anthropometric classification of fat distribution shown by computed tomography. *British Medical Journal* **290**, 1692–1694.

Baecke, J.A.M., J. Burema, J.E.R. Frijters, J.G.A.J. Hautvast and W.A.M. van der Wiel-Wetzels. 1983. Obesity in young Dutch adults II: Daily life-style and body mass index. *International Journal of Obesity* **7**, 13–24.

Baker, P.T., J.M. Hanna and T.S. Baker. (eds.) 1986. *The Changing Samoans: Behaviour and health in transition.* Oxford University Press, New York.

Beaglehole, J. 1962. *The Endeavour Journal of Sir Joseph Banks, 1768–1781.* Angus and Robertson, Sydney.

Beere, C. (ed.) 1990. Body image and appearances. In *Sex and Gender Issues—A handbook of tests and measures*, chap. 10. Greenwood Press, Westport.

Beller, A. 1977. Feast, famine, and physique. In *Fat and Thin. A natural history of obesity.* Farrar, Strauss and Giroux, New York. pp. 286–304.

Bindon, J.R. 1981. Breadfruit, banana, beef, and beer: Modernisation of the (American) Samoan diet. *Ecology of Food and Nutrition* **12**, 49–60.

Bindon, J. R., and D. Pelletier. 1986. Patterns of growth in weight among infants in a rural western Samoa village. *Ecology of Food and Nutrition* **18**, 135–143.

Birkbeck, J. 1981. Obesity, socio-economic variables and eating habits in New Zealand. *Journal of Biological Science* **13**, 299–336.

Björntorp, I., and P. Zimmet, *see* Zimmet and Björntorp.

Bray, G.A. 1979. Obesity. Disease-a-Month. Vol. XXVI, No. 1. Year Book Medical Publishers, Inc. Chicago, London.

Brown, P.J., and M. Konner. 1987. An anthropological perspective on obesity. R.J. and J. Wurtman (eds.), *Annals of the New York Academy of Sciences* **499**, 29–46.

Brumberg, A.B. 1988. *Fasting Girls.* Harvard University Press, Cambridge.

Cahnman, W.J. 1968. The stigma of obesity. *Sociological Quarterly* **9**, 283–299.

Cassidy, C. 1992. The good body; When big is better. *Medical Anthropology* **13**, 181–213.

Cockington, R.A. 1980. Growth of Australian Aboriginal children related to social circumstances. *Australian and New Zealand Journal of Medicine* **10**, 199–208.

Coyne, T., J. Badcock and R.J. Taylor. 1984. The effect of urbanisation and western diet on the health of Pacific island populations. South Pacific Technical Paper No. 186, Noumea.

Czajka, D., and E. Parham. 1990. Fear of fat: Attitudes towards obesity. *Nutrition Today* **25**(1), 26–32.

DeJong, W. 1980. The stigma of obesity: The consequences of naive assumptions concerning the causes of physical deviance. *Journal of Health and Social Behaviour* **21** (March), 75–87.

Drenowski, A., and D.K. Yee. 1987. Men and body image: Are males satisfied with their body weight? *Psychosomatic Medicine*, Pt. **49**, pp. 626–634.

Eaton, S. B., and M. Konner. 1985. Paleolithic nutrition. *New England Journal of Medicine* **312**, 283–289.

Ellis, W.H. 1831. *Polynesian Researches.* Reprinted, Tuttle, Honolulu, 1969.

Fischler, C. 1981. Food preferences, nutritional wisdom and sociocultural evolution. In D. Walcher and N. Kretchmer (eds.), *Food, Nutrition and Evolution.* Masson Publishers, N.Y.

Frisch, R.E., and J. McArthur. 1974. Menstrual cycles: Fatness as a determinant of minimum weight for height necessary for their maintenance or onset. *Science* **185**, 949–951.

Garn, S., and D.C. Clark. 1976. Trends in fatness and the origins of obesity. *Pediatrics* **57** (4), 443–455.

Gober, G., and G. Stemmermann. 1981. Hawaiian ethnic groups. In H.C. Trowell and D.P. Burkitt (eds.), *Western Diseases: Their emergence and prevention*. Harvard University Press, Cambridge.

Goldblatt, P.B., M. Moore and A.J. Stunkard. 1965. Social factors in obesity. *Journal of the American Medical Association* **192**, 1039–1044.

Hall, A., J. Liebrich and F. Walkey. 1983. The development of a food fitness and looks questionnaire. In P.L. Darby, P.E. Garfunkel, D.M. Garner and D.V. Coscina (eds.), *Anorexia Nervosa*. Alan R. Liss, Inc., N.Y. pp. 41–55.

Hallstrom, T., and H. Noppa. 1981. Obesity in women in relation to mental illness, social factors and personality traits. *Journal of Psychosomatic Research* **25** (No. 2), 75–82.

Huenemann, R.L., M.C. Hampton, L.R. Shapiro and A.R. Behnke. 1966. Adolescent food practises associated with obesity. *Federation Proceedings* **25**, 4–10.

Jaquiers, E. 1987. Energy utilisation in human obesity. *Annals of the New York Academy of Sciences* **499**, 73–83.

Keys, A. 1980. Overweight, obesity, coronary heart disease and mortality. *Nutrition Reviews* **38**, 297–307.

Keys, A., F. Fidanza, M.J. Karvonen, N. Kimuro and H.L. Taylor. 1972. Indices of relative weight and obesity. *Journal of Chronic Diseases* **25**, 329–343.

Knowler, W.C., D.J. Pettitt, P.H. Bennett and R.C. Williams. 1983. Diabetes mellitus in the Pima Indians: Genetic and evolutionary considerations. *American Journal of Physical Anthropology* **62**, 107–114.

Mann, G.V. 1974. The influence of obesity on health. *New England Journal of Medicine*. Part 1: **291**, No. 4; 178–184. Part 2: **291**, No. 4; 226–232.

Mayer, J. 1953. Genetic, traumatic and environmental factors in the etiology of obesity. *Physiological Reviews* **33**, 472–503.

Moore, M.E., A. Stunkard and L. Stole. 1962. Obesity, social class and mental illness. *Journal of the American Medical Association* **181** (No. 11), 962–966.

Neel, J.V. 1962. Diabetes mellitus: A "thrifty" genotype rendered detrimental by "progress"? *American Journal of Human Genetics* **14**, 353–362.

Norgan, N. 1987. Fat patterning in Papua New Guinea: Effects of age, sex and acculturation. *American Journal of Physical Anthropology* **74**(3), 385–392.

Parizkova, J. 1986. Body composition, food intake, cardiorespiratory fitness, blood lipids and psychological development in highly active and inactive preschool children. *Human Biology* **58**, 261–273.

Pollock, N.J. 1992. *These Roots Remain*. University of Hawaii Press.

Prior, I.A.M. 1976. Nutritional problems in Pacific Islanders. The 1976 Muriel Bell Memorial Lecture. Proceedings of the Nutrition Society.

Prior, I.A.M., and C. Tasman Jones. 1981. New Zealand and Pacific Polynesians. In H.C. Trowell and D.P. Burkitt (eds.), *Western Diseases: Their emergence and prevention.* Harvard University Press, Cambridge.

Roberts, D.F. 1953. Body weight, race and climate. *American Journal of Physical Anthropology* 11, 533–558.

Rolland-Cachera, M.R., and F. Bellisle. 1986. No correlation between adiposity and food intake: Why are working class children fatter? *American Journal of Clinical Nutrition* 44, 779–787.

Silverstone, J.T., R.P. Gordon and A.J. Stunkard. 1969. Social factors in obesity. *Practitioner* 202, 682–688.

Sobal, J., and A.J. Stunkard. 1989. Socioeconomic status and obesity: A review of the literature. *Psychological Bulletin,* 105 (No. 2), 260–275.

Stern, M.P., J. Pugh, S.P. Gaskill and H.P. Hazada. 1982. Knowledge, attitudes and behavior related to obesity and dieting in Mexican Americans and Anglos. *American Journal of Epidemiology* 115, 917–928.

Stunkard, A.J. 1977. Obesity and the social environment: Current status, future prospects. *Annals of the New York Academy of Sciences* 300, 298–320.

Stunkard, A., E. d'Aquili, S. Fox and R.D.L. Filion. 1972. Influence of social class on obesity and thinness in children. *Journal of the American Medical Association* 221 (No. 6), 579–584.

Trowell, H., and D.P. Burkitt. 1981. Hypertension, obesity, diabetes mellitus and coronary heart disease. In H.C. Trowell and D.P. Burkitt (eds.), *Western Diseases: Their emergence and prevention.* Arnold, London. (Harvard University Press, Cambridge.)

Turner, B. 1984. *The Body in Society.* Basil Blackwell, Oxford.

Vague, J. 1956. The degree of masculine differentiation of obesities: A factor determining predisposition to diabetes, atherosclerosis, gout and uric calculus disease. *American Journal of Clinical Nutrition* 4, 20–34.

Van Gennep, A. 1960. The Rites of Passage. London: Routledge and Kegan Paul.

van Itallie, T.B. 1986. Obesity: Adverse effects on health and longevity. *American Journal of Clinical Nutrition* 44, 2723–2733.

Withers, R.F.J. 1964. Problems in the genetics of human obesity. *The Eugenics Review* 56 (No. 2), 81–90.

Wooley, Susan C. and Orland Wooley. 1979. Obesity and Women I—Women's Studies International Quarterly 2, 69–79.

Zimmet, P., and S. Baba. 1990. Central obesity, glucose intolerance and other cardiovascular risk factors: An old syndrome rediscovered. In P. Zimmet and S. Baba (eds.), *World Data Book of Obesity,* Elsevier Science Publishers B.V. (Biomedical Division), *Excerpta Medica,* pp. 167–171.

Zimmet, P., and P. Björntorp. 1979. Adipose tissue cellularity in obese nondiabetic men in an urbanised Pacific island (Polynesian) population. *American Journal of Clinical Nutrition* 32, 1788–1791.

Zimmet, P., and S. Whitehouse. 1981. Pacific Islands of Nauru, Tuvalu and western Samoa. In H.C. Trowell and D.P. Burkitt (eds.), *Western Diseases: Their emergence and prevention.* Harvard University Press, Cambridge.

I

CULTURAL FATTENING PROCESSES

1

Food and Fatness in Calabria

VITO TETI
(Translated by Nicolette S. James)

In 1945 the writer Carlo Levi published *Cristo si è femato ad Eboli [Christ stopped at Eboli]*, a document in which he tells about his experience as a political exile in a little village in Lucania, Italy, during the period of fascism. He describes a "peasant civilization" almost unrelated to the modern world (Levi, 1984). The book shook the official Italian cultural world and provoked a lively debate amongst intellectuals, oscillating between nostalgia or, at least, the understanding of an ancient world, and the invitation and desire to go beyond Eboli (*see* Alicata, 1954, 1968; *see also* Rauty, 1976; Pasquinelli, 1977; Cirese, 1973; Teti, 1990a) and to leave behind a world whose values were considered archaic. Carlo Levi was able to gather, with such anthropological sensitivity and human understanding, the models and values of a crumbling world.

This famous painter and writer who, in the village of Lucania, exercised his profession of doctor, did not fail to notice the connection between poor and wretched food and the mentality and culture of the population. This is how Carlo Levi remembers Giulia, the woman with whom he lodged:

"Giulia considered me as her master, and would never have said no to any of my requests; or rather, with extreme naturalness, she took the initiative of serving me in small ways that I would never have thought of asking her for. She had had a large tub of enamelled iron sent from Bari to bathe in; and in the morning I carried it into my bedroom so that I could wash myself in it. ...This seemed very strange to Giulia who one morning opened the door, and without showing any sign of surprise at my nudity asked me how it was possible to have a bath without anyone soaping my back, and helping me to get dry ...Certainly after that I could not avoid having my back soaped and massaged by her strong rough fingers. The witch was amazed that I did not ask to make love with her ...She only praised my good looks: 'How good looking you are,' she said 'how nice and plump you are.' To be plump here is the first sign of beauty, as in Oriental countries; perhaps because to reach fatness, which is impossible for undernourished peasants, one has to be a gentleman and powerful" (Levi, 1984: 132–133).

In a world characterized by the insufficiency of things to eat, plumpness, which presupposed wealth and the availability of nutritious food like meat, was synonymous with beauty. Plumpness was the "aesthetic model" of the body of the individuals of traditional societies living in a state of chronic undernourishment, continually faced with the pangs of hunger, and having only on exceptional and ritual occasions had access to the products that supplied necessary animal proteins.

Many observers of life in the South of Italy have pointed out, at different periods, how plumpness came to be considered as a symbol of well-being and alimentary happiness, of beauty, wealth, power and dominance. The rich gentlemen, the barons, the ruling classes who exercised their power with violence and arrogance, are described and perceived as round, well-fed, fat. The English writer George Gissing, who visited Calabria in 1892, had the occasion to record the conflicts that existed in Calabria between the starving populace and the rich and fat mayors of the area. In Crotone he witnessed a popular demonstration against the "oppressive tax, called the "fuocatico," a tax on hearths, a tax on "every kitchen where food is prepared" (Gissing, 1971:86. *See also* Teti, 1976, 1989c).

"...the starving populace of Crotone didn't have enough energy to impose its will effectively; it limited itself to shouting: 'Down with the mayor!' and it broke up to go towards the taxed hearths for an almost imaginary service. I would like to have known if the Mayor and his imposing friend happened to be in their comfortable office during these disturbances; if they were, they were smoking their cigars as usual and continued to chat calmly. That was very likely the case. The privileged classes in Italy are slow to move and easily believe in the unlimited endurance of those beneath them. One day or another, undoubtedly, they will have a nasty surprise."

But it was Ignazio Silone in his famous novel *"Fontamara"* (1987) who described the "foods of hunger" (a few potatoes, beans, onions and maize) of the poor peasants and the abundant, sumptuous cooking flaunted by the rich. Old and new gentlemen are observed in their culinary showing off...Don Carlo Magna, an ancient gentleman, and Don Abbachio, the collaborating priest of the old and new powerful men, with their names (which are clearly nicknames for food insults that reveal the envy and scorn of the starving popular classes) are the representatives (and the metaphors) of a world dominated by people who stuff themselves and starve poor people.

Abundant and luxurious cuisine, banquets and the arrogance of the rich, their indifference to the starving poor, are lucidly observed by the women who in vain ask for justice.

"The smells from the saucepans reached us. The servant began to recount to us with lots of details how the banquet had gone. There had already been a fine toast by Don Circostanza. Then she talked to us about the dishes. She expressed herself in little words. She said: 'baby onions, a little sauce, tiny mushrooms, little potatoes, a slight aroma, a small flavour.'"

The banquet must have been drawing to an end because they were beginning to feel the effects of the wine already. "...The drunken voice of Don Abbachio said, with an ecclesiastical cadence:

"In the name of the bread, the salami and the white wine, amen!"

"A shower of laughter greeted the priest's bon mot. There was another pause. Then with his church voice Don Abbachio sang:

"'Ite, missa est.'"

"It was a signal for the banquet to end. The diners, in a group, started to go into the garden, as was the custom, to urinate. In front of all went the priest Don Abbachio, fat and puffing, with his neck full of veins, his face purple, his eyes half closed in a beatific expression. The clergyman hardly held himself vertical for his drunkenness and started to make water against a tree" (Silone, 1987:75–76).

Fatness, and consequently good food, strength, physical force, erotic capacity and beauty were models to be attained, forbidden dreams for the poor, starved, undernourished, thin people who wandered around like shadows and ghosts in the countryside, in the little villages, in the urban centres of Calabria in the nineteenth century and first half of the twentieth, when "hunger" not only meant the desire for the unobtainable food of the rich (such as meat and white bread), but also the condition of individuals who were prey to continual famines and food deprivation (Teti, 1990b; Sole, 1990).

From at least the end of the eighteenth century many foreign travellers, internal and external observers and writers contributed in their different ways to trace the image of the undernourished, thin, feeble, lazy, ill Calabrian, who was always exposed to the risk of malaria and other diseases linked to malnutrition and the lack of food (Teti, 1985–86, 1990b).

Different scholars and observers agree on the image of the melancholic Calabrian, and seem to put him aside in his melancholy ("black bile"), an almost natural characteristic of the people of that region. Melancholy is thus presented as a sort of culture of people used to living with natural and historic catastrophies (Teti, 1989a).

Robert Burton, the author of *The Anatomy of Melancholy*, showed, as Bruce Chatwin has also reminded us (Chatwin, 1988), that travelling constitutes a remedy to melancholy, to the depressing effects of sedentary life (Burton, 1981, 1983). It is well-known that the "choice of being a brigand," the "flight into the mountains" of the people of Calabria was also an escape from the "land of hunger" and the search for the land of plenty, of a world where there was abundance of food and well-being (Teti, 1987a, 1989a). The Mountains, for the Calabrian brigands, was a sort of (pre-Lenten) Carnival to be reached once and for all. The image of the Mountains as a sort of food Utopia has been sketched by various Calabrian writers.

In the play by Vincenzo Padula, *Antonello capobrigante calabrese*, written in 1850, the mayor says:

"... the brigands want to be extravagant. Ham, salami, dairy foods, packets of cigars, dessert, wine and jam are indispensable things" (Misasi, 1976:54).

The desire to "eat well" is also the desire for physical well-being, to be strong and vigorous, to be considered good looking and thus able to have beautiful women. Even the peasants described by the writer Nicola Misasi are obsessed by the food and alimentary behaviour of the gentlemen.

The peasant, who later would have chosen to become a brigand, had to be content with a soup made of herbs and potatoes, with rye bread, and knew only from listening to his father talking about "bread that was white like milk, soft as ricotta cheese," or meat, and the "things that they sell in the cafés and in the pastry shops" and which he had never been able to taste (Misasi 1976:368–369).

The flight of the peasant into the Mountains provided a temporary end to the usual food deprivation. According to Misasi, the brigand often "...took to the woods feeling himself...drawn to the life of a brigand by the irresistible need for independence, by an unrestrainable desire to live well ... For two, three, ten, or twenty years, like so many others, if the Madonna del Carmine protected him, he would eat the white bread, succulent meat, delicious cheeses, and drink the best wine, he would be the chick of all the peasant women, what did he care about all the rest?" (Misasi, 1976:371–372). Misasi's description reflects the popular myth of the brigand as a well-built man, handsome, courageous, strong, vigorous, desiring good food and beautiful women.

Fatness as a sign of alimentary well being, of health, wealth, power and arrogance, can be found in the works of Corrado Alvaro. In his writings, food and water are decreed as the constituent elements of identity, memory, the nostalgia of the Calabrians who escape, and of so many of his characters who are wandering, troubled, rootless, foreigners to themselves (Teti, 1985–86, 1990c). Calabrians travelling or in flight, Alvaro's emigrants, are recognisable by their slow way of chewing, by the bag of provisions which they carry, by the need to stop in railway stations to drink, by their search and nostalgia for the food of their country of origin. The return, real or dreamed of, by Calabrians to their birth place often happens through the recognition and reappropriation of childhood foods, which represent the return to a lost universe of smells, tastes, colours, links and affections. Food nostalgia is never, however, missing a world of misery and hunger. In his most beautiful and well-known story, *Gente in Aspromonte* (People in Aspromonte)(1930), Corrado Alvaro describes the suffering and hunger of the shepherds and the opulence and arrogance of the gentlemen of a village of Aspromonte (Alvaro, 1982).

And in *Calabria* (1931), Alvaro reports the song of the bandit Nino Martino who chose the mountains also to be able to eat white bread and to have something on it. Recalling the popular myth of the brigand, he concludes:

"How many of us have dreamed about these words: to leave, to see, to know. Out of the most ancient nostalgia of freedom, of the mountains, of the forest, of better living, emigration was born" (Alvaro, 1931:36–37).

Emigration,as we will see, will make the dreams come true that forced the population to become brigands. The writer Fortunato Seminara in his famous novel *Le Baracche*, written in 1934 and published in 1942, describes the miserable and painful life of the inhabitants of a depressing, immobile isolated Calabrian village (Seminara, 1942). The lord of the village is described as *surly* and *bilious* (1942:59). He is seen by the people as a "gouty ox" (1942:63).

In the works of Seminara, who describes a violent universe, fatness makes one think of rapacity, of gluttony, of the unmeasured behaviour of the powerful who live by sucking the blood of the poor. In other novels, *Il vento nell 'oliveto* (The wind in the olive grove) (Seminara, 1963), the main character, a rich landowner, writes about himself in his diary:

"Well, I'm thirty-five years old. I'm well built, of medium height; I have a ruddy complexion, grey eyes, brown straight hair. My age and a little plumpness have made my movements heavy" (1963:63).

Fatness as a sign of nutritional well-being and good health is found again in the works of other Calabrian writers, such as Pietro Familiari, *La vera storia del brigante Marlino Zappa* (The true story of the brigand Marlino Zappa). He describes the miserable condition of the peasants and other poor social classes in a Calabrian village during the fascist period (Familiari, 1971). The average life-span is not more than 40 years, and five out of ten babies die in the first few years of their lives. Only nobly-born people can have access to meat and the other foods that supply a fundamental nutritional basis. Familiari writes:

"The Marquis De Frigeros being well fed... referring to his florid complexion, the peasants said; 'The Marquis's flesh does not taste of cabbages as ours does, but of steaks and little cheeses made with butter'" (1971:86).

In the nineteenth and early twentieth century literature, members of the poor classes (such as peasants, labourers, shepherds, craftsmen) are all seen as starved, undernourished, longing for good food, weak, thin, physically debilitated, weak from a psychological point of view. The rich (landowners, barons, marquesses, doctors, lawyers, and the like) appear in all their opulence: well fed, of good colour, fat, tall. Handsome, their fatness or stoutness is seen as a sign of power, of arrogance and gluttony.

Fatness appears as the dietary and aesthetic model for the people who present in their bodies and minds the signs of hunger and of a precarious and poor-quality diet, almost entirely based on vegetables, that are considered not very nutritious, and rejected for that reason.

In the pictures of the "fat," "greedy," "gluttonous" master, described in many ways by various Calabrian writers, envy, dreams, desires, anger, scorn, are all present together with the denunciation and sarcasm of those belonging to the lower classes towards the powerful and never-satisfied gentlemen. Popular poetic texts (songs, proverbs, stories, prayers, Carnival farces, for example) reveal in a telling way the food, dietary and aesthetic models of those popular classes, and their scorn and irony towards those who had the chance to eat *"a scasciapanza"* (till their stomachs burst).

Oral literature gives evidence of the popular feelings towards the ungrateful and gluttonous:

> "You have ten dishes and I have none, eat nine of them and give me one";

> "You eat and drink till your stomach bursts and I weigh hunger with the scales." (*see* Teti, 1976:172).

The differences between the world of the "full stomachs" and that of the "empty ones" were also noted during the nineteenth century and the first half of the twentieth by various researchers, specialists on the South, and external and internal observers. I have concentrated on these aspects on other occasions (Teti, 1976, 1984, 1990b), and just wish to point out here how the authors of many surveys and enquiries into the social and economic situation in Calabria considered the lack of food, its monotonous and uniform quality, almost entirely vegetarian, as the cause of many endemic diseases, the high level of stillbirths, infant mortality and general mortality for cases linked to nutrition, the low stature of individuals, their physical weakness, their low ability to work and psychological debility. Thin, weary, weak, feeble, afflicted bodies, marked by hunger, fevers, malaria and other illnesses have populated the villages of hunger of Calabria.

If one looks at the height of the young Calabrians called up for military service who were born in 1900, 1939, and 1945 (average height 159, 165, and 165 cm, respectively) one notices that it is amongst the lowest with respect to the other regions of Italy (the national average was 162, 168, and 168 cm). This gap is also likely to be due to dietary deficiencies (Teti, 1976). Even Alessandro Niceforo, who at the beginning of the twentieth century tried to explain the differences between the Italians of the North and those of the South in racial terms, had to admit the nutritional conditions of the South were not satisfactory. The small structure of the Southern Italians was, for this researcher, attributed not only to racial phenomena, but also depended on physical degeneration caused by scant food and unfavourable environmental conditions (Niceforo, 1901).

In the course of the nineteenth century in Calabria various famines occurred which often led people to die of hunger (Sole, 1990). In 1931 Corrado Alvaro recorded a recent famine which had afflicted the inhabitants of the village of Africo, in the province of Reggio Calabria. Some of them were found wandering through Italy as far as distant as Emilia (about 1000 km).

> "A loaf of bread made of straw was taken to the head of the Government to witness the state of the population. The Government suggested that the inhabitants move down (10 km along the sea), to be in contact with the principal roads and civilisation. Africo remained where it was, and it didn't take much to relieve its condition" (Alvaro, 1931:28–29).

Africo has become the symbol of hunger, floods, wandering and the dispersion of the inhabitants of inland Calabria.

In 1946 Umberto Zanotti-Bianco published a book on the people of Africo, *Tra la perduta gente* (Amongst the lost peoples) in which he wrote:

> "The diet is insufficient both as regards quality and the lack of food. Bread, which constitutes for many families almost the only food for several months, is made with the mixture that the earth produces, in other words with lentil flour, with chickling [*Lathyrus sativus*] flour and barley which has an acid and bitter taste. After seeing the rolls I sent him, Giustino Fortunato wrote to me—'I saw the bread before 1860. In the Apulian-Basilicata area people have even forgotten the memory of it ... The bread is wretched ....'

> "There is no meat eaten, very few fats, few pulses, a poor quantity of goat's cheese... What the unfortunate population were reduced to last winter had to be seen to be believed. 'We ate cooked thistles like hermits,' they complained, 'and acorns, excuse the expression, like little pigs!.'

> "This poverty of foodstuffs has increased mortality, especially that of infants. Last year, 1927, against 41 births there were 41 deaths of which 25 [individuals] were under 4 years old. The majority of the children that I saw showed evident signs of malnutrition. ...The Town Council did nothing to improve the sanitary conditions in Africo—as is shown by the 225 cases of endemic goitre which I was able to see in the centre. The

people also suffered from tuberculosis, deforming arthritis and trachoma."(Zanotti-Bianco, 1946:13–14)[1]

In 1948 the photographer Tino Petrelli, in one of his famous series of documentary photographs, showed the huts, the misery, the hunger of the people of Africo. The pictures of the bodies and the faces which bear the "stigma of hunger" produced an outraged reaction from national public opinion which, at that time, was rediscovering, thanks to experts, film directors and democratic photographers such as Petrelli, the dramatic situation of the "Southern question" (Petrelli, 1990). The inhabitants of Africo left their village from 1949 onwards and moved to new houses built along the Ionian coast, to New Africo, a village that has become a metaphor for the recent breaking up and dispersion of Calabrian people (*see* Stajano, 1979).

Besides recalling briefly the pictures that accompany the research done by Umberto Zanotti-Bianco and those by Petrelli, I also want to draw attention to how photographs contribute, from the end of the nineteenth century, precious documentary evidence for learning about the health and sanitary conditions of populations. Above all, photographs show the distance between the undernourished, thin, poor and the fat and healthy rich. Recently Francesco Faeta (1984) republished one-hundred and ninety photographs of peasant and petit-bourgeois origins, taken by Saverio Marra, between 1914 and 1946 in S. Giovanni in Fiore, in the Sila and in the Marchesato. Amateur photographers belonging to aristocratic families have given us, at the beginning of this century, the interesting figures of other faces and other bodies which reveal economic and dietary well being (*see* Faeta and Miraglia, 1988).

It is not possible to discuss in detail the intensity of the ways in which aristocratic photographers looked at their families and the peasant world: the relatives of the photographers show an attitude, an expression, a physical appearance and a way of holding themselves that certainly reveal a special aristocratic culture, but also the signs of dietary and economic well-being. The robustness, height, full and coloured faces of the gentlemen are the other side of culture, the social and economic universe, that was otherwise peopled by starving, thin and undernourished men. The tall bodies and the plumpness appear as models of the different social classes of the popular traditional world. Very few were able to reach that model, most of them dreamed of it, desired it, envied it and sometimes, not being able to reach it, mocked and criticised it.

I have pointed out in other publications how, during the nineteenth century, different foreign visitors and Calabrian researchers worked in various ways to build up the picture, often mistaken and stereotyped, of the Calabrian as *"parco, sobrio, buon lavoratore, resistente alla fatica"* (parsimonious, serious, a good worker, able to withstand much effort) (Teti, 1984). This picture contrasts with the descriptions of misery, deprivation, hunger, illness, malaria and the mortality of populations often described by the same observers. It is a picture that obeys the myth of the "good peasant" and which makes some ways of behaving, which were dictated by necessity, appear as deliberate choices reminiscent of the Classical world. (for the connection between the food habits of the Calabrian population and the cuisine and food rituals of the Greeks and Romans, *see* Dorsa, 1983).

It is a picture in which those belonging to the Calabrian working classes did not recognise themselves. If their reality was *hunger*, their desires and dreams, and even their behaviour, tended towards abundance, to a cuisine that was rich and elaborate, possible only during festivals and exceptional occasions. When the economic conditions and availability of food allowed it, the popular classes were far from the frugality and sobriety of which external observers spoke. As numerous poetic and folklore texts witness, those belonging to the working classes in Calabria refused explicitly the ecclesiastical culture of fasting, which often tied in well with the interests of the dominating classes (Teti, 1984, 1990b). The Calabrian peasants and farm labourers expressed their scorn in different ways for nonfat food, vegetables, pumpkins and onions considered as not very nourishing. It is not so much a question of refusing the foods that were a fundamental part of their identity and nutritional awareness, as a dislike of the foods that they were forced to live on daily. Oral texts, above all proverbs and popular stories, reveal that the religious choice of fasting was often the rationalization of the scarce availability of food and money. Some foodstuffs were "good to eat" only because foods considered better, more nutritious and more tasty were lacking or in short supply (*see* Harris 1971, 1979, 1990). Fasting appears more the result of necessity and not of religious rules. The peasants were well aware that prolonged fasting led to physical weakness and psychological feebleness. Two proverbs say:

"an empty stomach cannot reason";
"Fasting holds the devil at its arse" (Lombardi Satriani, 1969:189; Spezzano 1970:101).

Folk literature of the period of Carnival affirms the scorn and rejection by the lower classes of fasting, abstinence, herbs, nonfat food. Lent, which meant undernourished, thin, enfeebled, ugly bodies, was the subject of people's irony and sarcasm. It was imagined and depicted as a nasty "witch," thin, ugly, dried-up, bent and old, who gave out fasting and herbs which made adults and children cry.

Many nursery rhymes, which were recited or sung by children in various places in Calabria, reveal people's anti-Lent feelings, the popular rejection of thinness:

"Lent has come—eat bread and lettuce";
"Lent has a dead look—Because it doesn't leave any leaves in the vegetable garden" (Lombardi Satriani, 1969:245).
"My Lent, how long you are,
How short this carnival was,
I was used to liver and meat,
And now eating green I feel ill"
(Lombardi Satriani, 1940:113).

In the contrast between Lent and Carnival, people had no hesitation about which figure they should choose and prefer. Still today the current expression *"pari Corajisima"* (he/she looks like Lent) refers to a person who is ugly, unpleasant, unwanted. Lent today is still a synonym for thinness, ugliness and forced abstinence. Thinness was the result of compulsory chronic undernourishment, not of a freely chosen diet. It is noticeable that in popular language the term diet, meaning a rationally chosen way of eating, is almost nonexistent (Teti 1982, 1990b).

Not uncommonly, the thin person appeared as a worrying figure, threatening and dangerous. The thin man, in general also ugly, brought bad luck. According to some popular beliefs, the people who practised witchcraft were ugly, dried-up and thin. Even the *"jettatore"* (person who puts a jinx on things or brings bad luck), who has been widely written about in the city of Naples and the provinces of the Kingdom of Naples, was depicted as a person who was slight, slender, thin. It is enough to mention here the famous work on *Fascino volgarmente detto jettatura* (The fascination vulgarly called *"jettatura"*), published in Naples by Nicola Valletta in 1787. The people who "infallibly cause bad luck" are, in general, "certain big men with horrible faces; or accidents, some emaciated and pallid ..." (Valletta, 1984:63). It is not difficult to see behind the fear and the scorn of the big men, and also the emancipated and pallid people, also an ancient terror, and rejection of physical and psychological decadence which was connected with a precarious existence.

Perhaps it is also worth remembering how the image of the vampire, recorded from the end of the seventeenth century until the second half of the eighteenth century, in various countries in central and eastern Europe, was reminiscent of situations characterized by hunger, epidemics, mortality. The belief in vampires who remained intact in their coffins and returned to suck people's blood (often of living relatives) and the belief that the dead continued to chew and eat in their graves and returned to their relatives to eat and drink, take one back to ancient concepts present in many traditional folk cultures, but also reveal the problems of hidden food desires of populations. They also give evidence of the fear of dying of hunger, or of epidemics and diseases linked to lack of food. The fat, round vampire and this thin, pale victim remind one of the opposition between fatness and thinness, Carnival and Lent, the desire to die for excess of food, and the terror of dying of hunger, that we find in various traditional societies.

To the radical rejection of "eating nonfat food" and the negative considerations of "thin bodies" in Calabria the praise of meat and fat foods, and the admiration of "fat bodies" corresponded. Meat was, together with wheat bread, the alimentary dream of generations of undernourished and starving people who only had access to them a few times a year. The interminable and exasperating list of food and drinks that we find in many popular songs and in several farces from carnival time reflect the unobtainable dreams of those who were obliged to eat "bread and knife," bread and nothing else, as the following verses show:

"I could eat six calves in a single morning,
and six sheep with all their wool,
a whole cauldron of vermicelli,
a whole ovenful of bread,
a vat of wine,
six thousand kilos of macaroni,
And still my stomach would not be full,
Because it goes flapping like a bell"
(Collected in Parghelia, Catanzaro. *See* Lombardi Satriani, 1932:156).

"Darling if I die I'll leave a message for you,
Don't put me with the other dead people;
Prepare a long narrow ditch for me,
Just big enough for my poor suffering body to enter;

And may the coffin be of fried eggs,
The little lid of fish and trout;
For a cushion, a nice ham,
And strings of sausages for candelabras,
And that the Holy Water be a good strong wine,
Then put me between two unmarried women:
Sing a requiem for me because I am dead"
(Collected in Cassano AlloJonio, Cosenza. *See* Lombardi Satriani, 1932:163–4).

These two comic songs allude to an interminable and inescapable hunger.

The desire for meat to eat and sexual desire went together, and that appears to confirm why the robust man, since he had eaten meat, was considered also handsome and erotic. Abundance and quality of food, fatness, height, the capacity to work, sexual performance, all stem from the same dietary concepts of the popular classes. The model, to which Bachtin drew attention when examining the work of Rabelais, is that of the "Carnival body" (Bachtin, 1979).

Carnival was considered a character that was light-hearted, joking, someone who loved eating and drinking. He was the Emperor of the poor who dreamed of pork and wine. During the acting and recitations that took place during Carnival, he died from having eaten and drunk too much. The popular longing to die from overeating reflected the fear and anxiety about the possibility of dying of hunger. The dream of the land of plenty was the imaginary escape from the land of hunger. Carnival allowed them access to meat and good food, even if only for a few weeks of the year.

Carnival was insatiable, greedy and fat, and was opposed to Lent who was thin, dried-up and long (*see* Frazer (*The Golden Bough*), 1978; Toschi, 1976; Camporesi, 1976; Burke, 1980. For Calabria, *see* Lumini, 1888; Teti, 1982). The Carnival body, model of well-being and health, was also in Calabria a body that was full, fat, cheerful that alluded to an inexhaustible capacity for food and great sexual powers. People looked to the body of the Emperor Carnival with satisfaction and admiration.

From the belly of the person who was dressed as Carnival, or more often from the dummy that represented Carnival, the "masked men" (usually men disguised as doctors and nurses) extracted, after the incorrigible Carnival had died from overeating, boiled bones, fresh sausages, meat balls, fried chops, cracklings. The irony towards the greedy and insatiable pig, which in some villages symbolised the ungrateful rich lord, revealed an irresistible nostalgia for a "full stom-ach," people's desire to become like the fat Emperor, who was so similar to the fat lord. It is not possible to devote much time to the nu-merous aspects of the complex Carnival rituals which, in different ways, took place in Calabrian villages, but mention should be made of the oral testimonies of an old "*farsaro*," a person who until the begin-ning of the 1950s organised the Carnival rituals.

It has not been sufficiently understood, in my opinion, that Carni-val celebrations, at least in some areas of Calabria, were above all food celebrations. Food, drinking and eating appear as central to the core of complex rituals which served a variety of functions. A long and inter-esting record written, at my request, by Salvatore D'Eraclea, is perti-nent to the present subject (*see* D'Eraclea).

Salvatore D'Eraclea stated:

"I remember that when I was still a little boy, ragged and eternally hungry, as Carnival got nearer, I felt within myself an indescribable joy, due above all to the fact that after months and months of forced absti-nence, one could finally, thanks to the kind hearts of friends, eat some meat, meat balls, cracklings and large rissoles (meat tarts), black pud-ding and dishes of macaroni with a nice sauce made with pork and plenty of cheese. These gifts from God lasted all the month of February, the month in which well-off families killed their pigs, the month which coincided with the celebrations of Carnival. The farces began with the first Sunday in February dedicated to friends, the second to godparents, the third to relatives and the fourth to him, the Carnival King.

"Already from the first Sunday, people began to feel the festive air. In fact at dawn, even before day broke, the first masks which accompanied the fanfare appeared; it seemed as if they wanted to give people the good news.

"Even today I cannot tell whether people made masks in the hopes of being able to eat afterwards, or if one ate in order to make the masks..."

The question remains: it's Carnival, "Was it a festival because one could eat well?" or "Did one eat well because it was a festival?" Many oral poems confirm that the people who had nothing to eat did not feel fes-tive, they did not *feel the festival* (*see* Teti, 1976).

The "*farsaro*" explains that in the farces the contrast was repre-sented between well-being and poverty, between the rich gentlemen with fat stomachs and round faces and the poor who wore masks that bore the signs of hunger. From D'Eraclea's words, however, the nature of Carnival does not emerge as a *separate festival* or of radical oppositions. Even the rich participated in the organisation of the Carnival rituals:

"...the farces spared no-one. Everyone was made fun of to some extent, including the rich, but to tell the truth the gentlemen watched with amusement. Besides, one must not forget that the clothes, the beautiful clothes of silk, of satin and brocade and the marvellous velvet hats full of feathers and ribbons were in fact taken out of their old wardrobes and still held the intimate perfume of the previous century which had just ended. Even the tail-coats, riding-coats, stove-pipe hats, top hats, and bowler hats, military uniforms, swords and scimitars which had belonged to their ancestors, were kindly lent to us by them. Thus, as can easily be seen, there was no hostility shown by the gentry to the masks; on the contrary, in a certain sense they collaborated, even if they knew very well that with those costumes the farces were directed at them or intended to denounce affluence and poverty. They set opposite their fat stomachs and their round faces other haggard masks, emaciated and painted yellow, to show hunger and misery" (D'Eraclea).

The celebrations of Carnival were the temporary triumph of fatness and fatty foods against thinness and nonfat foods, greens, compulsory diets. The *"farsaro"* continues:

"The last Sunday of Carnival was dedicated to him, the King, the Carnival chief...He made his triumphal entry greeting the acclaiming and applauding crowd. The gentlemen of the village followed him with their bulging stomachs and their round faces, on which one could read affluence and tranquility. Now it was the turn of the bishop with his mitre and crook. Under his forehead stuck out a nose like a pepper, vermillion coloured. This man, slightly shaking his hips, distributed benedictions to left and right. He was followed by some fat parish priests and canons, and a flock of well-fed nuns. The procession was concluded by the poor, the ragamuffins of the village who, in order to express their thanks and gratitude to the Carnival father, held between their hands either a pig's trotter, a bone, or a sausage. This grandiose ceremony ended in the square, where his eminence the bishop, with an appropriate sermon, extolled the paternal qualities and goodness of Carnival....

"Late on Monday afternoon, Carnival became ill and although numerous brilliant physicians and surgeons were called, no one was able to save him, and on Tuesday morning, the lavish and generous Carnival left us. The following day, the bishop would hold his funeral speech. Now the compulsory diet based on wild herbs returned, which made people's faces green like them. One needed to go into a long hibernation and wake up with the first sounds of the death rattle of the pig being killed, a year later..."

The gentlemen of the village, the clergy, priests, canons, nuns and bishop were obese. They were the object of people's irony and sarcasm. The poor ragamuffins felt gratitude and thanks for King Carnival, fat and majestic, but also humble and generous with the starving poor. Mocked or envied, scorned or praised, fat round people with full protruding stomachs represented the aesthetic models of undernourished people, who lived the anxiety of hunger.

Many Calabrian folk texts talk of the links between good food, strength and health, and mention fatness as a sign of physical well-being and good health.

"From good food comes strength";

"Eating well makes you well—working too hard wears you out" (Lombardi Satriani, 1969;277,174);

"An empty sack—can't stand up";

"A full stomach sings" (*See* Teti, 1976).

In peasant society and also in many primitive societies fatness was equivalent to strength and was of value because it meant the ability to work (*see*, for Guayaki Indians, Clastres, 1980:133).

Even women were considered beautiful when they were fat. I could quote many oral sources which confirm the appreciation of fat women, also because they showed a stronger resistance to work. The erotic dream of the protagonist of the novel *L'uomo nel labirinto (The man in the labyrinth)* by Corrado Alvaro is peopled by fat women (Alvaro, 1983). It was only half way through the 1960s—when food consumer goods finally had been extended to the vast majority of the population—that fat people, becoming more numerous, began to be considered as "ill." *Thinness* began to be proposed by the food industry, which invented the ideology of the "good" diet and of healthy eating, and by the fashion and show-business world, as a model of health and beauty.

Before the economic boom of the 1960s, when the "great exodus" had not yet taken place from Calabria, and grave food shortages continued, fatness was valued by both men and women. It was a common opinion that fat, robust people lived better and longer than thin people.

A Calabrian proverb states:

"During the time necessary for a fat person to get thin, the thin person has gone."

The thin man gets ill more frequently than the fat man. The former dies more easily than the latter. It is by now clear why fatness was a treasure for the undernourished. It is evident why individuals who left their villages of hunger sought food abundance and, initially, tried to become fat, beautiful and desirable like the rich gentlemen.

The brigand established himself, even if precariously and dangerously, at times becoming a legend. He was perceived as a fat, robust, strong and courageous man with food and women available to him. But it is also the Calabrian emigrant, from the second half of the nineteenth century, who continues to make explicit the dreams and desires of the brigand. And he manages to escape from his hungry village permanently.

Emigration which, between the end of the nineteenth century and the early years of the twentieth, depopulated the country, the villages and the urban centres of Calabria (Teti, 1989a), becomes, as Nitti maintains, the "chief cause of transformation" of the Calabrian society (Nitti, 1968). Nothing remains as before. As Nitti remembers in 1910:

"'The world is free', said the poor peasant of Lagonegro. And it is freedom that, determining this tremendous exodus of men, has been both the reason of severe torment and of profound renewal."

It was in America, as I have maintained elsewhere (*see* Teti 1990c) that the poor people of Calabria succeeded, even if at great and painful cost, in realizing their ancient dreams of food. The well-known expression "either a brigand or an emigrant," which represents the historical condition of the southern populations, explains the continuity, from an alimentary point of view, between brigands and emigrants. America can be read as the land of Plenty, or Carnival becoming reality (*see* Teti, 1990d).

Above all it was in the United States that the Calabrian emigrants gained access to those foodstuffs which they had been denied in their native lands. In America they realized their ancient dreams, ate meat, eggs, milk, fish, cheese, all those formerly unattainable items. The "Americans" who returned home, when interviewed by Nitti, insisted that in America it was possible to eat meat every day. As Piero Bevilacqua observes pertinently:

"For our vegetarian peasants it is here that there is a break in age-old traditions on the dietary, cultural and mentality level. We can go as far as to say that within one generation the Italian emigrants were subject to a sort of anthropological change" (Bevilacqua, 1980:75).

In 1937 Amerigo Ruggiero in *Italiani in America* (Italians in America) pointed out the great difference, from the physical point of view and from that of height and appearance, between the young Italo-Americans who were now being nourished on butter, milk, meat as well as the foods that were typical of Italian cuisine, as compared to their parents who had been brought up in Italy. Bearing in mind the numerous emigrants of Calabrian origin, he writes:

> "Certain young sons of Calabrians, for example, when they are tall in stature and with fair skin, do not differ from the descendants of Anglo-Saxons because of the dolichocephaly which they have in common" (Ruggiero, 1937:150).

American photographers and film-directors focus on the world of the immigrants of southern origin portraying the sense of the great anthropological, physical and cultural mutations undergone by these Italians from the south (*see* Riis 1971; Hartney and Troper, 1975). If the first pictures refer to emigrants who arrive at the port of New York, at Ellis Island, in rags, dirty, thin, sick, the pictures relating to the second generation portray, often with the intention of creating dissension, an Italian who is tearful, nostalgic, a delinquent, only interested in playing the guitar, organising crimes and eating (*see* Pacini *et al.*1982).

The American cinema contributes to the creation of the stereotype of the Italo-American as violent, pitiful, clannish, and involved in the Mafia. Only from the 1960s onwards, when directors, actors and screenplay writers of Italian origin emerged, was the life of Italo-Americans observed in its multiple social and cultural aspects.

The subject needs to be examined at length, but here I would like to suggest that the reader look at the image of the man involved in the Mafia as depicted in some of Scorsese, Coppola and De Palma's films (M. Scorsese, *Mean Streets*, 1973; *Raging Bull*, 1980; *Goodfellas*, 1990; F.F. Coppola, *The Godfather* I, II, III, 1972, 1974, 1990; B. De Palma *The Untouchables*, 1987). He appears as the confirmation of the idea of America, as the realization of the incarnation of Carnival and also of the place in which ancient dietary models and the desired body image of the peasant populations of Southern Italy were able to become flesh. The Italo-American Mafia man, for example, the protagonists of *The Godfather I, The Godfather II*, and *The Godfather III*, by Coppola, *The Un-*

touchables by De Palma, and of *Raging Bull* and *Goodfellas* by Scorsese appear as obese, fat, robust. Each seems to have achieved, in other contexts, the ancient values and models of the popular classes of the villages of his grandparents and parents. He has as his point of reference the culture of his birthplace, and the new culture of the emigrant world in which he was born and brought up, and he tries to affirm their needs and values, in every way, even with violence.

The food behavior and dietary and "aesthetic" choices of the Mafioso may appear as a distortion and exaggeration of the lifestyles which are also present for different reasons in the community of Italo-American emigrants (*see* Teti, 1985). Whoever has observed the community of Calabrian emigrants living in North America, Canada and the United States, will have noted their attempt to eat in the peasant way and how the cuisine of their home country becomes the focus of their memories, and a characterizing element of their new identity. But while they affirm the richer cuisine of their original villages, they do not have nostalgia for the hunger they suffered there. Their longing concerns smells, flavours, colours and the emotional links evoked by food. In this way the emigrants affirm, deny and transform ancient culinary habits and traditions in the New World. Moreover, it would be hard not to note the sacred dimension they confer on food and eating. The importance they give to cooking, which is seen as an occasion for being together, at family and community levels, lies behind their care and attention to details such as specific peasant recipes. The obesity which is frequently noticeable even in emigrants of the second and third generation ought to be more carefully interpreted in relation to the dietary models of their society of origin. Mention should also be made of the long historical and cultural processes which send forth voices of chronic hunger, of people forced to eat weeds, who died dreaming of meat and wheat bread, of ill and undernourished individuals who longed to become beautiful and fat like the gentlemen of their villages.

And the emigrants, the "Americans," who returned to Calabria, started to eat like gentlemen. Meat, eggs, coffee, liquors began to appear in the diet of those who "returned" and their relatives who "remained." This profound change, partial and debated, did not take place without the resistance, irony, and concern of the dominant classes. If, in the course of the nineteenth century, observers had built up the image of the Calabrian peasant as parsimonious, sober, frugal and a good worker by the end of the last century, in the space of a few years the figure appears of the "American" who overturns the ancient stereotypic food models. And the landowners, the gentlemen, the "men of honour" cry scandal. The "Americans" are depicted as being spoilt, lazy, restless and insatiable. Stereotypes are born about "Americans" as presumptuous, exhibitionists, stupid, cuckolded. These images reveal, however, the profound transformations that had taken place in the fabric of society and in the cultural and mental spheres of the population (see Teti, 1987b). De Nobili writes in 1909: "Between the class of men of honour and the poor, a new class has recently grown up in Calabria, the class of the returned men, the Americans" (Taruffi, De Nobili and Lori, 1909:870).

The *American* introduces new values and new behaviour. He introduces new foods and asserts standards and models that formerly were only allowed to the rich. He shows off his affluence, wears new clothes and carries a watch on his waistcoat. He presents himself—and is observed—with a robust and well-coloured physique. Fatness is one of the signs of his wealth, of his new status, which is different from that of the "men of honour" to which he formerly looked with envy and resentment. The American tries to realize the ancient dreams of the popular classes and to reach the affluence of the rich. Corrado Alvaro, with his usual attention to the changes that took place in Calabrian society with emigration, remembers how the emigrant presented himself with a new physical image that revealed a changed economic and food status, as well as the assertion of a new mentality.

"Angelino returned one day, sent back by America to his native village like a criminal. In Argoni people discussed for a long time whether Angelino was truly to be considered a criminal born in our village, or whether instead had become a criminal there where he had landed as a boy before his character was formed. ...

"I hugged him without any hesitation whatever, first of all because we are cousins, and then because in our country a criminal is not such only because the law defines him as one. The mortality of poor countries has nothing to do with what is universally accepted on the presupposition that everything is just and everyone has the same rights. Angelino had become a man, tall, robust, almost fat, and in this he resembled no one in Argoni, and not even anyone of his own family, like a plant that was seen to grow with difficulty initially and then developed beyond measure because it found the right fertile soil" (Alvaro, 1955:486).

I have written that emigration involves the death of the ancient village which is reborn in another place. The village is duplicated. The "village number one" and the "village number two," one the shadow of the other (see Teti, 1989a). The original village and the village born in the New World are both inseparable and unable to join up again, they maintain very strong links between themselves, influence each other reciprocally.

It has been seen how the long dietary history and culture of the original village can condition the food choices, constructions, inventions, and nostalgia of Calabrians in the places to which they emigrate. And it has been suggested how precisely the emigrants who return to their native country introduce new foods, break with a diet that had been predominantly vegetarian, overturn the image of the peasant as a sober and frugal man, and show off new behaviour revealing the attainment of a new status. The "Americans" present themselves as a "new class," with a new culture, new values, new ways of perceiving themselves, of showing off and asserting themselves.

The Italo-American Mafia was born for defensive reasons and also to assert a power and control between the communities of the emigrants and in the larger society. It addresses itself to overturning and modifying the original culture of the emigrants, bearing in mind the "honoured society" already existing in the traditional agropastoral world until the end of the nineteenth century and in some villages of the province of Reggio Calabria. The Sicilian Mafia or the Neopolitan Camorra are a different matter. The actor and filmmaker Sergio Leone has frequently maintained that Italy sent peasants to America and America sent back Mafiosi (Once upon a Time in America, 1984). There is some truth in this provocative observation. In many Calabrian villages, where no delinquent organizations or "Honoured society" existed, the return of the "Americans" meant the establishment or reinforcement of the "Ndrangheta" (Calabrian equivalent of the Mafia): It is well-known that, from the beginning of this century, the native village and the community of emigrants over the ocean would communicate through members of the "Ndrangheta" and the Mafia.

I certainly do not mean that it was emigration that determined the birth of the "honoured society," but wish to underline that experts have not paid sufficient attention to the closeness, at times the confusion, between the figure of the "American" and the member of the "Ndrangheta" in many Calabrian situations. Both the "Americans" and the members of the "honoured society" behave as members of rising social classes. They come from the "popular world," from which they try to distance themselves in order to rebel against the power of the ancient lords, very often substituting themselves for the latter. In many villages the "American" and the man of the "*Ndrangheta*" are the same person.

The Calabrian men of letters were the first to realise this link: Antonio Margariti in *America! America!* (1979); in 1973 *La Famiglia Montalbano* by Saverio Montalto was published; in the autobiographical novel *Il previtocciolo* by Luca Asprea (1971).

The American, who had been initiated as a Camorrista (member of the Camorra) in New York, with a brigand's moustache, tall, handsome, agile, robust, admired by women, seems to be the personification of the dreams of generations of poor Calabrians, who set out on their journeys, first to the Mountains, then to America.

America is Carnival made flesh: the affirmation of abundance, of fatness and the beauty of the large Carnival body which had attracted and fascinated the feeble inhabitants of the villagers of hunger. Being elegant, tall, robust like the wealthy, are the signs of a new status attained by both the *Americans* and the members of the *Ndrangheta*, who have some links with the world of emigration.

Certainly one must not forget the high prices that people paid to attain better living conditions. In Calabria in the first half of this century, situations of grave food discomfort continued, when there were not cases of real famine. Only after the 1950s, when the exodus started again and with the economic boom which touched Italy, did the food standards of the Calabrians really improve from the point of view both of quality and quantity.

I underline only that pasta, meat, wheat bread are no longer the forbidden dreams of the population. There is by now a progressive and significant rejection of the "vegetarian regime," and of the "Mediterranean diet," which from both necessity and choice had characterized the Calabrian food history. Thinness is no longer a sign of starving and undernourished bodies.

In conclusion, a contradiction should be pointed out with regard to food abundance, and fatness, which appears to be its expression. This contradiction reflects the ambiguous relationship to tradition, which at times is asserted, at times denied, at times invented.

From a recent survey on food consumption carried out by the National Food Institute, it appears that today Calabrians eat well and abundantly, and that they have discarded the old way of eating (*see* Saba *et al.*, 1990; *see also* Collaridi, 1990; Teti, 1989b). But does not this distance from their earlier eating habits indirectly reflect the assertion of ancient food needs and desires? Do people perhaps not eat too much nowadays because in the past they did not eat enough or ate badly? Referring to that cultural inheritance, they hold the conviction that "to eat in the traditional way" (when in fact they eat in the way people dreamed of eating in the past) means the end of the ancient miserable and wretched diet. Abundance, which is affirmed and praised, is the end of the ancient hunger. Nowadays throughout the population, irony is expressed towards diets or fasting imposed by doctors, the latter being considered as old-time preachers. A protruding stomach, the sign of continual overeating, is regarded with much more indulgence than in areas where the ideology of controlling appetite has triumphed. Many still continue today to want to put on weight as if to ward off the times of hunger and enforced fasting, to forget a past full of thin, weak, ill bodies.

However, new behaviour and food models, imposed from outside, by the food industry and alternative cuisines, tend to stress the idea of fatness as an illness and as physical ugliness. "Fatness is half an illness" says a proverb that shows the penetration of a new dietary concept among the less well-off classes. A fat stomach comes to be considered the sign of poor nutrition, of greediness, of scant consideration for one's own body. Today, now that everyone can be fat, fatness is no longer a model as when it signified wealth, power, affluence, beauty. A fat body is no longer fashionable, indeed it is negatively perceived. The valued body image of the newly rich is no longer that of the past wealthy classes. There are many reasons to affirm that new dietary distances are being created between the rich and today's lower classes. The latter, if they are no longer dying of hunger, are kept a long way away from the new luxuries and outside trends which can make people die of excess food, of malnutrition, of bad quality and poisoned foods. The criticism of "the good old food days" must mean also some recognition of the values that were, however, present in the traditional diet, and may dictate a critical attitude towards today's basic diet of tasteless, colourless, sophisticated, tainted foodstuffs which create in people a "thinness" that, even if different from the past, seems to be the prelude to an ever-possible and imminent end.

NOTES

Vito Teti (San Nicola Da Crissa, Catanzaro), is Associate Professor of Popular Literature in the Faculty of Letters and Philosophy of the University of Calabria, Italy. He is the author of tracts on the anthropology of nutrition and on emigration, on feasts, pilgrimages and Carnival in Calabria. He has written on ideology of nutrition in the lower classes, myth, folklore, poetry and traditional music in Calabria, and is author or editor of books on some of these topics.

1. Goitre, of course, is due to iodine deficiency, not unsanitary conditions, but knowledge of these scientific facts may not have been widespread in the 1920s, when they became better known north of Africo.

REFERENCES

Alicata, M. 1954. Il meridionalismo non si puó fermare ad Eboli, *Cronache Meridionali:i* i(9), 585–603.

Alicata, M. 1968. *Scritti letterari*, Il Saggiatore Milano.

Alvaro, C. 1931. *Calabria*. Nemi Firenze. (new ed., 1990).

Alvaro, C. 1955. *Angelino, in 75 racconti*. Bompiani, Milano.

Alvaro, C. 1982. *Gente in Aspromonte*. Garzanti, Milano. (1st ed., 1930).

Alvaro, C. 1983. *L'uomo nel labirinto*. Bompiani, Milano. (1st ed., 1926).

Asprea, L. 1971. *Il previtocciolo*. Feltrinelli, Milano.

Bachtin, M. 1979. *L'opera di Rabelais e la cultura popolare. Riso, carnevale e festa nella tradizione medievale e renascimentale*. Einaudi, Torino.

Bevilacqua, P. 1980. *Le campagne del Mezzogiorno tra fascismo e dopoguerra. Il caso della Calabria*. Einaudi, Torino.

Burke, P. 1980. *Cultura popolare nell'Europa moderna*. Mondadori, Milano.

Burton, R. 1981. *Malinconia d'amore*. Rizzoli, Milano.

Burton, R. 1983. *Anatomia della melanconia*. Marsilio, Venezia (originally published in 1621).

Camporesi, P. 1976, *La maschera di Bertoldo. G.C. Croce e la letteratura carnevalesca*. Einaudi, Torino.

Chatwin, B. 1988. *Le vie dei canti*, Adelphi, Milano.

Cirese, A.M. 1973. *Cultura egemonica e culture subalterne*. Palumbo, Palermo. (1st ed., 1971).

Clastres, P. 1980. *Cronaca di una tribú. Il mondo degli Indiani Guayaki*. Feltrinelli, Milano.

Collaridi, P. 1990. *Aspetti dei consumi alimentari in un'area Mediterranea: la Calabria*. Thesis for an undergraduate degree. Facoltá di Scienze Matematiche, Fisiche e Naturali, Corso di Perfezionamento in Scienze dell'Alimentazione, Universitá di Roma "La Sapienza," Roma.

DeMartino, E. 1976. *Sud e magia*. Feltrinelli, Milano. (1st ed., 1959).

D'Eraclea, S. undated, *Carnevale*, unpublished text, personal records of Vito Teti, San Nicola Da Crissa (Catanzaro).

Dorsa, V. 1983. *La tradizone greco-latina negli usi e nelle credenze popolari della Calabria Citeriore*. Forni, Bologna. (1st ed., 1884).

Faeta, F. 1984. *Saverio Marra fotografo. Immagini del mondo popolare silano nei primi decenni del secolo*, Electa, Milano.

Faeta, F., and M. Miraglia (eds.) 1988. *Sguardo e memoria. Alfonso Lombardi Satriani e la fotografia signorile nella Calabria del primo Novecento.* Mondadori—De Luca, Milano-Roma.

Familiari, P. 1971. *La vera storia del brigante Marlino Zappa.* QualeCultura, Vibo Valentia.

Frazer, J.G. 1978. *Il ramo d'oro,* 2 vol., Boringhieri, Torino (originally published in 1922).

Gambino, S. 1990. *Fischia il sasso.* QualeCultura—Jaca Book, Vibo Valentia, Milano.

Gissing, G. 1971. *Sulle rive dello Ionio.* Cappelli, Bologna.

Harris, M. 1971. *L'evoluzione del pensiero antropologico. Una storia della teoria della cultura,* Il Mulino, Bologna.

Harris, M. 1979. *Cannibali e re. Le origini della cultura,* Feltrinelli, Milano.

Harris, M. 1990. *Buono da mangiare. Enigmi del gusto e consuetudini alimentari.* Einaudi, Torino.

Hartney, R., and H. Troper 1975. *Immigrants. A portrait of the urban experience, 1890–1930.* Van Nostrand Reinhold, Toronto.

Levi, C. 1984. *Cristo si è fermato ad Eboli.* Einaudi, Torino. (1st ed., 1945).

Lombardi Satriani, R. 1932. *Canti popolari calabresi,* Vol. III. De Simone, Napoli.

Lombardi Satriani, R. 1940. *Canti popolari calabresi,* Vol. VI, De Simone, Napoli.

Lombardi Satriani, R. 1969. *Proverbi in uso in San Costantino di Briatico.* Peloritana, Messina. (1st ed., 1913).

Lumini, A. 1888. *Le farse di Carnevale in Calabria e in Sicilia.* Nicastro, Nicotera. (new ed., 1977).

Margariti, A. 1979. *America! America!* Casavelino Scalo (SA), Galzerano.

Misasi, N. 1976. *Il Gran Bosco d'Italia,* In (ed.), Cosenza, Pellegrini. *In Calabria,* pp. 368–369.

Montalto, S. 1973. *La famiglia Montalbano,* Frama's, Chiaravalle Centrale.

Niceforo, A. 1901. *Italiani del Nord e Italiani del Sud.* Bocca, Torino.

Nitti, F.S. 1968. *Scritti sulla questione meridionale, Vol. IV: Inchiesta sulle condizioni dei contadini in Basilicata e in Calabria,* parte I, Bari, Laterza (1st ed., 1910).

Pacini, M., G. Rondolino, G.C. Bertolina and D. Candeloro 1982. *Integrato Metropolitano. New York, Chicago, Torino: tre volti dell emigrazione italiana.* Fondazione Giovanni Agnelli, Torino.

Pasquinelli, C. (ed.) 1977. *Antropologia e questione meridionale.* La Nuova Italia, Firenze.

Petrelli, T. 1990. *Tra la perduta gente. Africo 1948.* Marina di Belvedere, Grisolia.

Rauty, R. (ed.) 1976. *Cultura popolare e marxismo,* Editori Riuniti, Roma.

Riis, J.A. 1971. *How the other half lives.* Dover Publications, New York.

Ruggiero, A. 1937. *Italiani in America.* Treves, Milano.

Saba, A., A. Turrini, G. Mistura, E. Cialfa, and M. Vichi 1990. Indagine nazionale sui consumi alimentari delle famiglie italiane (1980–84). *Rivista della Società Italiana de Scienza dell'Alimentazione*.4, Anno 19: 53–65.

Seminara, F. 1942. *Le Baracche*. Rizzoli, Milano, (new ed., 1988).

Seminara, F. 1963. *Il vento nell'oliveto*. In *Il vento nell'oliveto, Disgrazia in casa Amato, Il diario di Laura*. Einaudi, Torino.

Silone, I. 1987. *Fontamara*, Mondadori, Milano, (1st ed., 1949).

Sole, G. 1990. Santi, grani e carestie nella Calabria Citeriore dell'800, "*Daedalus*" 5, 85–127.

Spezzano, F. 1970. *Proverbi calabresi*, Martello, Milano.

Stajano, C. 1979. *Africo*. Einaudi, Torino.

Taruffi, D., L. De Nobili and C. Lori 1909. *La questione agraria e l'emigrazione in Calabria*, Barbera, Firenze.

Teti, V. 1976. *Il pane, la beffa e la festa. Cultura alimentare e ideologia dell'alimentazione nelle classi subalterne*, Guaraldi, Rimini. (new ed., 1978).

Teti, V. 1982. Carnevale é ancora una festa? "*Calabria Sconosciuta*" no. 20, pp. 27–34.

Teti, V. 1984. La carne e le cipolle. Note di storia dell'alimentazione calabrese: menzogne colte e desideri popolari, "*Miscellanea di Studi Storici*," IV, Universitá della Calabria, pp. 141–164.

Teti, V. 1985, *Beni alimentari. Cosnervazione e innovazione nella comunitá calabrocanadese a Toronto*. In *Beni culturali della Calabria*. Roma-Reggio Calabria, Gangemi-Casa del Libro, Vol. II, pp. 627–649.

Teti, V. 1985–86. Acque, paesi, uomini in viaggio. Appunti per un'antropologia dell'acqua in Calabria in epoca moderna e contemporana, *Miscellanea di Studi Storici, V. Universitá della Calabria*, pp. 73–118.

Teti, V. 1987a. La cucina calabrese: caratteri romantici di un modello e di un mito alimentare. In P. Falco (ed.), Cultura romantica e territoria nella calabria dell'Ottocento. *Periferia, Cosenza*. pp. 347–380.

Teti, V. 1987b. Note sui comportamenti delle donne sole degli "americani" durante la prima emigrazione in Calabria. "*Studi Emigrazione*", no. 85, pp. 13–46.

Teti, V. 1989a. *Il paese e l'ombra*, Periferia, Cosenza.

Teti, V. 1989b. L'invention d'une cuisine regionale. Le cas de la cuisine calabraise. In S. Peltre and C. Thonevenot (eds.), *Alimentation et Regions*, Nancy, pp. 411–421.

Teti, V. 1989c. *Taverne, trattorie e alberghi in Calabria nel XIX secolo negli scritti dei viaggiatori stranieri*. A report presented at the International Conference, "Les restaurants dans le monde á travers les ages," Université de la Sorbonne, Paris, 9–12 October 1989, in press.

Teti, V. 1990a. Il folklorista e il cuculo. Splendori e paradossi delle ricerche sula poesia popolare. Il caso della Calabria. In V. Teti and G. Plastino, *L'acqua di Gangá. II: Note sulla poesia e la musica tradizionale in Calabria*, Vibo Valentia, Milano, QualeCultura-Jaca Book, pp. 13–274.

Teti, V. 1990b. Fame, digiuno, dieta nella storia e nella cultura folklorica della Calabria. In M. Di Rosa (ed.), *Salute e malattia nella cultura delle classi subalterne del Mezzogiorno*. Guida, Napoli, pp. 89–134.

Teti, V. 1990c. La teoria di uomini. Pellegrinaggio a Polsi e viaggio nelle opere di Corrado Alvaro, Fortunato Seminara, Francesco Perri. In Sanctuary of Santa Maria di Polsi and the Deputazione di Storia Patria per la Calabria (eds.), *S. Maria di Polsi. Storia e pietá religiosa*, Laruffa, Reggio Calabria, pp. 527–601.

Teti, V. 1990d. Pane e fantasia. Da una ricerca su "Il mangiare di una volta," In L.M. Lombardi Satriani, (ed.), *Le perle della memoria*. Roma, 50&Piú, pp. 21–74.

Teti, V. 1990e. New York: Mito e specchio della Calabria. In M. Mattia and S. Piermarini, *Lo sguardo di New York*, La Casa Usher, Firenze, pp. 121–190.

Toschi, P. 1976. *Le origini del teatro italiano*, Boringhieri, Torino, (1st ed., 1955).

Valletta, N. 1984. *La jettatura*. Longanesi, Milano. (1st ed., 1787).

Zanotti-Bianco, U. 1946. *Tra la perduta gente (Africo)*, Le Monnier, Firenze.

2

Physique of Sumo Wrestlers in Relation to Some Cultural Characteristics of Japan

KOMEI HATTORI

INTRODUCTION

Physiques of athletes differ from sport to sport. Professional Sumo wrestlers are in a special position within the Japanese sports society, and the peculiarity of their physiques is remarkable. In the entire industrialized world there has been a recent trend toward healthy living and away from obesity. Sumo wrestlers, with their extremely large bodies, seem to be living anachronisms in a lean world.

Their physiques may be mainly due to the competitive nature of the sport of Sumo. However, we cannot ignore the potential effects of the unique society to which Sumo wrestlers belong. This society, moreover, is accepted by the general population of Japan. The Sumo society, with its unique norms and role expectations, is an important part of Japanese society.

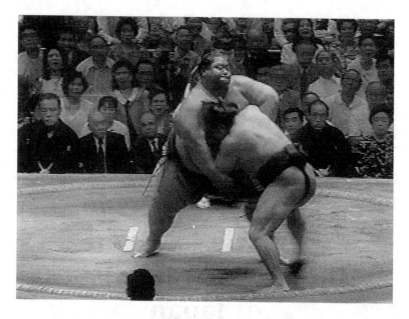

Figure 1.   Sumo wrestlers during a Sumo match. The lighter wrestler is trying to get both his arms on the inside and firmly grasp his opponent's belt. This technique gives a wrestler commanding control. The traditional hairstyle and the belts of the Sumo wrestlers are unusual.

The purpose of this paper is to review the physique of Sumo wrestlers in relation to some unique cultural characteristics of Japan.

CULTURAL ASPECTS OF SUMO AND THE SUMO SOCIETY

Sumo has a 2,000-year-old history that qualifies it as the national sport of Japan. Sumo became a professional sport almost 300 years ago, and although it is practiced today in many amateur clubs (Thayer, 1983), it has its greatest appeal as a professional spectator sport (Figure 1). There are at least three monthly Sumo magazines which are presently distributed throughout Japan. Entire tournaments are broadcast as television programs by NHK (Japan Broadcasting Association). In a recent tournament, the playoff by the three most popular wrestlers recorded an audience rating of 66.7% (66 million viewers). The extent of the diffusion of Sumo into Japanese society can be seen in newspaper cartoons depicting political figures as Sumo athletes (Figure 2).

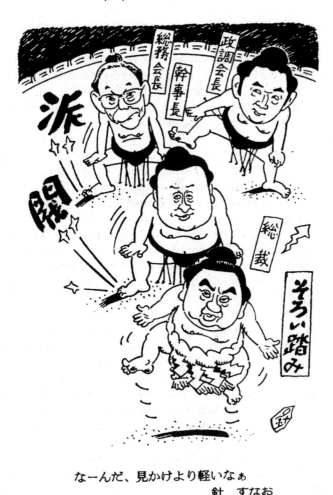

なーんだ、見かけより軽いなぁ
針 すなお

Figure 2. Newspaper cartoon depicting political figures as Sumo athletes.

The Sumo society has many old-fashioned and feudalistic elements, and the cultural makeup of Sumo society is rather complicated. Sumo is vaguely associated with Shinto, which is the earliest
and most distinctive of the Japanese religions (Reischauer, 1992). Every aspect of professional Sumo is controlled by the Japan Sumo
Association, which is run by 105 retired wrestlers who are qualified as

the members. Although the wrestlers control the sport, there are some other working ranks which are essential for the maintenance of Sumo.

The wrestlers who wear only *mawashi* (loin cloths) step into the ring after each wrestler's name is called by the ring steward (*yobidashi*) for the bout. The names are announced using an unique tone, and this creates a solemn atmosphere in the arena. Another typical characteristic of the wrestlers is the traditional hairstyle and topknot inherited from the 18th century.

The referee (*gyoji*) is a trained professional who has had no special career as a wrestler. Referees are promoted step by step, and only one person can become the top-ranked referee who can officiate at a grand champion bout. Referees wear dignified traditional costumes and their basic actions are systematically formalized.

The five judges (*shimpan*) sit around the ring and have a right to overrule the referee's decision of victory or defeat. They are all ex-wrestlers and members of the Japan Sumo Association.

All wrestlers belong to various training establishment stables called "*heya*." Each *heya* is rigidly ruled by a single individual (*oyakata*), who must be an ex-senior wrestler and a member of the Japan Sumo Association. The *heya* are heavily influenced by Sumo tradition and are therefore, quite resistant to change. The basic training style is almost identical in all stables, because the following three traditional exercises are considered as the absolute basics of Sumo: *shiko* (raising one leg sideways as high as possible and then stamping it down), *teppo* (slamming one's open hands against a pole), and *matawari* (sitting with legs spread as wide as possible and leaning forward until the entire upper body is pressed against the ground).

Everybody has a chance to be a Sumo wrestler if he has the potential. Recruits are usually 15 years of age or have finished junior high school. Recently, many college graduate wrestlers who have had successful careers in their amateur leagues, and foreign wrestlers found by talent scouts, are registered at various levels of the league (division). Thus, the home towns of wrestlers are located throughout Japan. Usually people support the wrestler coming from their home town, and each competitive wrestler is supported by his fan club.

Facilities and tools for Sumo are quite unique. The ring (*dohyo*) is the bouting spot, but it is also considered a sacred place which must be purified by a scattering of salt by the wrestlers. The *dohyo* is a 4.55 meter diameter circle of special clay packed hard and sprinkled with sand. The border of the *dohyo* is defined by the tops of bales of straw bags filled with earth and sunk in the clay. There are two dividing lines in the middle of the circle about 90 centimeters long, which face each other about 120 centimeters apart. It is at these lines that the two wrestlers meet to glower at each other during their psychological buildup for the match. They finally leap at each other in the initial charge (*tachiai*).

CHARACTERISTICS OF SUMO AS A COMPETITIVE SPORT

The six major Japanese Sumo tournaments are held in Tokyo, Osaka, Tokyo, Nagoya, Tokyo and Fukuoka every other month. Each tournament takes fifteen days to complete.

After the two opponents step up to the ring for their match, there are roughly two main stages, the initial buildup stage (ritual preliminaries) and the actual fighting stage. The initial stage takes about 4 minutes and involves a bewildering ritual of stamping, squatting, puffing, glowering and tossing salt in the air. All the processes are determined following a systematic order. The bout is initiated by a sign from the *gyoji* after the final quadruped position with the wrestlers glaring at each other. In order to win a Sumo bout, wrestlers are required to maintain a standing posture within the *dohyo*. Following the initial charge, the wrestler must attempt to eject his opponent from the ring or cause him to touch the surface of the *dohyo* with any part of the body other than the soles of his feet.

In Sumo, the most important factor for winning is the momentum which can be produced by the multiplication of the wrestler's body mass and velocity of his charge. This is the reason why wrestlers place a great amount of stress on the initial charge with the opponent.

A Sumo match usually only lasts for several seconds. If it lasts for more than one minute, it is called a "great bout." Since the match time is so short, the main physical quality needed is anaerobic power. The ability to transport oxygen to working tissues (that is, aerobic power), is therefore lacking, and this deficiency has been reported by several authors (Ogawa *et al.*, 1972, 1973; Nagatomo *et al.*, 1979).

With respect to the short duration of the Sumo bout, it should be noted that the characteristic "conciseness" is not unlike the conciseness seen in other forms of Japanese art, language and technology. *Haiku* is a form of poetry which is characterized by simplicity and conciseness. It is an entire poem occupying a very small space. The Japanese language—particularly that part adopted from the Chinese (for example, *kanji*)—is also very concise since its information is conveyed

Height
Upper limb length
Weight
Neck girth
Chest girth
Waist girth
Hip girth
Upper arm girth
Forearm girth
Wrist girth
Thigh girth
Calf girth
Ankle girth
Subscapular skinfold
Abdominal skinfold
Triceps skinfold

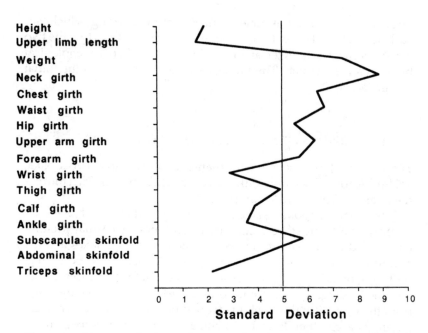

0   1   2   3   4   5   6   7   8   9   10

Standard Deviation

Figure 3. Diagram of relative deviation of anthropometric dimensions for Sumo wrestlers (*sekitori*).[a] Norms for Japanese males of corresponding age are adopted as the standard.
[a]Ogawa *et al.* (1973).

pictorially. Finally, many technological innovations which have come from Japan have been characterized as being "neat," "tidy," or "compact." All these concepts are embodied in a Sumo bout. All the wrestlers' abilities are concentrated into a brief moment of confrontation in a small ring. It is this simplified style of exertion which seems to have such great appeal to the Japanese Sumo fan.

THE PHYSIQUE OF SUMO WRESTLERS

As mentioned above, the essential constitutional requirement to be a Sumo wrestler is a large body mass. Figure 3 shows the relative deviations of 16 body dimensions of Sumo wrestlers compared to Japanese norms for males of the same age. Body weight and girths (especially neck girth) of Sumo wrestlers are at the extreme upper end of the population norms.

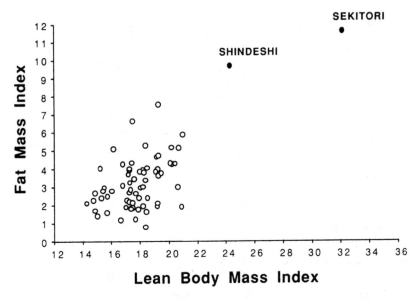

Figure 4.   Body composition chart for Sumo wrestlers (•) and ordinary Japanese males (○) of corresponding age.

The candidates for acceptance into the sport must also exceed additional height and weight standards which are set by the Japanese Sumo Society. The standards for screening potential applicants have been revised several times, with the levels being increased each time. As of this writing, the height and weight standards are 173 cm and 75 kg, respectively. It must also be stressed that any candidate who meets these minimal standards is acceptable. In other words, no attention is paid to body proportion or body composition.

Candidates who exceed the minimal height and weight standards are called "*shindeshi*" or apprentices (pupils). Although their body size is already very large, they are expected to increase it during the period of their apprenticeship. A wrestler who fails to gain weight throughout his apprenticeship is not likely to be promoted, and many apprentices in this position voluntarily quit the sport. The most recent mean height and weight measures of the "*shindeshi*" are 178.3 (plus or minus 4.60) cm and 107 (plus or minus 18.01) kg, respectively (Hattori, unpublished data).

Table I shows data from "*shindeshi*" and "*sekitori*" (highest league) class wrestlers. Detailed inspection of this table reveals that there are

TABLE I. Physique and body composition of top league class wrestlers (*Sekitori*) and apprenticed wrestlers (*Shindeshi*)[a]

	Top league class wrestlers (N=7)		Apprenticed wrestlers (N=19)		
	Mean	S.D.	Mean	S.D.	
Age	29.9	4.41	19.5	3.39	**
Weight (kg)	140.2	19.56	108.9	20.42	*
Height (cm)	179.1	5.46	179.1	5.19	
Upper arm length (cm)	33.6	2.37	32.8	1.61	
Forearm length (cm)	26.3	1.38	25.7	1.38	
Upper thigh length (cm)	41.9	1.21	41.4	1.98	
Lower thigh length (cm)	40.4	1.81	41.2	2.18	
Fat (kg)	37.1	14.19	31.0	11.48	
LBM (kg)	103.1	6.48	78.0	10.27	**
Fat%	25.7	7.04	27.6	6.38	
Body mass index #	43.7		34.0		
Lean body mass index #	32.1		24.3		
Fat mass index #	11.6		9.7		
Cross sectional muscle area:					
Upper arm (cm^2)	67.6	7.9	51.2	11.9	**
Forearm (cm^2)	60.8	7.0	49.8	8.0	**
Upper thigh (cm^2)	204.6	22.4	200.7	28.8	
Lower thigh (cm^2)	112.9	18.5	87.9	11.6	**
Cross sectional bone area:					
Humerus (cm^2)	4.5	0.3	3.7	0.6	**
Radius (cm^2)	2.2	0.3	2.1	0.3	
Ulna (cm^2)	2.3	0.3	2.5	0.5	
Femur (cm^2)	6.6	1.0	6.5	0.8	
Fibula (cm^2)	1.3	0.3	1.3	0.3	
Tibia (cm^2)	10.3	1.9	7.4	0.9	**

[a]From Wada, S. (1987). *Tokyo Ika Daigaku Zasshi* **45**(3), 317–324.
**(*) Significant at 0.01 (0.05) level.
Calculated from means of height, weight, lean body mass and fat mass.

considerable physical differences between wrestlers of the *"shindeshi"* or apprenticeship class and wrestlers of the *"sekitori"* or champion wrestler class. Figure 4 is the graphic representation (body composition chart) of lean body mass index and fat mass index for Sumo wrestlers with data for the general population (Hattori, 1991). Their physiques are located out of the range of the general population, showing an extreme adipo-muscular type. This tendency is strikingly seen in the *"sekitori"* wrestlers. Tanaka *et al.* (1979) also reported that the champion wrestlers have a greater lean body mass (LBM) than do the apprentice candidates. Suda (1957) and Ogawa *et al.* (1973) have presented data showing marked girth increments from the apprenticeship period to the top class period. While some of this increase in girth may be due to increase in fat, the data in Table I suggest that it is likely due to increases in LBM. In other words, in order to be successful the *"shindeshi"* need to change their physiques by adding both more fat and more lean body mass.

The reason for this apparent body composition change from the apprenticeship period to the top class wrestler period is that wrestlers who gain weight through an increment of LBM possess two advantages in the creation of momentum. First, the mass which has been added through an increase of LBM is heavier than that which could have been added through an increase in fat. Secondly, the increased weight of LBM tissue can be moved with greater velocity than the increased weight of fat tissue, since the tissue itself (that is, muscle) is useful in creating increased velocity. Since momentum is the main physical requirement of Sumo, increasing both mass and velocity through increase of LBM is more advantageous than increasing mass at the expense of velocity.

Previously published reports concerning the physiques of Sumo wrestlers (for example, Kohara, 1965; Nakajima *et al.*, 1979) have suggested that there are secular trends which have affected the sport. Height and weight are steadily increasing. With respect to height, Nakajima *et al.* (1979) have shown that this trend has paralleled that of the general population. Weight of Sumo wrestlers, however, also showed a marked increase in the 1970s, far exceeding the normal range of ordinary men (Nakajima *et al.*, 1979).

It is interesting to note that the 1970s were years which marked the levelling off of the Japanese economy after twenty-five years of very high growth. In addition, the decade was associated with rapid accumulation of television sets by Japanese consumers and a corresponding increase in audience participation.

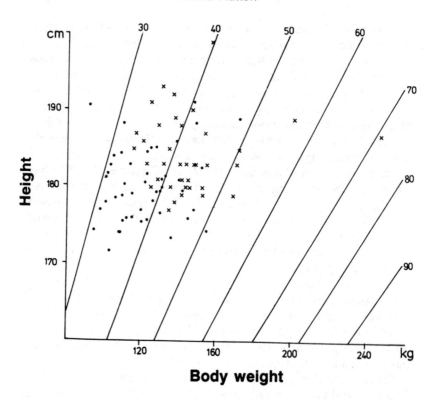

Figure 5.   Scatter diagram of body weight and height of Sumo wrestlers (*sekito-ri*) in 1970 (•)[a] and 1988 (x)[b]. The lines and the numbers represent the body mass index.
[a]Ogawa *et al.* (1973).
[b]Japan Sumo Association (1988).

Sumo wrestlers' nutritional situation must be improved. Figure 5 is the scatter diagram of height and weight for Sumo wrestlers in 1970 and 1988. The oblique lines represent the body mass index (BMI). The present wrestlers are inclined to be heavier than wrestlers of earlier years, and there seem to be clear differences in height between the two groups as well. Also, although the average BMI for Japanese males of the same age is 20.87 plus or minus 2.67 (Hattori, unpublished data), all the present wrestlers' BMIs exceed 30. In one extreme case the BMI is close to 70. Most wrestlers retire from this rigorous sport in their early thirties.

DISCUSSION AND CONCLUSION

The recent economic development of Japan has been mainly associated with the development of engineering in, for example, electronics and cars. This industrialization seems to have dramatically changed Japanese lifestyles. However, although the products of industrialization have improved their daily life, the national traits of Japanese people which have been fostered for several hundred years during Japan's period of isolation probably can not be changed in such a short period. Reischauer (1992) pointed out that modernization in Japan has not necessarily been achieved in the form of westernization, but has rather proceeded on the base of traditional culture. Since most of the outward appearances of daily life have been westernized, Japanese people tend to remember traditional costumes with fondness. Sumo may be a whole unit of life in which is packed the main essence of Japanese traditions. It is also associated with Shinto, which continues to be a part of Japanese life. The Sumo wrestlers are representatives upon which the Japanese can project their original national hopes. They are expected to be elegant, strong, manly and sacred.

The vast majority of Japanese people are quite familiar with the organization of Sumo society. In point of fact, the populace is content with the present system, since it is widely believed that it is the best system for developing Sumo wrestlers.

In addition to possessing the necessary power to defeat their opponent, each Sumo wrestler is expected to exhibit all the characteristics of traditional Japanese culture and manners. This latter requirement is quite different from cultural requirements in other western fighting sports such as boxing. It may be one reason why Sumo does not prevail outside of Japan. Moreover, the skills (and physiques) which are required in Sumo are performed in a closed society. Like other activities which are performed within the confines of specifically determined actions (for example, the tea ceremony), Sumo serves an aesthetic purpose which is independent of its sport function, as shown in the grand champion's ceremonial entrance into the ring. This ceremony has Shinto overtones.

The concept (and shape) of Sumo wrestlers has been used as a model in many fields of Japanese drawing, sculpture and doll making. The "pear" shape associated with Sumo is therefore not perceived to be unattractive in Japan (see Chapter 16). While obesity in general is not perceived positively in Japan, obesity in Sumo wrestlers is not only tolerated, but perceived quite positively. It is, therefore, quite difficult to conceive of a fundamental change in the body proportions of Sumo wrestlers being possible in the short term.

ACKNOWLEDGMENTS

I would like to express my great thanks to Dr. Yukinari Kohara of Rikkyo University and Dr. K. Yuasa of Chukyo University for helpful suggestions with this paper. Thanks also to Dr. Richard Danielson of Laurentian University for his invaluable comments on the text.

NOTES

Komei Hattori, Ph.D., graduated from Tokyo University of Education in 1965, is a Councillor of the Anthropological Society of Nippon, and is currently Professor of Anatomy and Physical Activity Sciences of the Faculty of General Education, Ibaraki University, Mito, Ibaraki 310, Japan.

REFERENCES

Hattori, K. 1991. Body composition and lean body mass index for Japanese college students. *Journal of the Anthropological Society of Nippon* 92(2), 141–148.

Hattori, K. Unpublished data. Relative variation of lean body mass for Japanese young adults.

Kohara, Y. 1965. Anthropometry of Sumo wrestlers. *The Heredity* 19, 16–21 (in Japanese).

Nagatomo, M., K. Tanaka, H. Kato, K. Kikuchi, H. Nakajima, H. Shibayama, H. Ebashi, Y. Nishijima, M. Matsuzawa and S. Ogawa 1979. Characteristics of respiratory functions in "*Shindeshi*" Sumo wrestlers. *Bulletin of the Physical Fitness Research Institute* 43, 41–55 (in Japanese with English abstract).

Nakajima, H., H. Shibayama, H. Ebashi, Y. Nishijima, M. Matsuzawa, K. Tanaka, H. Kato, M. Nagatomo, K. Kikuchi and S. Ogawa 1979. Some considerations on the physical fitness of "Shindeshi" Sumo wrestlers. *Bulletin of the Physical Fitness Research Institute* 44, 29–46 (in Japanese with English abstract).

Ogawa, S., Y. Furuta, K. Yamamoto, N. Nagai and H. Nakajima 1972. Physical fitness studies in Sumo (Studies on the physique and physical fitness of *Shindeshi*). *Japanese Journal of Physical Fitness and Sports Medicine*. 21, 118–128 (in Japanese with English abstract).

Ogawa, S., Y. Furuta, K. Yamamoto and N. Nagai 1973. Studies on the physical fitness of Sumo wrestlers. Report II. Physical fitness and development of the Sekitori. *Japanese Journal of Physical Fitness and Sports Medicine* 22, 45–55 (in Japanese with English abstract).

Reischauer, E.O. 1992. *The Japanese Today. Change and continuity.* Charles E. Tuttle Company, Tokyo, Japan. pp. 395–412.

Suda, A. 1957. Physique of Sumo wrestlers. *Anthropological Reports* 18, 259–286 (in Japanese with English abstract).

Tanaka, K., H. Kato, K. Kikuchi, M. Nagatomo, H. Nakajima, H. Shibayama, H. Ebashi, Y. Nishijima, M. Matsuzawa and S. Ogawa. 1979. Anthropometric and body composition characteristics of *Shindeshi* Sumo wrestlers. *Japanese Journal of Physical Fitness and Sports Medicine* 28, 257–264 (in Japanese with English abstract).

Thayer III, J.E. 1983. Sumo. *Encyclopedia of Japan.* Kodansha Ltd. Tokyo. pp. 270–274.

Wada, S. 1987. Comparison of body weight and composition between Sumo champions and beginners. *Tokyo Ika Daigaku Zasshi* 45, 317–324 (in Japanese with English abstract).

3

Sociocultural Aspects of the Male Fattening Sessions among the Massa of Northern Cameroon

IGOR de GARINE

INTRODUCTION

Observing fatness and obesity in a culture where it is neither frowned upon nor considered conducive to psychological unrest (Cassidy, 1991: 191) and a passport to early death (Bray, 1987), might allow us to run free of the western world yardstick (Sobal, 1991) and stereotypes, and have a fresh outlook on their psychological, social and biological consequences. Such observation might permit different views to be formed as to the psychological, social and biological correlations involved.

In many societies, fatness among women is associated with the capacity to bear children (Huss-Ashmore, 1980) and is valued aesthetically and sexually (Sheik Nefzaoui, 1964; Ley, 1979). Among men, overweight is less appreciated and usually appears as a symbol of

45

economic affluence and power (Brown and Konner, 1987: 42). This used to be the case among Polynesian chiefs (Prior, 1976) and is still true among traditional African kings. In contemporary Cameroon, being unable to fasten one's shirt collar because of a fat neck—"le cou plié"—is an external sign of success among civil servants.

Although systematic overfeeding of women is done in a number of societies, for example, in Djerba, Tunisia (Laplantine, 1981), among the Tuaregs (Hildebrand *et al.*, 1985), or the Moors of the Sahara (Abeille, 1979) with a view to marriage, there are very few present-day examples of fattening sessions among men, if we except the Sumo wrestlers of Japan (Nakajima *et al.*, 1979), and Chapter 2, this volume). The Massa of Northern Cameroon and Chad, together with their neighbours, the Tupuri, the Kera and, more recently, the Mussey perpetuate an institution—the *guru*—which aims precisely at making the men plump ... or obese.

Anthropological aspects have recently been published (Garine and Koppert, 1991); the present paper will deal with the cultural significance of this institution.

GENERAL DESCRIPTION OF THE *GURU*

The Massa terms used are: *guru*—collective fattening session; *gurna*—participant in the collective fattening session; *guru walla*—individual fattening session; *gor walla*—participant in the individual fattening session. (The same word designates both singular and plural forms.)

At different periods of the year, men spend most of their time taking care of the cattle, the most valued asset in the culture since they are used as bridewealth. They live with the herd, drink its milk and receive a more abundant diet than the rest of the villagers. They dance and wrestle to display their strength and beauty, and to affirm the affluence of their village.

There are two kinds of *guru*. One is individual, the *guru walla*. During the sessions, which last two months, the participant remains secluded and ingests very large quantities of food, mostly milk and red sorghum porridge. In 1976, the first participant observed consumed daily about 10,000 kilocalories (Garine and Koppert, 1991), which is a world record for daily intake over such a long period and is higher than what has been achieved under experimental conditions among Caucasian volunteers (Sims *et al.*, 1968).

In 1988–1989, a detailed energy balance study including food intake, body weight, body composition and activity carried out on 9 volunteers over a period of 65 days reached lower results than those obtained in 1976 (Pasquet *et al.*, 1992). Average daily energy intake was around 7,500 kcal (SE = 22) and daily mean energy intake was 127% of baseline intake (3,249 kcal)—range 56% to 217%; average body weight increase was 17kg (SD = 4) with two star subjects reaching respectively 20.2 and 23.2 kg. After two months of a very sedentary life, the participant has made spectacular fattening progress—in 1976 we observed an increase of 34 kg (Garine and Koppert, 1991). At the end of the *guru walla*, the subject is ready to resume normal life and, most often, to join the second kind of fattening session, the collective *guru*. Only about 5% of the male population participate in the *guru walla*, but most men take part several times during their lives in the collective *guru*.

There are different types of collective *guru*, of which the most common are the *guru sarmana* ("of the fresh grass"), which takes place from September to January, and the *guru fata* ("of the sun"), between February and May. In the collective *guru*, the participants (whom we shall call *gurna* from now on) lead a more active life. They take care of the cattle and participate in the seasonal activities of the village. They demonstrate their physical fitness and their skill in dancing, singing and wrestling, and are a credit to their lineage, whose dynamism and prosperity have enabled them to achieve such fitness. The *gurna* spend a good deal of their time training and grooming themselves in order to be beautiful. They consume mostly cows' milk and sorghum porridge and receive about 3,500 kcalories daily (about 1,000 kcal more than the male villagers) and a larger amount of animal proteins (83 g instead of 45 g) and lipids, both from milk. They appear at all seasons to be 7 kg heavier than the other villagers.

CULTURAL VIEWS

What is the cultural viewpoint with regard to this institution? Men are supposed to enter the *guru*, literally "eat *(ti)* the *guru*," in order to drink *(ci mira)*, to become beautiful *(naa*—actually good and beautiful) and to grow *(nya*—increase, grow [for animals, plants and objects]) (Figure 1).

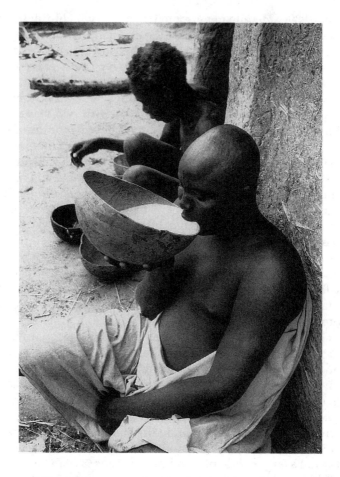

Figure 1.   (Photo A) Participant in the individual fattening session, gorging on milk.

References in the Oral Literature

Dauzats (1938) mentions a myth according to which: "...Two wealthy heads of family had beautiful children, but in one of the families they constantly died and only one boy was left. The father told his son to go, with some lactating cows, to his maternal uncle, saying 'Go, you are the last one and I hold you for dead.' After a few years, the young man had become strong and fat on the milk of his cattle."

In the foundation myth of the Gumay clan, among the Northern Massa: "... The ancestor, Regassa, was used as a herder for a rich man, Malam, the father of four daughters. After heavy rain and high flooding, Regassa could not go back home and settled his cattle on a patch of emerged land. He stayed there quietly drinking milk. His landlord sent his daughters to find out what was going on. They reported that Regassa was doing well so Malam decided that his daughters would take his daily staple to the herder. After a few months, the girls became pregnant and populated most of the Gumay region" (Dumas-Champion, 1983). A similar story exists in the Walia clan. It is possible that these myths help to justify the adoption of sedentary cattle herding by the Massa. The sexual episode is interesting and refers to one of the deep characteristics of the *guru*, sexual desirability. Actually the oral tradition does not offer anything decisive to explain the *guru*. We are luckier as regards the relation of milk drinking to beauty, strength and sexual desirability, all closely entwined.

Beauty. If we skim though the tales, we can quote a few examples concerning beauty and desirability (*naana*):
"Three brothers decided to go out to choose a wife. Two were twins, the other a single child. The latter decided to drink milk beforehand. He drank milk for a long time and grew fat. He put on a leopard loin skin, one of his brothers a gazelle skin and the other that of a bush antelope. They had taken their food with them: milk, water and sorghum cake. After walking for a long time, they came across a group of women. 'Ladies, tell us which of us is the most beautiful.' They answered, 'You are all beautiful but the one with the leopard skin is the most handsome!' The twins thought it was because of the leopard skin and stripped their brother of it, but it was always the same, he was still declared the most handsome."
"A chief had ten wives and many children. One of the children was the only offspring of his mother. He put himself to drinking milk for a long time and became very fat and strong. One of his father's wives asked him to go to bed with her. He refused. Another day she met him again and said: 'I want to go to bed with.' He refused and got into a lot of trouble..."
Referring to the esteemed body shape (see below Table V and Figure 3), the Massa value a protruding stomach and buttocks (*rodom calia*—protruding stomach; *gerda*—pot belly), and a full figure with smooth, shining skin with no scars or scratches. These prized features are specific to the Massa and severely mocked by the neighbouring

Mussey "...Their buttocks are fat and they make a noise when they walk, and they stink." The full features appreciated by the Massa are achieved when a small and well-distributed layer of fat is acquired. This is valued not only among men but also among women, and is one of the reasons why a newly-married bride is given milk in order to adapt herself to her husband's group and become beautiful.

Morality.   *Naana*, beauty, is also a quality. It goes deeper than physical appearance. As in many traditional societies, among the Massa size and weight are associated with strength and prosperity, power and majesty. Most traditional chiefs in Massa country (chef de canton) are tall and fat; they are not necessarily good and peaceful. The Massa believe that the *guru walla* is a learning session: *a gor walla*, while putting on weight, also gains at the same time those moral and psychological characteristics which are usually attributed to fat people. The *gurna* is good in all senses of the term, powerful and serene. He does not quite become a "bull" as the neigbouring Gula say (Pairault, 1966), with all its characteristics, but he is bound to be kind and lenient although powerful, and does not have to demonstrate his strength. His size and composure dictate a certain attitude from other people. He is respected. The benevolence associated with milk drinking is rather reminiscent of the equanimity associated with the cow in India.

The *guru* institution is the only occasion for a Massa man to be submitted to a strict discipline. During the *guru walla*, he has to follow blindly the feeding schedule imposed. In the collective *guru*, he has to obey the camp chief and be totally reliable when taking care and watching over the cattle. He is heavily punished for any mistakes.

The term *naana* also refers to what fits the custom. A *gurna* listens to recommendations (*hum gatna*), he obeys his elders (*hum bumna*), he is proper—"a nice young man," and conforms to tradition.

Love.   As we saw in the *guru walla*, the participant has to save all his strength in order to eat and become fat. To do so, he respects chastity. In the collective *guru*, on the contrary, the participants do all in their power to accumulate love affairs, although sexual intercourse (impure) is forbidden near the cattle. A large number of the themes of *gurna* songs deal with love, including the very delicate relationships uniting lovers prior to their wedding or outside marriage bonds. *Bananda, cilena, yagina*, there are many terms to designate permanent lovers, and special names and coded terms allowing them to communicate intimately, although publicly: "... My darling, what is happening to us? You did not look at me, what is happening to us? I would like to run away with you and take a 'plane to N'Djamena [the capital of Chad]." Or, more realistically: "... I put my hand on the clitoris of my beloved. I put my hand in her pubic hair, which grows strongly...."[1]

Strength and wrestling.   Milk drinking is also related to becoming strong, heavy and powerful, and to wrestling. The tales are full examples: "The son of God drinks milk in the *guru walla*. He becomes very fat, nobody is strong enough to wrestle with him."

"A chief put his daughter in a hut in the *guru walla* to drink milk. A very strong man, Guyu, came to wrestle. She threw him on the ground. His parents took him back and put him also in the *guru walla*. He became so fat that he filled the hut. They told him to go back to the girl, but he was so heavy that they had to dig his feet out of the ground. He went to wrestle with the girl. She hit him and pushed him strongly but he did not fall ..."

In another version: "... the girl said that she would marry the man strong enough to throw her in wrestling. The lion tried his chance and, at first, was unsuccessful. He also went to the *guru*, won the contest and married the girl."

It appears from the analysis of the oral literature and from interviews that fatness is linked to strength and makes men desirable to women. However, two physical types are distinguished. The first one, pertaining to the collective *guru*, is plump and muscular. The second, the *gor walla*, is obese and hardly able to move—at first view not a very functional type in a population which has to be constantly active in the pursuit of its subsistence through agriculture, fishing and herding in a very hot environment.

TESTING ATTITUDES TOWARDS BODY SHAPE

We next tried to look into the Massa's opinion regarding the body shape of the two types of *gurna* as compared to that of thin and undernourished adult males. We were not equipped to use photographs showing a gradient from thin to very fat, as done by Massara (1980) among U.S. Puerto Ricans. We utilized a set of 9 photographs showing various types of Massa body shape:

Photo 1, A skinny man (Figure 2),

Photo 2, An undernourished man,

Igor de Garine

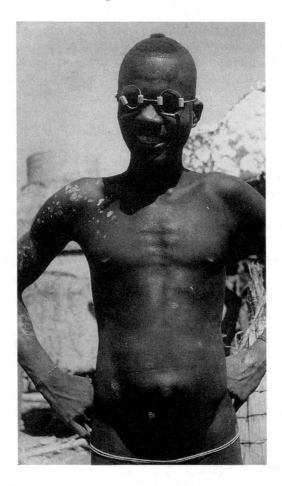

Figure 2. (Photo 1) The thin-skinny body shape, negatively appraised.

Photo 3, Three rather thin collective *gurna*,

Photo 4, One fat *gor walla*, just coming out of his fattening session,

Photo 5, A very fat *gor walla*, in the middle of his session (Figure 3),

Photo 6, An extremely fat man,

Photo 7, Four collective *gurna*, in good body shape for wrestling (Figure 4),

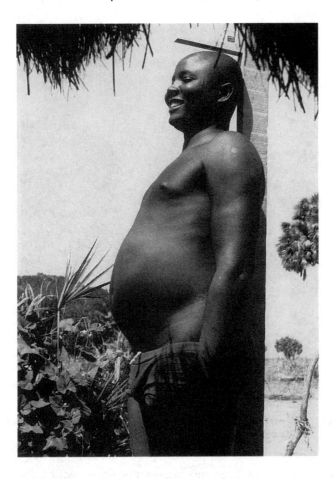

Figure 3.   (Photo 5) The fat body shape most valued. Same individual as in Figure 1 having increased his weight from 65 to 96 kg through the two kinds of fattening sessions.

Photo 8, Participants in each kind of *guru*, in very good shape (Figure 5),

Photo 9, Four Tupuri collective *gurna* at different stages of fatness.

Adult subjects were invited to comment on the photos. How did they name this type of body composure? Did they like it? For what

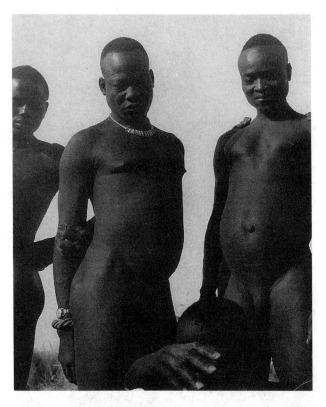

Figure 4.   (Photo 7) The fit, slightly plump body shape appreciated by all.

kind of activity was it appropriate—working, wrestling, love-making, for example?

It is not an easy task to apply this type of test in an illiterate society, and one has to make sure that the picture is correctly read. It also arouses many side comments, and should therefore be considered as a starting point for an interview rather than as a test. Twenty-two answers from males and 7 from women were reliable and allowed us to obtain a rating of the various body shapes (Table I), which can be regrouped in three categories (Table II): thin, Photos 1 and 2 ; very fat, Photos 4, 5, 6, 9; fit, Photos 3, 7 and 8. It appears that the attitude towards fatness, beauty and fitness has more nuances than we expected. It remains obvious that eating abundantly and the resulting fatness are valued. We expected that the obese *gor walla* (Photos 4, 5 and 9)

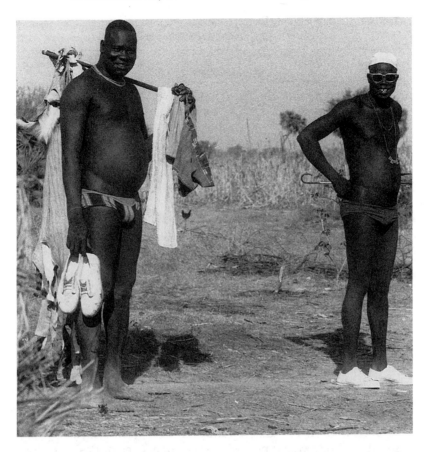

Figure 5.   (Photo 8) The two ideal types. On the left, the fat participant in the individual *guru*. On the right, a well-proportioned participant in the collective *guru*.

would be selected unanimously, but this was not quite the case (Table II).

Thin individuals (Photos 1 and 2; Figure 2) were the most often rejected. They appear skinny and weak. They are said to look tired, scraggly, not getting their share of food. They are poor and shamefaced (17 male opinions). Their body shape is ugly and ridiculous ("like ground squirrels"). Men considered them as miserable and too weak "to work in the sun" or to fight. Women thought they were dis-

TABLE I. Rating of body shapes based on photographs among the Massa (N = 22 men and N = 7 women)

	Rating			
Photo	Fat without specification	In shape for wrestling and love-making	Thin	Disproportioned
1.	1 = M1[a]	0	8 = M8	9 = M2 + 7W
2.	4 = M1	0	9 = M9	5 = M5 + W2
3.		21 = M17 + W4	0	2 = M2
4.	12 = M10 + W2	0	0	7 = M6 + W1
5.	13 = M10 + W3	3 = M3	0	12 = M8 + W4
6.	13 = M10 + W3	1 = M1	0	15 = M8 + W7
7.	2 = M2	22 = M16 + W6	0	1 = W1
8.	0	27 = M20 + W7	0	0
9.	19 = M15 + W4	0	0	5 = M2 + W3

[a]M= Men's opinion, W = Women's opinion.

proportioned, with rough skin through which bones and veins protrude (15 opinions, of which 9 were expressed by females).

A fat *gor walla* (in Photos 4, 5, 6 and 9; Figure 3) were selected both as positive and negative types, which was unexpected. Positive com-

TABLE II. Rating of main body types among the Massa

	Opinions			
Photos	Skinny (weak)	Very fat (passive)	Disproportioned (ugly)	Fit (muscular)
Thin (Fig. 2)	17 M[a]		7 M, 9 W	
Fat (Fig. 3)		52 M, 16 W	24 M, 15 W	
Fit (Fig. 4)			4 M, 4 W	53 M, 17 W

[a]M= Men's opinion, W = Women's opinion.

ments referred to the fact that they were ideal *gor walla*, having consumed much food and been successful in their attempt to gain weight (68 opinions, of which 16 were expressed by women). The men, especially those who had undergone the *guru walla* themselves, considered them to be attractive to women and strong for wrestling. But 24 males and 15 females mentioned the fact that they were somehow disproportioned. As Fallon and Rozin (1985) remarked with regard to U.S. students, the evaluation differed according to the sexes. The women found them too heavy, easily out of breath—and consequently bad lovers, besides which they looked difficult to feed. They appreciated them as sons, not as lovers or husbands. Both sexes pointed to the need for a *gor walla* to put on weight but to keep his body "well in hand," harmonious, and not to let his food overwhelm him (Photo 6). He should be ready to come back to a slimmer and better-fitting shape during the *guru sarmana*. Both sexes pointed to a number of functional disabilities in relation to increased weight: lack of breath, not being able to work in the sun, too heavy to wrestle.

A positive aspect in relation to fat body shape is the fact of having been provided with a large amount of prized food: "That man, he certainly has drunk milk and sorghum porridge!" (Photos 5 and 6; Figure 3), which demonstrates the affluence of the sponsors, an important aspect of the institution. Strength is considered to go together with size; being big, and heavy but firm, is valued, but the wrestler type belongs to the collective *guru*, "upright in his footsteps, with thighs like millet stalks." (Photos 7 and 8; Figure 4). "These men have just the right amount of flesh around their body, they hold their body well in hand." They are successful dancers, wrestlers, good workers and unsurpassable lovers (opinions of 53 males and 17 females). They need to be muscular with a full and firm figure and smooth, shiny skin. Tables III, IV, V and VI provide details about the traditional terminology applied to body shape in terms of volume, strength, beauty and fitness. Finally, in order of preference, Photos 3, 7 and 8 were selected as representing the most beautiful types.

Many of the comments made by the subjects interviewed referred to harmony, being in good shape and not having skinny legs, an asymmetric posture, a flabby stomach or buttocks (Photo 6). So we end up with two desirable fat body shapes: On one hand, a very fat (obese by western standards) individual, passive, chaste, living a secluded life in the framework of a well-watched household. On the other, a slightly beefy athlete who makes the most of every occasion to demonstrate

TABLE III.   Main categories relating to body appearance among the Massa
BODY VOLUME

Positive aspects	
Categories	Comments and expressions
Big = *nolo*, not only physically but also in relation to age and affluence	His flesh is a little around his body
	His flesh is growing, taking shape
	His flesh will soon be sufficient
Fat = *dorayna*, having purposely done something about it	He is slightly fat
	He fattens and grows well
	His stomach not too big
	He is fat
	His flesh is large and strong
	He is so fat that women don't leave him in peace
	He is very fat, on the obese side
	He is so fat you cannot see his eyes
	He is so fat that his skin will wrinkle when he loses weight.

Negative aspects	
Small = *goro*, not only physically but also in relation to age and affluence	The flesh his mother gave him at birth is skinny
	His food has not been sufficient
Thin = *fetna*	His neck is like that of the white-faced teal (*Dendrocygna viduata*)
Skinny = *noka*. Also tired	He looks like the wasp with too thin a waist
	His flanks are like those of the ground squirrel
	His chest is like that of a dove

his efficiency as a dancer, singer, wrestler and lover outside the community (Figure 5).

How is it possible to reconcile these opposed but enviable roles? Table VI shows their complementarity. In practice, the *guru walla* appears to be the preparatory stage to the collective *gurna* and a transition from the "closed" rainy season to the "open" dry one. After gorging on milk, the *gor walla* usually joins the *guru* "of the fresh grass" camp of his lineage, in which he will parade and appear as a star. A participant may consciously seek overweight in order to defeat a specific rival in wrestling competitions. Progressively he loses weight, becomes an efficient wrestler and a prized dancer and love

TABLE IV.   Categories relating to body appearance among the Massa
STRENGTH

Positive aspects	
Categories	Comments and expressions
Strong = *denoo*	This man, his strength is good
Strong, courageous = *bayna*	He is standing like a manly wrestler
Powerful = *ganarana*	His arm is very strong
Strong at wrestling = *gujuna*	His thighs are strong like millet stalks
(like a lion)	A bludgeon cannot affect his body
Negative aspects	
Weak and thin = *fetayna*	Small
Small = *goro*	Tired
	So thin that his children can wrestle with him
	His chest is so small that his breathing is killing him
	A man with such a bad weakness

partner. However, the two types of *guru* contrast in many ways, as Table VII shows.

ROLE OF THE COLLECTIVE GURU

The role of the *gurna* is rather transparent—they act as the spearhead "warriors" of their kinship group and demonstrate the power of their group through their physical fitness, their beauty, their aggressivity towards men and seductiveness towards women. They display the demographic weight and fighting ability of their clan on the occasion of funeral feasts. Whilst enjoying a pleasant life in the camp, they are also taught discipline and respect towards the elders. They also contribute to the general social control by public stigmatizing of reprehensible individuals in their songs. In practice, they take good care of the cattle, prevent them from eating the crops and, most of all, from being stolen, which could imply bloodshed. They accumulate prestige for their own lineage, for their fathers and for themselves, and may use it for their own economic and matrimonial strategies. They travel outside their territorial community and, being sexually attractive, spread their genes and secure wives from very different genetic

TABLE V.   Categories relating to body appearance among the Massa
BEAUTY

	Positive aspects
Categories	Comments and expressions
Beautiful = *naa*, not only physically but good morally	He is very beautiful and very good
	His flesh is beautiful
	He is beautiful like the girls
	His fatness is smooth and well distributed
	His body has become plump and smooth
	His flesh is smooth like that of the catfish (*Clarias*)
	His flesh is smooth like that of the dogfish (*Hydrocyon*)
	His meat is smooth like okra
	His cheeks are full
	His navel is nicely protruding
	His stomach is firm
	His buttocks are well up
	His loins are sloping down nicely
	The socks looked good on his legs
	Negative aspects
Ugly and bad = *joo*	Your eyes don't want to see his body for his ugliness
	He is ugly to my eyes
	His stomach is very hollow and veins show in his body
	He has scars
	His veins are showing

groups. Their role in taking care of the cattle, with which the bride-wealth is paid, and the active way in which they seduce women, may be regarded as contributing to expansion of the population to which they belong. The stocks of fat they accumulate afford them a better resistance to the shortage periods than the rest of the group. They also keep a permanent supply of energy in reserve, eventually for heavy tasks. These aspects are adaptive (Huss-Ashmore, 1980).

On the negative side, the privileged use of milk by men may be seen as jeopardizing access of the women and children to one of the best protein-rich foods available in the Massa's diet. As milk is about the only source of protein during the rainy season, when food shortages

TABLE VI.   Categories relating to body appearance among the Massa
FITNESS

Positive aspects

No single concept
sa ciw gita = somebody [with] his
    flesh perfect (just as it should be)

sa ciw wan kalamu = somebody [with
    his] flesh on himself well
    distributed

sa koy twan ir boyna = somebody
    with his body well in hand in
    front of the women
jif iria = very alive

His flesh right enough
His flesh well distributed
His flesh well around him
His flesh good at his body
His stomach full and firm
Upright in his footsteps, his flesh under
    control
Standing upright like a true male
Well posed
His loins moving well behind him
That one, when he runs, the game he will
    kill it right away
When you play with him, his sperm comes
    fast

Negative aspects through excess weight

No single concept
dorey joo = fattens badly

Disproportioned or impaired
Badly poised
Having flaccid flesh like the puffer fish
    (*Tetrodon*)
His stomach sticks out badly
Having a flabby stomach
Having a big stomach without eating (in
    the *guru walla*)
Having his flesh distributed at random
Having his bottom drooping down through
    flabbiness
His flesh moves in a flabby way
His flesh moves when he is in motion
He runs with his stomach flapping about
He has stretch marks on his body
He has been overwhelmed by his eating
He cannot wrestle
He can't work out in the sun
He eats too much
He is so full that his breath hardly comes
    up through his throat
He is so fat that his sperm doesn't come out
He is too fat for love-making

Negative aspects through excess weight and strength

His flesh is like dust
Fat but not heavy
His body is sickly
He cannot work out in the sun

TABLE VII. Comparison between the two types of *Guru* among the Massa

Positive aspects		
Individual *guru* (*guru walla*)	Common to both *guru*	Collective *guru*— *guru sarmana, guru fata*
Rainy season		Mostly dry season
Short duration (2 months)		Long (2–6 months and more)
Once or twice in a lifetime		Often, if possible every year
Inside the village		Outside the village
In the host's household		Moving around the village according to grazing opportunities
Village – Culture		Bush – Nature
In a compound, inside a hut		In a cattle camp, mostly
In the shade, in the dark		outside
Isolated, secluded	Cows	In the sun
	Milk	In a group, outside
"Closed"	Red Sorghum	"Open"
Inactive (saving energy) activities,		Very active (technical dancing, wrestling
Female style ("like a new bride")	Overeating	Masculine style ("like a lion")
Naked		Groomed and decorated
Fat		Firm
Submissive	Beauty	Aggressive
Observing chastity	Discipline	Sexually very active
Magic and religion	Goodness	Profane, success in competitions
	Collective prestige (for the organizers)	
Health		No bad deaths
	Individual fame (for the participants)	
	Affluence	
	Supernatural protection	
Affluence, health as supernatural protections		Wealth in cows as a result of material strategies

Individuals moving from the *guru walla* to the *guru sarmana* as the seasons move from the rainy growing period to the dry harvest time.

occur, they may contribute indirectly to the level of morbidity and mortality in women and children during that period (Garine and Koppert, 1991: 23), which can be seen as counteradaptive.

ROLE OF THE INDIVIDUAL GURU

The benefits derived from the *guru walla* are not so easy to determine, although those who have participated in it consider it to be a very positive and prestigious experience. The *gor walla* appear to be beautiful mostly in their own eyes and in those of the person who financed the session. The experience is painful because the novices are obliged to swallow all the food they are offered although their stomach is not yet distended, even if they have vomited. It is boring, implies chastity and is considered uncomfortable.

Undergoing a *guru walla* session is also interpreted as symbolically dangerous. The participant is believed to be much envied and a target for witchcraft from frustrated humans and supernatural beings. This is one of the reasons why he is secluded, and has to bury his faeces to avoid being bewitched. Informants also stress similarities between his condition and that of a new bride, kept inside to lose her shyness while drinking milk.

Being usually outside his own family enclosure, he should take very good care of the vessel out of which he drinks, as it is associated with his own soul. Before being allowed to circulate freely outside the compound in which he was shut, he must put his soul in a safe place. This is why he first brings back his calabash (and his soul) to his father's house. As with all dangerous processes, the *guru walla* pollutes progressively and the *gor walla* has to be purified—"to push his head forward" (*van yan goyo*). He does so by attending a funeral feast, circling in beautiful array (carrying his special bludgeon) around the dead person's compound and touching as many people as possible to get rid of his impurity before leading a normal life.

Nutritional Aspects

Traditional beliefs in relation to the *guru walla* are not devoid of objective nutritional knowledge. As the aim is to acquire weight rapidly, the participant has to abstain from energy expenditure and remain secluded indoors. Overfeeding during a hot period is considered dangerous (Stini, 1981, quoting Robinson) and the *guru walla* has to stop as soon as the participants perspire abundantly indoors (October) for fear of dying.

Skinny young girls are sent to the *guru walla* in order to fatten, to reach puberty faster and be ready for marriage so as to bring in wealth in the form of cattle to their fathers. This suggests that the relation between fatness and feminine maturity, and possibility fecundity, is perceived (Huss-Ashmore, 1980). Male and female *gor walla* are also believed to retain the ability of increasing weight easily if they have the opportunity to do so once they have undergone a session (Faust *et al.*, 1978).

Seasonal variations in food availability and level of energy expenditure allow the *gurna* to eliminate the fat they may have accumulated. *Guru* and *guru walla* fatness and obesity, unlike what we witness in modern western society, should both be interpreted as transitory bouts, not as a dooming, inescapable physical and mental pathological state, unadapted to current lifestyle.

Conspicuous Consumption

Both forms of *guru* are intended to demonstrate the affluence of those who organize them and provide the food—parents, friends or affines—as well as the prestige and popularity of the individual taking part in them. They also illustrate the supernatural protection enjoyed by the organizers and, in the case of the *guru walla*, the participant. In both cases, the aim is to eat—to become plump and handsome for the *gurna*—very fat and imposing for the *gor walla*, who may be viewed as a bag of food symbolizing the material and supernatural success of those who supported him (a good role for a son, not for a lover).

Ambiguity of the *Gor Walla*'s Role

Of course, eating abundantly is a cultural ideal among the Massa (their average daily per capita consumption is around 2,500 kcal) but, in a society submitted to frequent food shortages, is not overeating in order to become obese, as is the case of the *gor walla*, likely to appear as an ambiguous pursuit? Isn't it hoarding food? Informants remark that fat people may be bad people. There are two conspicuous examples of evil fat people in ordinary life: the local county chiefs (*Lamido*), who literally fatten themselves on the backs of the tax-payers under their jurisdiction. Chiefs are perceived as cunning and greedy individuals; they respond to the general stereotype of the "bad, greedy fat man"

(Fischler, 1987: 269). In the oral literature they are represented by a nasty lord, *Mul Kabraw*. Secondly, one of the principal characters in the oral literature is a fat glutton (*Hlo*) who is constantly stealing and hoarding food, and to whom many misfortunes occur as a consequence.

The *gor walla* is perceived in a positive manner because he becomes fat not through his personal initiative but because he is ordered into it and has to follow a very rigid and painful traditional procedure. The *gurna* and the *gor walla* symbolize the affluence and success of their kinship group, but the latter adds a new dimension to the rather profane and easy-going collective *guru*. The transformations sought through the two types of *guru* are not only material but also moral, and correspond to the pursuit of an ideal type. In the collective *guru*, the participant is increasingly socialized into respecting the traditional hierarchy. In the *guru walla*, he is believed to reach, through his diet and seclusion, a certain level of purity. That is why he is given sour milk and bitter tree bark such as *Gardenia erubescens* to make him vomit and empty his bowels before beginning his diet of God's blessed foods: red sorghum ("the cultural superfood" Jelliffe, 1967) and milk which make him strong, gentle, placid and good-humoured.

Magico-religious Aspects

The *guru walla* takes place at a period when milk is available but when the cereal shortage is at its peak. It is a typical case of conspicuous consumption: the *gor walla* puts on weight at the time when everybody else is on a restricted diet. This corresponds to the period following the weeding, when fields should be left in peace to grow, when many animals, such as kites and ducks, are out of sight, brooding and "shut in," just like the *gor walla*, before coming out at the onset of the dry season.

Perhaps we witness here something like a "prosperity magic": the *gor walla* is growing at the same time as the sorghum crop (Dumas-Champion, 1983). This symbolic link is corroborated by the fact that a *guru walla* session can never go on beyond the time when the sorghum canes are cut in the field after the harvest. This would mean the death of the participant. The *gor walla* appears to be filling an ambiguous function at the level of his community: symbolically demonstrating by his fatness during the seasonal shortage period that there is no lack of food, that the group nourishing him has the power to defy the seasons and has things under control. At the same time, feeding the *gor walla* may also correspond to taking care magically of the crop and helping it to grow. In this way, the *gor walla* is rather like the symbol of his kinship group's material success and of the help bestowed on the group by the supernatural powers. Attention should be drawn to the similitude between the *gor walla* and the role of the Earth Priest in neighbouring populations such as the Guisey Massa and the Tupuri. There, the traditional priest is like a hostage in the hands of his people. He is a symbol of their health and wealth, which is why he should not endure a long sickness and is killed when he becomes seriously ill.

Guru and Class Aspects

Economic aspects are obviously pertinent to the institution. It is based on the ownership of lactating cows and the ability to divert a large part of the milk yield to feed the *gurna*, thus jeopardizing the growth of calves. Wealthy Massa have more chances to take part in the *guru*, but it should not be interpreted as a class institution, creating some kind of better-fed elite.

According to the bridewealth system (ten heads of cattle to obtain a wife), wealth is transitory. Procreating girls, for whom a brideprice will be received, is the key to success. Having male offspring, for whose marriage a brideprice will have to be paid, rapidly cuts one down to size.

The *guru* provides the opportunity to boost the individual qualities of the participants, who also have to be congenial and popular. Outside their ascribed social status (as sons or friends of wealthy cow owners) they may acquire personal prestige through their beauty, strength, humour, ability to wrestle, dance, sing and compose songs. Very few Massa men die without taking part in the *guru*. It should be noted, that mourning for a close relative interrupts for at least one year participation in the *guru*. Rather than a permanent asset for the privileged, the *guru* allows Massa males as a whole to benefit from an institution which boosts their prestige, their biological fitness and, in a Darwinian perspective, helps them to spread the genes of the Massa population. As the participants say, this is the time for beauty, love and mating: "... I went to dance at a funeral feast. I was handsome, I met a girl, she was beautiful. We talked to each other and we got married." Family heads remember the *guru* as the best time of their life and want their children to experience it too, which ultimately contributes to increasing social cohesion between age groups. Temporary pursuits which enhance individuals' status are in the long run beneficial to the Massa population as a whole.

CONCLUSIONS

The *guru* of the Massa is a complex and rather exceptional institution, setting in motion most aspects of social life. It is actually the crux of the Massa culture.

In the changing world of Northern Cameroonian societies, the *guru* institution appears as a means of enhancing cultural values and of allowing individuals to achieve status according to standards which are not borrowed from the invasive Muslim and negro-urban values. On the contrary, becoming a plump and happy *gurna* and limiting work to dealing with prestigious cattle is appealing enough nowadays for *guru* camps to be maintained in most Massa villages, to the despair of modernizing agents. Even the neighbouring Mussey are converting to the system.

Individual and collective *guru* are complementary aspects of an attempt to integrate the Massa society in a heavily seasonal environment, subject to food shortage and in which food anxiety is latent (Garine and Koppert, 1990). In such a context, temporary induced fatness and obesity appear to be biologically functional. Obesity due to the *guru walla*, as a symbol of material and supernatural success, should be considered as the preliminary stage to a more functional muscular and plump body type admired in the collective *guru*. Materially, having fat stores allows seasonal food variations to be endured more successfully. Symbolically, overfeeding the *gor walla* during the shortage period and catering for a *guru* camp (like supporting a successful sporting team in western society) the year around demonstrates the affluence and ability of a society to maintain some control over food uncertainty. It creates a feeling of well-being which has behavioural consequences and might ultimately contribute to biological success.

It is also worth considering that psychological stress and the material pathological consequences of overweight are likely not to be the same in a society where it appears comforting as in one in which it is considered a disgrace.

Observing overweight in a rather candid population may shed light on a kind of "adaptive fatness" to which authors such as Prior (1976), Pagezy (1983) and Cassidy (1991) have alluded, and which is

68   Igor de Garine

increasingly accepted by biologists (Stini, 1991: 225). It can no longer
be witnessed in contemporary urban societies, but is probably as
normal to man, and acknowledged to be so, as the culture-bound
syndrome (Ritenbaugh, 1982), stigmatizing overweight in an industrialized world dominated by Max Weberian cultures, not prone to
indulging in food, and in which the "scientific" dietetic discourse is
not totally free from fashion and vested interests.

NOTES

Igor de Garine received his Doctorate of Ethnology from the Sorbonne. He is
currently Director of Research at the Centre National de la Recherche Scientifique (CNRS) in Paris, Chairman for the International Comission on the Anthropology of Food and Nutrition of the International Congress of
Anthropological and Ethnological Sciences (ICAES), and in charge of the Research Group on the Anthropology of Food, Maison des Science de l'Homme,
Paris. Among his many publications is *Coping with Uncertainty in Food Supply,*
which he co-edited with G.A. Harrison (Clarendon Press, (1988).

1. A hairy pubis is considered to be a beauty asset among women.

REFERENCES

Abeille, B. 1979. *A Study of Female Life in Mauritania.* Office of Women in De-
    velopment, Agency for International Development, Washington, D.C.
Bray, G.A. 1987. Overweight is risking fate. Definition, classification, preva-
    lence and risks. In R.J. Wurtman and J.J. Wurtman (eds.), *Human Obesity.*
    Annals of the New York Academy of Sciences 499, 73–83.
Brown, P.J., and M. Konner. 1987. An anthropological perspective on obesity.
    Annals of the New York Academy of Sciences 499, 29–45.
Cassidy, C. 1991. The good body: When big is better. *Medical Anthropology,* 13,
    181–213.
Dauzats, N. 1938. Etude commerciale des mouvements du bétail de la subdi-
    vision de Yagoua. Archives du Poste de Yagoua, Cameroun. Multi-
    graph.
Dumas-Champion, F. 1983. *Les Massa du Tchad: Bétail et société.* Cambridge
    University Press, Cambridge. Editions de la Maison des Sciences de
    l'Homme, Paris.
Fallon, A.E., and P. Rozin. 1983. Sex differences in perception of desirable
    body shape, *Journal of Abnormal Psychology* 94, 102–105.
Faust, I.M., P.R. Johnson, J.S. Stern, and J. Hirsch. 1978. Diet-induced adipo-
    cytes number increase in adult rats: A new model of obesity. *American
    Journal of Physiology* 235, 279–286.

Fischler, C. 1987. La symbolique du gros. *Communications, Ed. du Seuil* **46**, 255–278.

Garine, I. de, and G.J.A. Koppert 1900. Social adaptation to season and uncertainty in food supply. In G.A. Harrison and J.C. Waterlow (eds.), *Diet and Disease in Traditional and Developing Countries*, Cambridge University Press, Cambridge. pp. 240–289.

Garine, I. de, and G.J.A. Koppert 1991. *Guru-fattening sessions among the Massa. Ecology of Food and Nutrition* **25**, 1–28.

Hildebrand, K.A., S. Hill, S. Randall, and M.L. Van Den Erenbeemt 1985. Child mortality and care of children in rural Mali. In A.G. Hull (ed.), *Population, Health and Nutrition in the Sahel*. Routledge and Kegan Paul Inc. London.

Huss-Ashmore, R. 1980. Fat and fertility: Demographic implications of differential fat storage. *Yearbook of Physical Anthropology* **23**, 65–91.

Jelliffe, D.B., 1967. Parallel food classifications in developing and industrialised countries. *American Journal of Clinical Nutrition* **20**, (No. 3), 273–281.

Laplantine, F. 1981. La Hajba de la Fiancée à Djerba (Tunisie), *Revue de l'Occident musulman et de la Méditerranée* **31**,(1), 105–118.

Ley, P. 1979. Psychological, social and cultural determinants of acceptable fatness. In M. Turner (ed.), *Nutrition and Lifestyles*. Applied Sciences Press, London. pp. 105–118.

Massara, E.B. 1980. Obesity and cultural weight valuations: A Puerto Rican case. *Appetite* **10**, pp. 291–298.

Nakajima, H., H. Shibamaya, H. Ebashi, M.A. Nishiji, K. Kikuchi and S. Ogawa 1979. Some considerations on the physical fitness of "*Shindeshi*" Sumo wrestlers. *Bulletin of Physical Fitness Research Institute* **44**, 29–46.

Nefzaoui (Sheik) 1964. *The Perfumed Garden*. Lancer Books, New York.

Pagezy, H. 1983. Attitudes of Ntomba society towards the primiparous woman and its biological effects. *Journal of Biological and Social Sciences* **15**, 421–431.

Pairault, C. 1966. *Boum-le-Grand, Village d'Iro*, Institut d'Ethnologie, Paris.

Pasquet, P., L. Brigant, A. Froment, D. Bard, I. de Garine, and M. Apfelbaum. 1992. Massive overfeeding and energy balance in man: The *Guru walla* model. *American Journal of Clinical Nutrition*. **56**, 483–490.

Prior, I. 1976. Nutritional Problems in Pacific Islanders. The 1976 Muriel Bell Memorial Lecture. New Zealand Nutrition Society, Proceedings.

Ritenbaugh, C. 1982, Obesity as a culture-bound syndrome. *Culture, Medicine and Psychiatry* **6**, 347–361.

Sims, E.A.H., R.F. Goldman, C.M. Gluck, E.S. Horton, P.C. Kelleher, and D.W. Rowe 1968. Experimental obesity in man. *Transactions Association of American Physicians* **81**, 153–170.

Sobal, J. 1991. Obesity and socioeconomic status: A framework for examining relationships between physical and social variables. *Medical Anthropology* **13**, 231–247.

Stini, W. 1981. Evolutionary aspects of human body composition. *Karger Gazette* **42, 43,** 1–4.
Stini, W. 1991. Body composition and longevity. *Medical Anthropology* **13,** 215–229.

4

Fertility and Fat: The Annang Fattening Room

PAMELA J. BRINK

INTRODUCTION

White, middle- to upper-class North American women give every appearance of being obsessed with their weight. Women's magazines, sold at every check-out counter in supermarkets, regularly feature articles on dieting, especially before the summer. Women are frequently heard saying "You can never be too thin." Yet researchers have found that women can indeed be *too thin.* When a Caucasian woman falls below 18% body fat, she stops menstruating, is unable to conceive and carry a child, cannot develop enough breast milk to breastfeed, loses the ability to store estrogen, and develops osteoporosis. Yet, in North America, the woman who has very low amounts of body fat is envied by other white women who feel somehow guilty if their bodies are not as thin.

In contrast, the Annang of Nigeria, similar to Sierra Leoneans (MacCormack, 1982), value a "woman of substance" as both beautiful and healthy. The Annang have the tradition of "fattening up" girls before marriage to make them "fat and beautiful." To do this they put a girl in seclusion, refuse to allow her to do physical work of any kind, hire a

71

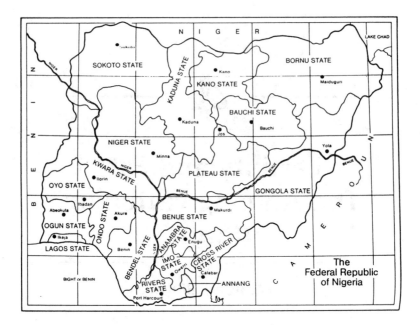

Figure 1.   Map of Nigeria, showing location of the Annang. (K. Enang, 1979).

small child to fetch and carry for her to keep her from any unnecessary physical exertion, and feed her whatever she wishes to eat. Her primary goal is to become fat.

This paper is the result of three field visits to the Annang of Akwa Ibom State, Nigeria. The primary purpose of the most recent visit (1989) was to determine whether the Annang still retained the custom of the fattening room, and if they did, what form and function it took.

One reason for studying the Fattening Room custom in Nigeria was to obtain a controlled sample of women who were deliberately "fattened" as opposed to the North American experience of "accidental" or nonpurposive fattening. Information on these women adds to our general knowledge about obesity as a "culture-bound syndrome" (Ritenbaugh, 1982; Cassidy, 1982). The North American value placed on obesity is negative whereas the Annang view on obesity is a positive one. They see "fat as beautiful."

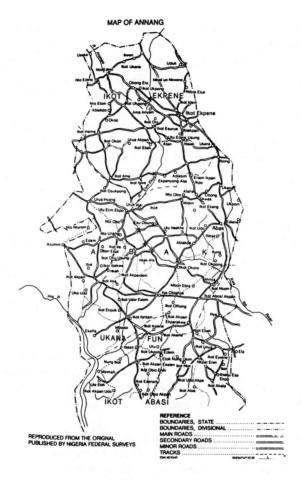

MAP OF ANNANG

REFERENCE
BOUNDARIES, STATE
BOUNDARIES, DIVISIONAL
MAIN ROADS
SECONDARY ROADS
MINOR ROADS
TRACKS

REPRODUCED FROM THE ORIGINAL
PUBLISHED BY NIGERIA FEDERAL SURVEYS

Figure 1.   (Continued)

Population and Setting

The Annang, also known as the Anang-Ibibio (Brink, 1977, 1989, foot-notes; Messenger, 1957), are a patrilineal, patrilocal, slash-and-burn, hand-hoe subsistence farming group living in the Palm Belt of south-eastern Nigeria (Udo, 1970) in Akwa Ibom State within the Cross River Basin area (Enang, 1979, Figure 1). They are linguistically and culturally related to the Efik (Welmers, 1968) and the Ibibio (Talbot and Mulhall, 1962). According to Annang oral tradition, the Annang and Ibibio originate from Arochuku (Enang, 1979:5), and the Ibibio are descended from the Annang (Brink, field notes, 1974–75). Both the Annang and Ibibio have lived in their particular areas for a very long time, so no definite statement can be made as to which is the parent stock.

There are 33 distinct Annang clans and 652 villages (Enang, 1979:12) bounded on the west by the Ngwa and Ndokki Igbo; on the north by the Isurogu Igbo; and on the east and south by the Ibibio (Messenger, 1957, 1959:279). Each clan occupies a specified geographical land mass which was increased or decreased by warfare. If a member of one clan farmed the lands of an adjoining clan, warfare would result. Whichever clan won the war won the land. From the time of British rule, clan warfare has been discouraged and clan size has remained comparatively unchanged.

The area is characterized by lush vegetation, heavy annual rainfall, a variety of palm trees (particularly raffia palm, oil palm and coconut), and twenty-three varieties of yam. Most families, except the poorest, have their own farms and have gardens around their compounds. Nigeria is based upon a cash economy, so the rural Annang often sell their produce at market. In addition, a small income is to be made in harvesting and processing of palm kernels for palm oil, the tapping and selling of palm wine (from raffia palm) and its fermented derivative "native gin" (akaiakai), and wage labour (Martin, 1956; Udo, 1970).

Houses are of wattle and daub construction with thatch roofs ranging in size from single small two- to three-room residences, to a large one- or two-storied multiroomed cement house. Each compound (husband and wife/wives) is surrounded by a dense vegetable garden. In 1989, many houses were of cement with tin or asbestos roofs. The simplest home was a two-room construction—one room for the husband, one room for the wife and children. There was an opening between the rooms and each room had a door to the outside. Older and more established men, who either had more than one wife or whose senior son was married, would have additions to this basic form to house all the family. In this case there would be a central parlour next to the head of the household's room in a central building. The senior son would have a room in his father's house. Separate from this building and behind it would be separate housing for each wife and her children. The household head would probably also house his widowed mother. If he were the senior son, he would be expected to house his father's other wives and to educate their children.

Men are responsible for the care of the family's palm trees and for slashing and burning the land in preparation for planting. The women and children are responsible for garden maintenance. Women and children are also responsible for bringing firewood and water from the streams to the household. Annang women work hard in the family farms, stooping over to plant, weed and harvest. They work hard at home carrying food and water long distances (there is no water, electricity, telephone, or health care in the villages) and bearing children. The Annang are characterized by small and lean stature. The fattening room experience is their only time of rest and relaxation, and this happens once in their lives, if at all.

The Annang are a very spiritual people who believe in an Eternal God (*Abasi*) who has many attributes. Although *Abasi* is masculine, God has a mother (*Eka Abasi*) who is perhaps even more powerful. Because God and His mother are very busy, God has spirits (*ndem*) to help Him, who are found everywhere (Enang, 1979). The Annang believe that every human has four souls; three souls reside in the body while the fourth soul lives on the surrounding land in trees, rivers, brush, or rocks (Enang, 1979). These four souls, in conjunction with the belief in supernatural powers, are the foundation for the ceremonial year, social control, healing, kinship solidarity, and etiquette. For example, no food is eaten or liquid drunk that is not first shared with the ancestor spirits, one of the three souls that resided in the body during life.

All men of the village are related to a central ancestor via the male line. (Although a man may live in his mother's village, he would always identify himself as a member of his father's village.) To maintain the integrity of the lineage, the senior male is responsible for propitiating the ancestors at all seasonal changes. If the ancestors are mistreated, or if any of the *ndem* who populate the village are mistreated, an individual or the entire family may fall ill and die. If all male offspring die, the ancestors have no one to care for them. The male line must be safeguarded. To *ensure* the continuation of the lineage, therefore, a wife must conceive and bear male issue. Although girls are welcome, only men continue the line. Fertility is a major driving force in Annang life.

The Annang diet is composed primarily of cassava (manioc, *Manihot utilissima*, as *garri*, a source of complex carbohydrate with low vitamin and mineral content), that is prepared by putting it into hot

water until it forms a thick paste, and then dipping it into a thick vegetable soup. This forms the basic morning and evening meal. Pounded
or boiled yam is periodically substituted for *garri*, as is boiled rice.
Other foods: eggs, dried and fresh fish, chicken, goat, fruit (including
bananas and plantains) contribute to this basic diet.[1] High status
guests are served fried plantain, eggs and dried fish in a soup (*otong*),
or if they cannot stay, are given food to take away with them. Men are
served first, followed by women and children. When asked what they
have had for a meal, the Annang will respond with the starch (*garri*,
yam, rice), in contrast to the American who will respond with the protein (beef, pork, chicken).

Martin (1956:43) estimated the distribution of calories from
"starchy" foods as 89% (she included bananas and plantain under
starchy foods) with 11% derived from protein foods. There is almost
no animal fat in the daily diet; the major source of fat is palm oil, which
is used primarily in cooking. Depending upon the wealth of the family and the size of the farm holdings, Martin (1956:43) estimated the
daily intake to be between 1,509 – 2,479 calories (kcal) per person per
day. Children under 3 were calculated as one fourth of a person and
children under 15 were considered one-half a person. Yet, the Fattening Room did create distinctly obese girls, judging from the size of one
young woman seen coming home from her "outing ceremony" at the
market. Most physically active persons would not gain weight on a
daily intake of 1,500 kcalories. The Fattening Room had to have a different activity level and calorie intake to produce fat girls.

THE FATTENING ROOM AMONG THE ANNANG

The custom of the Fattening Room as a preparation for marriage was
once widely practised among both the Annang and their neighbours
the Ibibio (D. Talbot, 1915; P.A. Talbot, 1912, 1914; Malcolm, 1925; Messenger, 1957; Andreski, 1970; Udo Ema, 1940; Nzekwu, 1959). Every
young girl, except perhaps the daughters of the poorest, expected to
be *Mbobo* (fattening room girl). *Mbobo* was a part of the traditional
religious system and was associated with marriage and the custom of
bride price.[2]

The fattening room was a specific, designated, place in the parent's
compound: either a barricaded portion of her mother's room or a separate room of her own in her mother's house.[3] The point was to se-
clude her away from everyone's view. If a man had more than one

daughter in the fattening room at a time, each girl had her own "room" and her own attendant. There were usually more than one *mbobo* in a village at a time, but each was housed separately from the others in her parent's compound. She slept on a bare bamboo bed in the belief that the bamboo would "soften her up," or soften up her muscles and replace them with fat. She was completely naked while she was in seclusion so that one might observe her fatness. A special, secluded place was created with palm fronds, near her room, just for her toileting. If her room was not large enough for her to bathe there, she should bathe in her toileting area. She was fed whatever she wished to eat. She did no physical work and was assigned a small child to fetch and carry for her.

Traditionally, the Fattening Room was a period of seclusion and feeding of young girls before marriage, the stated purpose being to "fatten her up." A girl entered the "Fattening Room" with some form of ceremony; and when she left the "Fattening Room," it was a major social event, including feasting and dancing, for the entire village. The fatter the girl, the higher the bride price that could be asked (Malcolm, 1925; Messenger, 1957, 1959; Talbot, D., 1915; Talbot, P.A.. 1912, 1914, 1923, 1967; Udo Ema, 1940) During the period of fattening, a girl was taught the womanly arts of pleasing her husband, of child care and domestic arts. This fattening room was simply for fattening—to make a girl fat and beautiful, to make her desirable as a choice of wife, to show all the villagers how wealthy her family was in being able to produce such a fine fat girl.

A second purpose was to ensure the girl's ability to conceive, carry, bear and suckle her first child (Brink, 1989). Informants stated that fattening created broad hips which were requisite to providing a large enough birth canal so that babies could slide out easier. This fattening room experience lasted as long as the family could afford to support a nonworker. The length of stay and the degree of obesity of the girl all contributed to the status of the family (Brink, 1989).

There was another type of fattening room, however, not limited to premarital girls. The second form of fattening was requisite to entrance into secret societies. Each secret society had an initiation period in which the initiate learned the rituals, songs and paraphernalia of the society. To learn what it meant to become a member, the initiate was secluded away from the village, placed in an isolated area with a society member in attendance, and "fattened up." This place of seclusion could be a room in one's own home or in another person's home, but the point was that the initiate was to receive no visitors except the instructors and attendants. The initiate was excused from all manual labour during the period of seclusion and the only effort needed was toileting, eating and learning. Adults had their entire bodies shaved during this period as a sign of ritual cleanliness. Then they were bathed and oiled. This fattening room experience was time-limited. They have been described elsewhere (Brink, 1989); they too contribute to the status of the family.

Becoming Mbobo

To become an *mbobo* (a fattening room girl) one must first be initiated into the two women's secret societies (*ndam* and *ngwongwo*). The first society a girl must join is *ndam*. Little girls as young as seven years of age can be initiated into *ndam*, as well as women as old as grandmothers. As a secret women's society, *ndam* is desired as an end in itself, or can be prescribed by a diviner or fortune teller (*idiong*) as a treatment for intractable headaches. There are two stages in *ndam* (raffia) requiring two periods of confinement of one week each separated by a one week rest in between. Initiates came out of seclusion on the same day one week later. *Ndam* represents the mother's side of a girl's family.

As with *ndam*, young girls or married women could join *ngwongwo*, the second secret society. *Ngwongwo* could be prescribed by the *idiong* (diviner or fortune teller) for persons who suffered from extreme headaches, protracted thinness, sleeplessness and/or infertility. Intractable thinness was the symptom most influential in directing the prescription of *ngwongwo*. Unlike *ndam*, *ngwongwo* requires a minimum of three weeks of seclusion. Just as *ndam* represents the mother's side of the family, *ngwongwo* represents the father's side of the family. I was told by my informants that if a wife was barren, the cause was sought from her mother's side of the family first. She was treated, first, with *ndam*. If she did not conceive, then the cause of her barrenness was believed to be on the husband's side of the family. The treatment of choice would be *ngwongwo*. Therefore, *ngwongwo* was considered to be "more serious" than *ndam*.

For initiation into these societies, the girl or woman was placed in seclusion on specific days. *Offiong*[4] day was the day of initiation into *ndam*. *Ngwongwo* was initiated on *editaha* day and seclusion was terminated on the same day three weeks later unless she was to begin *mbobo*. During the vigil of her initiation into *ngwongwo* she was circumcised. (If *ngwongwo* had been prescribed as treatment of an illness, then the girl or woman did not have to be initiated into *ndam* first.)

Mbobo has only one function: it is the simple fattening process before marriage. *Mbobo*, although not itself a secret society, requires that the fattening room girl must be initiated into both *ndam* and then *ngwongwo*, if she hasn't been before. A second requirement for *mbobo* was that a girl must be a virgin. (A woman who had conceived a child could not be a *mbobo*, no matter how wealthy her family or her husband's family might be.) Her virginity was examined in secrecy before the final coming-out ceremonies. If *mbobo* was found to be not virginal, she was shamed and was not considered virtuous enough for a proper marriage. Her only recourse was to become self-supporting through prostitution. In addition to establishing her virginity by examination, she was commanded to swear a solemn oath on the eve of her coming-out ceremony that she had not known a man. If she lied, she would die within six months.

All *mbobo* from the same village leave seclusion on the same day (*uruabom*). There is only one coming-out day a year, and that occurs in September. (If a young girl does not leave the fattening room on that day, she must wait until the next year. Or if a girl entered the fattening room in July or August, she had to complete all stages of the secret societies to "come out" in September). *Mbobo* are paraded nude[5] in the village square to show off their fatness and beauty and go to their husbands following this display.

The Fattening Room Today

Today there is very little talk of *Mbobo*. The practice may be either dying out or becoming an underground practice, particularly among Christian and/or Catholic families. *Mbobo* is considered to be "old fashioned" by some Annang, and is associated with bride price, which is illegal. It is also too expensive for most families. There are more girls going to school, and schooling determines how long a girl will be in the fattening room, since a girl will usually remain in seclusion only during school holidays. In some cases, the custom has become Christianized, modernized, and given a different name, but remains very much a social custom for the daughters of wealthy women.

Major informants and prior field contacts stated that they were not aware of any Fattening Room girls during my three field visits. They said they believed that the practice had died out. Yet, in 1989, one informant stated that he knew of five fattening room girls. In the end, however, he was unable to obtain permission for me to visit them.

While visiting in one village on another matter, I was told by my village sister that there was a fattening room girl in the next village and that we could visit her. We did indeed visit her and observed her in the "fattening room," but were told that we could not photograph her or stay unless we paid her a lot of money. In essence we were all chased away. Yet, this girl was living in the village of my major informant (a senior male in the village who would be expected to know what was going on), who said he did not know of any *mbobo*. One night after dark, again in 1989, as the field team were leaving an informant's compound, we saw a Fattening Room girl on the highway accompanied by two older women. She was—by her body decorations, hair style and lack of clothing—a fattening room girl (*ngwongwo*) returning from the market where she had been on display all day, yet, no one had informed us of her presence. Finally, in obtaining permissions from the various chiefs and heads of office, we were told about the fattening the chiefs had for their own daughters just three years before (Brink, 1993).

The practice of fattening and women's secret societies continues to exist but, judging from the degree to which the girls were protected from my seeing them, they are much more hidden and protected from strangers than in former times. There are possible explanations for this secrecy. First, all Catholics are banned from this practice by their Bishop. These may have been Catholic families. Had I known about them, I might have told the Bishop, and the families might have had sanctions against them that they did not wish to experience. This explanation may explain why I was not told about the first *mbobo*. Second, since I am not Annang, and since these are village-based secret societies, only a woman friend of mine who belonged to the society would have invited me to meet the girl, her family and her society members. In 1980, I was introduced to a little girl being initiated into *ngwongwo*. I was taken there by a friend, who was herself a member of the secret society in that village. Without that direct connection, I would not be taken to see such an event. This satisfies the second incident (Brink, 1991).

There may be fewer *mbobo* due to the requirement that all must remain in seclusion until the annual "coming-out ceremonies." In addition, this degree of fattening is very expensive. On the other hand, *ngwongwo* does not require the same length of seclusion. A girl does not have to "come out" in three weeks but may remain longer. This length of seclusion is more controllable by the family wealth. In addition, *ngwongwo* is a specific treatment for infertility. The six young women who were in the fattening room the summer of 1989 were all married women sent there by the *idiong* (the diviner). All were perceived as being infertile (none had conceived). I never met any of these women.

My informant, who offered to introduce me to five of these young women, was a young male, without status in his village. He did not have the authority to invite me to meet these girls. He did, however, introduce me to his father, who was an *idiong* man. I shared the information (about my invitation) with my informant's employer who was a Catholic priest (as well as an anthropologist), assuming, that as an Annang from that area, he knew all about it. The family may have experienced some negative consequences as a result of my revelations. Or, they may simply have feared negative consequences and decided I was not safe.

A family could impoverish itself to maintain a Fattening Room girl as is evident in the following example. One man, a taxi driver, had sold his taxi to pay for his wife's fattening room experience. The taxi was his only means of earning money for the family. His wife could not conceive and they had been married several years. They were both Christians and had exhausted the fertility-producing recommendations of physicians. The need to produce a male offspring was uppermost in the minds of these families. The husband was not considered to be infertile, the entire emphasis was upon the fertility of the wife.

Function of the Fattening Room

There has been a significant shift in the use of the fattening room for *mbobo*. In traditional times, *mbobo* served a health-promotion function. A girl was to become fat to ensure that she could conceive, that her baby would be healthy and that she would have an easy birth. In 1989, the fattening room appeared to serve as a treatment for infertility. We found six young women in the fattening room—ranging in age from 15 to 27. All of these young women were married but unable to conceive a child. There were no young women in the fattening room as a prelude to marriage, although the clan head said his daughter had been in the fattening room three years before. He did say, however, that she had been diagnosed with severe headaches and extreme thinness.

One informant, an Annang state registered nurse, was appalled that a 15 year old girl would be placed in the fattening room to assist her to conceive. She was positive the treatment would fail. She insisted that Annang girls did not begin to menstruate until they were 17 or 18 years of age. Given the very slender, underdeveloped physique of many of the village girls I met, I would tend to agree with this informant.

In a very compelling argument, MacCormack (1982) points out the relationship between degree of body fat and onset of menarche in West African and Pacific girls. She cites Malcolm (1966) as stating that the onset of menarche among the Bundi of Papua New Guinea was 18.8 years of age on average, in contrast to 12.4 to 13.5 years in affluent societies (Marshall and Tanner, 1974). These figures seem somewhat dated, as it is no longer uncommon for North American mothers to announce the onset of menses of their 10-year-old daughters. Sixth grade school teachers cite example after example of their obviously blossoming school girls. MacCormack states that Frisch (1975, cited in MacCormack, 1982) recommended between 20 to 22% body fat as a required minimum for a girl to become fertile.

MacCormack's argument is extended in a paper by Townsend and McElroy (1992) in which they place fertility, lactation and pregnancy in an ecological context. They refer to studies of the !Kung San of southern Africa in which "Conception is most likely to occur between June and August, when food supplies are greatest and women's weight is at a maximum. During the season of minimal weight, women are not ovulating" (1992:18). They document the precise amount of kcal needed to carry a pregnancy (an extra 300 kcal/day) and breastfeed (500 kcal/day) infants over one year. They posit that the ritual fattening, as described in this paper, "can be interpreted as storage of energy for the demands of pregnancy and lactation" (1992:21).

Although the Annang do not have access to recent research reports on the corollaries and consequences of obesity and anorexia, they appear to have come to similar conclusions about the need for an optimal level of weight for fertility. This information has been part of traditional Annang culture and has not changed. The change in the use of the fattening room from *prevention of infertility* prior to marriage, to a *curative function to treat infertility* may be a reflection of the economic situation in Nigeria. Times are hard in Nigeria. The national shift from agriculture to cash economy and governmental dependence upon oil as the sole income-producing export has left Nigeria in serious financial difficulties. Oil revenues are not stable, and oil cannot be eaten. Other cash crops, that were once part of the national economy (palm oil, rubber), no longer produce sufficient revenue.

The people are forced back upon their own subsistence farming efforts, which produce very little additional cash—a necessity for health care and schooling. Yet, producing sons to carry on the lineage remains a priority and producing enough children to assist in subsistence farming has become, once again, a necessity. Fertility of women is basic to the survival of the people. The fattening room is the only remedy they have.

ACKNOWLEDGMENTS

Funds for the 1989 field visit were provided by the Alberta Foundation for Nursing Research, the University of Alberta Central Research Fund, and the University of Alberta Small Faculties, Funds for the Advancement of Scholarship. I wish to express my gratitude to Father U. E. Umoren, Christopher and Regina Udomesiet, and Emanuel A. Sade for all their assistance in this and prior field visits; to my sister, Veronica Obong Godwin Akpan; and to my research assistant, Coral Paul. I dedicate this paper to my long-time friend, Christopher Ebong, who was always supportive of my research among the Annang, and who died shortly after my last field visit.

NOTES

Pamela Brink, RN, Ph.D., FAAN, is Associate Dean of Research in the Faculty of Nursing at the University of Alberta, Edmonton, Canada.

1. Part of the Annang diet is palm wine, which when it is fermented and sits becomes a native gin or *akaiakai*. Men climb trees to tap the wine, and women frequently are responsible for distilling it. Although alcohol is part of a man's daily caloric intake, men control women's intake of alcohol in any form. Women cannot drink palm wine on certain days of the week, and cannot drink palm wine from certain trees on certain days of the week. *Akaiakai* is usually reserved for formal social visits or ceremonial occasions when every member of the group present will taste or "kiss" the *akaiakai*.

2. There is now a national law against the payment of bride price, but there are ways in which bride price can be accomplished other than the payment of a lump sum. The groom may have to buy cloth for all the girl's relatives, provide service to her father, pay for the Fattening Room expenses, or contribute to the expense of the social occasion in which the girl leaves the Fattening Room.

3. The wealthier an Annang man was, and the more wives he had, the more "houses" he had on his compound, as each wife had her own two-room house for herself and her children. In some cases, a man might add a room to his wife's house to accommodate the need for privacy of the *mbobo*.

4. The Annang have an eight-day week. Certain days of the week are pre-scribed for initiation into secret societies and for the final display of the successful candidate to the village.

5. The girls were covered in body paintings, had beads woven into their hair, beads about their neck and wrists, had a string of bells around their waists and ankles. Although they were "technically" nude, they did not appear naked.

REFERENCES

Andreski, Iris 1970. *Old Wives Tales: Life stories from Ibibioland.* Schocken Books, New York.

Brink, P.J. 1977. Decision making of the health care consumer: A Nigerian ex-ample. In Marjorie V. Batey (ed.), *Communicating Nursing Research: Nurs-ing research in the bicentennial year.* Western Interstate Commission for Higher Education, Boulder, Colorado, pp. 351–362.

Brink, P.J. 1989. The Fattening Room among the Annang of Nigeria. Anthro-pological approaches to nursing research, *Medical Anthropology* 12(1), 131–143.

Brink, P.J. 1991. The Fattening Room in Nigeria. *The Canadian Nurse* 87(9), 31–32.

Brink, P.J. 1993. Studying African women's secret societies: The Fattening Room of the Annang. In Claire M. Renzetti and Raymond M. Lee (eds.), *Researching Sensitive Topics.* Sage Publications, Inc., Newbury Park, Cali-fornia. pp. 235–248.

Cassidy, Claire 1982. Protein-energy malnutrition as a culture-bound syn-drome. *Culture, Medicine and Psychiatry* 6, 325–345.

Enang, K. 1979. Salvation in a Nigerian background. *Afrika*, Serie A, Band 19. Verlag von Dietrich Reimer, Berlin.

MacCormack, C. 1982. Ritual fattening and female fertility. In T. Vaskilampi and C.L. MacCormack, (eds.), *Folk Medicine and Health Culture: Role of folk medicine in modern health care.* Proceedings of the Nordic Research Symposium, 27–28 August, Department of Community Health, Univer-sity of Kuopio, Kuopio, Finland.

Malcolm, L.A. 1966. The age of puberty in the Bundi people. *Papua New Guinea Medical Journal* 9, 16–20.

Malcolm, L.W.G. 1925. Note on the seclusion of girls among the Efik of Old Calabar. *Man* 25 (69), 113–114.

Marshall, W.A., and J.M. Tanner 1974. Puberty. In J.A. Davis and J. Dobbing (eds.) *Scientific Foundations of Paediatrics*. Heineman, London.

Martin, Anne 1956. *The Oil Palm Economy of the Ibibio Farmer* Ibadan University Press, Nigeria.

Messenger, J.C. 1957. *Anang Acculturation: A study of shifting cultural focus*. University of Michigan, Ann Arbour. Ph.D. dissertation, University microfilms.

Messenger, J.C. 1959. Religious acculturation among the Anang-Ibibio. In W. Bascom and M. Herskovits (eds.), *Continuity and Change in African Cultures*. University of Chicago Press, Chicago. pp. 179–299.

Nzekwu, Onuora 1959. Iria Ceremony. *Nigeria* 63, 341–352.

←→ Ritenbaugh, Cheryl 1982. Obesity as a culture bound syndrome. *Culture, Medicine and Psychiatry* 6, 347–361.

Talbot, D.A. 1915. *Women's Mysteries of a Primitive People: The Ibibios of Southern Nigeria*. Cassell and Company, Ltd., London.

Talbot, P.A. 1912. *In the Shadow of the Bush*. W. Heineman, London.

Talbot, P.A. 1914. Some Ibibio customs and beliefs. *Journal of the African Society* **XIII** (No. LI April), 240–257.

Talbot, P.A. 1923. *Life in Southern Nigeria: The magic, beliefs and customs of the Ibibio tribe*. Macmillan and Co., Ltd., London.

Talbot, P.A. 1967. *Tribes of the Niger Delta: Their religions and customs*. 2d edition. Frank Cass & Co., Ltd., London.

Talbot, P.A., and H. Mulhall 1962. *The Physical Anthropology of Southern Nigeria*. Cambridge University Press, Cambridge.

←† Townsend, P.K., and A. McElroy 1992. Toward an ecology of women's reproductive health. *Medical Anthropology* 14, 9–34.

← Udo Ema, A.J. 1940. Fattening girls in Oron, Calabar Province, *Nigeria* 21, 386–389.

Udo, R.K. 1970. *Geographic Regions of Nigeria*. University of California Press, Berkeley.

Welmers, W.E. 1968. *Efik*. Occasional Publications, No. 11, Institute of African Studies, University of Ibadan Press, Ibadan.

5

Social Fattening Patterns in the Pacific—the Positive Side of Obesity. A Nauru Case Study

NANCY J. POLLOCK

INTRODUCTION

Obesity in the Pacific has become legendary, with chiefs in Hawaii and Tahiti the most commonly cited examples. Captain Cook began the record, as he was impressed by the size of both the men and women amongst the nobility he met on his visits to various Pacific islands (Beaglehole, 1962). Subsequent writers have maintained the legend so that these people's extraordinary body size is cited in many texts on health issues and diet (for example, Beller's *Fat and Thin*, 1977).

More recently Nauruans have been widely publicized in accounts of their obesity associated with a high rate of diabetes and glucose intolerance, as a result of a series of epidemiological studies. Per capita consumption of 7,500 kcalories by adult males and 5,000 kcalories by adult females has been reported (Zimmet, 1979;148). The research base has been extended to cover many of the island societies of Polynesia, as well as some in Melanesia and Micronesia, with an aim to reach some understanding of the link between obesity and diabetes.

In all this research obesity is considered a disease itself, along with the diabetes with which it is associated. It has strong negative connotations according to medical thinking, so the aim of the research is to identify steps that can be taken to ameliorate the condition, in order to counter this so called "disease of modernisation" (Zimmet *et al.* for Kiribati, 1984). The question as to whether it is a genetic or an environmental problem is still hotly debated (*see* McGarvey, 1991), as it affects the remedial treatment.

In this chapter I will demonstrate that large body size is a very positive attribute, actively encouraged in certain people, in Pacific societies. It does not have the negative attributes found in other parts of the world. Body shape is culturally enhanced, whether by external adornment or ritual encouragement of particular shape. In many Pacific societies strong social honours and ritual were devoted to the accomplishment of large body size. And the fattening processes were also closely associated with lightening skin colour as two linked standards of beauty. Such cultural fattening processes and the strong belief in the beauty of a fat body were in practice long before Europeans visited their shores, and may even be part of the Polynesian evolutionary heritage as protection against the cold on the open ocean during the period of voyaging (Baker, Hanna and Baker, 1986; Houghton, 1991; McGarvey, 1991). The epidemiological studies fail to take account of these early cultural values scattered throughout the ethnographic literature.

In this chapter I will argue that fattening processes have been an integral and vital means of demonstrating key cultural values. They represent another value of food, not for itself, but as a symbol of well-being and social pride. The body thus becomes a symbol of two aspects of society. Respect and pride pertain not to the individual who is fattened, but rather to the society's members who bring it about. And the large body size is recognized as a symbol of well-being between societies. So it will be argued that cultural values fit closely alongside biological values, so must be understood together.

I will examine the case of Nauru in some detail, as it has been so widely cited in the epidemiological and popular literature as an extreme example of obesity in the population in recent (modern) times. By close consideration of the environment in which Nauruan society has developed, the cultural practices they used to ensure well-covered women, and the historical events that have altered that environment and also threatened the very survival of their population, we have a broader social and temporal framework within which to gain an understanding of obesity as a positive factor in their lives.

BACKGROUND

Nauru is a single small island just fifty miles (92.6 km) south of the Equator in the central Pacific. Its nearest neighbours are the Marshall Islands to the north, Kiribati to the east and the Solomons a long way to the west. The greatest cultural contacts have been with Kiribati and the southern Marshalls, from where Nauru's legendary figures, such as Tabuarik, came (Pollock, 1987). Since 1906 phosphate has been mined on the island, bringing many outsiders to take up temporary residence (Ellis, 1936).

Ocean Island just 200 km (108 miles) to the east lies between Nauru and Kiribati; it was formerly inhabited by Banabans whose lives were interwoven with those of their Nauruan neighbours, particularly through marriage and voyages. Ocean Island was depleted of its phosphate in 1946, leaving no land on which the Banabans could live, so they were relocated to Rabi, an island in the Fiji group (*see* Silverman, 1971, for a detailed account of the effects of mining on Banaban society). Their history provides a salutary lesson for Nauruans.

The people of Nauru speak a language that does not fit closely with either East Micronesian or Polynesian (Bender, personal communication). Culturally they differ from other populations in the Pacific. They have maintained a strong matrilineal link to this day, so that the clan of a newborn child or a dead person is noted in birth and death announcements in the *Nauru Gazette*. Nauruans are proud of this distinct heritage, but still consider themselves an integral part of the Pacific.

The island is shaped like a hat, with a narrow shoreline brim, above which rises an interior crown, known as topside, about 100 meters (328 feet) above the shoreline. The small size of the island, just 20 km (12.4 miles) in circumference, and its limestone base mean a lack of diversity of resources, particularly soil and water, and a high degree of vulnerability to vagaries of the weather.

The island soils were unsuitable for the root and tree crops which provided the starch staples in such abundance elsewhere in the Pacific. Instead Nauruans relied for food on pandanus and fish. Pandanus produces large (10–15kg) globular fruit, of which the drupelets are edible, but it is a seasonal crop, bearing between October and early February, and it requires human intervention to select the type that produces edible fruits. Thus the people had been forced by circumstances to extend their food supply both by exchanging with their neighbours varieties of pandanus that would extend the season, and by preserving the excess fruit at the end of the season, making it into *edongo* paste by the process of drying.

Fish are plentiful around the island, but since it has a very narrow sheltering reef, there are periods of the year when it is unsafe to launch a boat and shore fishing is difficult. A small internal lagoon, Buada, located topside, fed from the sea by underground channels, is the source of an alternative fish supply. *Ibija* fish (*Chanos chanos*) have been farmed under strict cultural protocol by certain families who have hereditary rights to specific areas of Buada lagoon. Supplies of fingerlings were brought back from islands in the Kiribati group, tended in the household and introduced to the lagoon when they were big enough to survive. These provided an alternative supply of fish, highly prized, which were designated mainly for feasts and ceremonial occasions (Stephen, 1936:55).

Coconut trees were plentiful around the coastal rim in the early decades of this century, due to encouragement by German colonial authorities for their copra trade operating through Jaluit in the southern Marshalls. Coconut meat did provide a useful accompaniment to the diet, as well as a source of cash, but the number of trees has diminished drastically, as sale of phosphate is much more lucrative, and housing and plant associated with the mine took over coconut land (Pollock, 1987).

The central Pacific has long been subject to both cyclones and droughts, the latter being more frequently recorded on Nauru by early visitors. The drought could last two or three years, killing off much of the vegetation and reducing the already meagre supply of fresh water in the springs (Hambruch, 1914–15).

Nauruans had thus become accustomed to an irregular food supply. When pandanus and fish were available they took advantage of the bounty, but when neither was available they might have only a little water to drink. The pattern of a starch and its accompaniment which marked the diet of other Pacific island people (Pollock, 1985) was available for only part of the year, as long as the preserved *edongo* paste lasted, and fish could be caught. The breadfruit tree was introduced, probably from the Marshalls or Kiribati, to provide another starch resource, and bananas grew well if well watered and not battered by a cyclone. Feasts, which were an integral part of ceremonials and special events as elsewhere in the Pacific were marked by an abundance of whatever food was available, plus the *Ibija* fish and noddy terns which were caught in the trees on topside. The lifestyle was thus one of famine and feast, where people ate what was available, and survived until the next eating occasion. Strategies to maintain a small population at a level that was within the bounds of those resources were vital.

Before Europeans regularized their food supply through importing food in empty phosphate ships, Nauruans had devised a number of these strategies, whether consciously or unconsciously we cannot tell. A well-covered body was one; that was particularly important for women at the beginning of their reproductive years. Land division was another that enabled family groups to support those families, using the entire island's resources. A hierarchical social structure may have been another, particularly one which differentiated Nauruans themselves from newcomers, the latter having to work for the indigenous people until they gained land of their own. The *temonibe* and *amenengame* people as the nobility of the land controlled the resources, while the *itsio* class consisted of strangers and those without land.

FATTENING PRACTICES

Fattening practices were directed primarily at young women of rank. The first menses of young women of *temonibe* (chiefly) rank were celebrated by a big feast lasting three days for everyone on the island with gifts brought to her family. The girl herself was expected to perform the *Ibija* fish dance in which she wore the largest fish from the lagoon in her hair, one in her mouth, and others tied around her waist (*see* Dobson Rhone, 1921:21 for a photograph of one such girl wearing her fish; I estimate she may have weighed 85 to 95 kg (187–210 lbs). This event marked the conjunction of two facets of the island's fertility.

The celebration was followed by a seclusion period in a specially built hut for up to six months. During this time women of her family stayed with the young girl to ensure her every comfort and to feed her. Other relatives brought large amounts of whatever food was available, always observing strict food tabus, and drawing on the meagre resources through kin networks. The girl was not expected to work, or to go outside, and her every need was met as far as possible. This se-

clusion ended with another large celebratory feast at which two
groups of women performed a special dance in which men sometimes
joined. Wedgwood (1936) was told that this represented a sort of war
dance, reminiscent of the fight between the mythological heroes,
Araimin and Abonoque, the flow of blood symbolizing the female
equivalent of men shedding blood in battle. This final ceremony was a
chance for members of a high-ranking girl's extended family to show
off her body size, and her light skin, to other members of the community, and thereby gain prestige (Kretzschmar, 1913).

Girls from the other two classes were also secluded in a specially
built menstrual hut, situated on the inland side of their parents'
house, for four to five days every month. During this time the maternal grandmother taught the young girl the art of lovemaking, as was
noted also in the Marshalls (Mason, 1947).

A woman from any class was under special care from her family
and the community during her pregnancy. She was expected to stay in
a hut specially built for her, and she was not allowed to work. Her
food was subject to increasing tabus during the period of her confinement. These limited not only what she could eat, but who could touch
and carry her food. She was not allowed to eat fish caught from a ca-
noe for fear of offending the gods, and to ensure her child would be
beautiful. For a chiefly woman, her eldest son, father, mother and
daughter could not touch her food, so she had to rely on the help of
other relatives and friends. A violation of this prohibition was said to
wake up the child who would then harm the mother (Kretzchmar,
1913:18). For second ranked women the prohibition applied only to
the pregnancy with her oldest son. These restrictions became more
strict as the pregnancy progressed.

Her husband was not allowed to work during the pregnancy so he
too was fed by his relatives. He could resume normal life after the
birth, but she was not allowed to do heavy work for three months, and
the fish prohibition continued for three years (Wedgwood, 1936:27).

The custom of designating certain people to take responsibility for
feeding the menstruating or pregnant woman ensured that she was
fed at crucial points in her reproductive years. By drawing on a network of relatives throughout the island, she was assured of whatever
food supplies were available. The process was reciprocal, so that all
young girls were given this physical and moral support and families
shared resources at a critical point in the development of the next generation. The highest ranking was the centre of more attention at a feast
that mobilized an even wider network of food contributions. But giv-

en the small size of the population, such major celebrations of a *temonibe* girl's puberty would have occurred only once every ten years or so.

The restriction of a girl to a menstrual hut where she was not allowed to work or move around served to conserve her energy and thus her personal fat store. It also meant that her close kin recognized her special status and thus her readiness for reproduction, so that they could take whatever steps were deemed right for meeting her needs and those of her husband during the pregnancy. Thus a girl entered her first pregnancy in the peak of physical condition both to conceive and to nourish the fetus through parturition, whatever irregularities might occur in the food base.

These fattening practices had a dual focus. They nurtured the strength of the young woman herself at the time she was becoming and adult, and they also supported her in her role in the production of new life for the community. It seems likely that, based on past observations, the Nauruan elders drew a close association between a woman's fat body and her survival well into adulthood, overcoming the physical stresses of a number of pregnancies. The success of such a fattening programme was thus not only in the number of young women who lived to bear several children and the survival of those children themselves, but also in the prestige they brought to the whole clan. The continuity of the matrilineal line depended on such means of cultural support. It provided many new members for a clan group, and thereby strengthened the opposing units of Nauruan society.

A large body was not just a successfully functioning unit. Fat was a sign of beauty in Nauru, as Stephen, a long time resident and the father of six Nauruan children, observed (Stephen, 1936:46). It made a girl sexually attractive, and thus brought renown to her family for nurturing her so well. Several names cited by Hambruch (1914–15) reflected this very positive attribute; *Babu* meaning round, *Etibat* meaning she is fat, and *Ebabou*, meaning obese one. Whether these names were given at birth to encourage the owner's family to ensure the child lived up to them, or whether they were given at a later point in the child's development when the success of fattening practices began to show, is not clear. Hambruch's photo of *Babu* shows her to be a most successful representative of her clan's efforts, as she must have weighed some 150 kg (300 lbs).

All of these safeguards of a woman during her menses and pregnancy were forms of cultural recognition, in both material and symbolic terms, of the importance of women's contribution to the continuation of the clan and thus ultimately of Nauruan society as a whole. As a matrilineal society, ties through the mother were the means by which the newborn gained access to a nurturing kin group, and also to the land, which was the source of their group support. So it is to be expected that on an island where the food resources were marginal, culturally devised means were put in place to ensure the success of a woman's reproduction.

Children were much loved by all their relatives, so a new birth was a welcome event particularly for the mother's matrilineage. The newborn was cared for by the mother's mother and the mother's oldest sister. These women carried out practices such as dropping sea water in its eyes, rubbing its body with coconut oil to assure it would be healthy, and feeding it coconut water to cleanse its system. Babies were and still are fed on demand.

Three children was the average, according to Hambruch (1914–15), but his genealogies, and Stephen's own testament of pride in his six children, indicate that some women bore eight or ten. The baby was not fully recognized as a member of society until a month after its birth, when it was given a name at a special feast on its behalf. This practice of not giving the child full social status for the first month of life was a pragmatic response to the fragility of life in these islands, as Marshallese mothers explained a similar practice to me (Pollock, notes, 1967).

For women who could not bear children or bore only one there was a considerable stigma. They could undergo special treatments by the local female doctor to try to rectify this social calamity. The Nauruan view was that each pregnancy renewed a woman, so a woman who had no children was considered unhealthy. She brought shame on her family, who took every step they could, including fattening and massage, to rectify sterility.

Nevertheless, it is clear from Hambruch's detailed genealogies that a number of women did bear no children. Some of these may be recording errors, but I noted a similar phenomenon in my genealogies for Namu atoll in the Marshalls; there, in the very large families of ten to twelve siblings, one at least of the females was reported as never having borne children (Pollock, field notes, 1967). What caused the sterility is unclear; it could have been due to some infection, such as venereal disease. Or those women may have been unable to carry enough fat to nurture the fetus through to parturition—the fattening process had failed. Alternatively the fattening process may have been too successful so that a woman was too fat to conceive, as Frisch and McArthur (1974) have argued.

Another explanation of this sterility phenomenon may be a genetic propensity to limit the size of progeny from a sibling set and thereby lighten the impact on restricted resources—an inbuilt population control. Another may be a form of sterility passed from mother to daughter that was brought about by unsanitary birthing conditions, or a genetic mutation (*see* Rallu, 1990 for such arguments to account for the high rate of sterility in the Marquesas between 1885 and 1911). A third and more likely explanation in the case of Nauru and the Marshalls is that the sterility and infertility were caused by an inadequate food supply before and during the pregnancy.

The fattening customs noted above were recorded during Hambruch's visit in 1911 when the island was green and well-watered and food plants were growing well. But Stephen (1936) records long periods of drought, over two or three years, when rainfall was very light and much of the vegetation died. He does not tell us what they ate during these times, but the poor food supply must have had a toll on women's reproductive capacity. Only those women who carried sufficient body fat, that is, had undergone the cultural fattening practices at puberty and for an earlier pregnancy, would have had enough bodily reserves to nourish a fetus during those long, hard nine months.

Thus we are arguing that the process of fattening was both a genetic and a cultural mechanism that ensured the continuity of the population. The celebrations recognizing that a young girl has reached puberty indicate that at some time in the past it may have been fairly common for women not to menstruate, either because of being undernourished or because they were sterile due to mutation or disease. Genes alone would not be sufficient to enable a woman to put on weight on a resource-poor island such as Nauru. The supporting cultural practices were thus essential to ensure a woman had enough fat for herself and for the next member of the clan.

DISRUPTIONS IN DEMOGRAPHY AND HISTORY

The cultural fattening practices that enabled women to achieve a reasonable reproductive success were part of a larger process for the maintenance of the Nauruan population as a viable entity. Nauruans have long held a major concern that their population should reach the magic figure of 1,500, but that has been a struggle. In some years births were low and deaths were high; for example in 1908 Hassert reported 50 births and 169 deaths (cited in Underwood, 1989:9). Not only was the population declining but also some clans died out. Between Hambruch's visit in 1910 and Wedgwood's fieldwork in 1933, two clans had disappeared due to the lack of women to carry on the line (Wedgwood, 1936).

While we do not yet have a detailed reconstruction of the genealogies based on census data that Rallu has used to explain depopulation in the Marquesas between 1886 and 1921 (Rallu, 1990), we do know that in the 1880s women of Nauru were much more numerous than men, and the ratio of children to adults was increasing, but disease epidemics took their toll (Underwood, 1989:7). Women were reproducing, but not fast enough to maintain population growth above the rate of mortality due to new introduced diseases.

We can however draw on the early descriptions for some evidence. That the fattening processes described in the last section were effective is evidenced by statements such as that by Simpson in 1844 that the men he saw were "about middle size, but not robustly made," while the women were "rather good looking with a good figure, rather inclined to be stout though they appeared naturally graceful and easy in their manner" (Simpson, 1844:100). The ethnographic reports by Hambruch (1915), Kayser (1918), Delaporte (1920), Dobson Rhone (1921) and most particularly the photographs taken by Hambruch and Dobson Rhone indicate that the adults were robust, the women being generally larger than the men. Some of the young women in the photographs may have weighed 150 kg (300+lbs). How many were this heavy and may be categorized by what we would call today "overweight" or "obese" by western standards, may not even be a relevant question. No record of diabetes or heart disease was reported in the annual reports on health to the League of Nations officials for the years 1920 to 1940.

From the tables of population size (Underwood, 1989, Table 1) it is clear that the population did not grow much between 1889 and 1919, hovering around the 1,300 mark. But there also were no major setbacks, as the Fatal Impact thesis would have us believe. In the 1920s and 1930s Underwood estimates that "between 50 and 60 live births each year were produced by an effective maternal breeding pool of no more than 200–250 adult women" (1989:10). Infant mortality, however, was high in this period. The magic figure of 1,500 was reached in

1932, a demographic landmark still celebrated today that honours the mother, Mrs. Amram and her child, the 1,500th Nauruan.

That success was short-lived. From a high of 1,848 in 1942 the population suffered a major setback during World War II. Exile of two thirds of the population by the Japanese, from which only 800 returned, and deaths due to American bombing and to starvation during the American blockade of the Japanese garrison between 1943 and 1945 reduced the population again (Pollock, in press). By December 1946 only 1,369 had survived that calamitous war. Miraculously the figure of 1,500 was again reached in 1949, from which time the population has continued to grow to an estimated 5,700 in 1989 (Nauru census).

This chequered demographic history represents a strain on women's reproductive powers. Any genetic potential for fat deposition that epidemiologists consider lies behind the obesity patterns of the 1970s was sorely tested in the Nauruan case; historical events and demographic processes have served to highlight Nauruans' concern for the reproductive powers of their women, and thus are an indirect holdover of traditional ideas of fat as a sign of beauty, health and the strength of the community. While we do not yet have for Nauru in the 1880–1920 period a detailed reconstruction of the genealogies based on census data, we do know that in the 1880s women were much more numerous than men and the ratio of children to adults was increasing, but disease epidemics took their toll (Underwood, 1989:7). Women were reproducing but not fast enough to maintain population growth above the rate of mortality due to newly introduced diseases.

PHOSPHATE MINING

With the commencement of phosphate mining in 1906, several new factors were introduced into the picture of body size on Nauru. Firstly, food became available on a regular basis from the local stores. And secondly, a western-style medical system became widely available. Thirdly, new values arrived along with the outsiders, so new health ideas were proselytised as well as new ideas of beauty.

At the same time that imported food became available, and Nauruans could buy small amounts from the trader if they had the money, they also lost the land from which they had derived some food supply, particularly pandanus. Phosphate mining reduced the area from which the meagre local food resources were obtained, as all vegetation was stripped from the land on topside to reach the phosphate in the soil beneath. Pandanus trees were torn out and coconut trees on the shore-line were reduced as the new administration drew on "coconut" land for phosphate plant and associated buildings. By 1921 Nauruans were still using some local resources to make their *edongo* paste from pandanus and catching fish, but increasingly their food supply was derived from store-bought imported foods (Dobson Rhone, 1921).

The food supply became more varied after World War I when Chinese labourers brought in to work in the phosphate mine took to planting small gardens of imported foods for sale to the Europeans or anyone who wanted to buy them, as well as for their own household use.

The Nauruan diet thus changed, but the value of food underwent very little change. The long lean periods of food shortage that had been such a feature of their social existence became a thing of the past. In addition, the Congregational (religious) mission condemned the amount of feasting and uncivilized practices such as puberty ceremonies, with their fattening processes, and polygamy (Wedgwood, 1936).

But missionaries could not entirely stamp out the deep-seated Nauruan love of food. Food was the greatest means by which to express generosity and assistance to relatives and others, including visitors. The exchange of food at feasts was more than just an exchange of material goods. It marked the status of the individual in the community, as a member of that community who had land, and a share of Buada lagoon, from which to draw gifts to be presented at the feast. Food was thus a mark of prestige, and was used to convey social messages at public events. This is a social hallmark that Nauru shares with other Pacific societies (Pollock, 1992a). Large-bodied members of the family were thus a personification of this value of generosity with food.

At the same time that new food was being introduced, so also were new forms of social organization being developed and new cultural practices. The status system differentiating the *temonibe* and *amenengame*, the chiefly classes, from the *itsio*, commoners/slaves and all outsiders, was being replaced with new social forms of differentiation, such as cash income and education, and living outside Nauru. When these classes disappeared the puberty ceremonies and fattening processes diminished in importance even beyond the missionaries' attempts to stamp them out. But the value of food still remained and was transferred to the new foods available.

Land became even more precious, and identity as a Nauruan was carefully delineated from that of the newcomers on the basis of access to land. Outsiders cannot gain rights to land. The means by which mining rights were taken without Nauruans' consent is still the subject of legal contest in the International Court of Justice in the Hague (Weeramantry, 1992). The British Phosphate Commission which took over administration of Nauru in 1919 from the German administration introduced new forms of social organization such as allocating a chief per district, and thereby creating a new direct association between chiefs and specific areas of land. It is ironic that under the terms of the Nauru Agreement (1919) whereby the League of Nations handed over the caretaker responsibilities for Nauru to Australia, Great Britain and New Zealand as the British Phosphate Commissioners (BPC), there was no discussion with Nauruans, nor was any Nauruan party to the Nauru Agreement. Mining was thus allowed to continue for the profit of the BPC at the expense of the Nauruans (Pollock, 1992b).

WORLD WAR II

Those former cultural fattening processes also enabled Nauruans to withstand another historical event and demographic disaster, World War II. When the Japanese invaded the island in 1941 to provide a base for their push into the South Pacific, they began to build up their personnel on Nauru to reach some 7,000 by 1943, probably the greatest density the island had ever known. The 1941 Nauruan population of 1,827 people was too large for the island according to Japanese thinking, so some had to be moved out to make space for Japanese forces. 1,200 Nauruans were moved in two groups of 600 to Truk in 1942 where they suffered many privations, including starvation, while being forced to work for the Japanese building military installations, or growing sweet potatoes, an entirely unfamiliar task. By 1946 when they were repatriated to Nauru, only 800 had survived, 400 having died in exile (see Pollock, 1991).

To stem the Japanese advance the United States forces attacked Nauru relentlessly from the air, aiming to "bomb the island out of existence" (see Pollock, 1991, for details). Out of the 600 Nauruans left on Nauru, some Nauruans (and many Chinese) were killed in those bombing raids, while the rest had to work for the Japanese. The United States bombing raids were so effective they blockaded the island for two years so that no Japanese supply ship could get through and the entire population received smaller and smaller rations of rice. As a result those Japanese, Nauruans and Chinese left on the island were reduced to eating pumpkins grown in oil drums of night soil, together with whatever fish they could catch. The Australian armistice party was amazed at the good physical condition of the people despite the appallingly filthy condition of the island (Ellis, 1950). Once reunited with those transferred from Truk in 1946, the Nauruan population totalled 1,369.

How had Nauruans survived these privations? We can credit that survival to an earlier fat patterning and a resilience to adversity and starvation. Those who still had the cultural and genetic strength to draw on any body fat built up in the good years before 1940 made it through to 1946, while those who lacked this body fat succumbed to the privations.

We do not know the fate of any conceptions by Nauruan women during this time, but we do know that by 1949 the population again reached 1,500, for an average of 75 births per year from 1946 to 1949. Some deaths would have resulted from the privations of the previous three years, and some due to old age and sickness. But the women's ability to conceive successfully and bear to full term so soon after their bodies had been severely undernourished must indicate that amenorrhea due to undernutrition stopped as soon as a regular food supply was available. The rapid revival process indicates both a very strong cultural force supporting those women during that pregnancy, as well as a physical store of body fat to nourish the fetus. The population of Nauruans has continued to grow since 1946, reaching 2,328 in 1960, with 120 births in 1959 and only 20 deaths.

Nauru continues to have a positive population policy to this day. The government encourages families to have children with a child support programme. There is also a very low rate of out-migration by Nauruans on a long-term basis, some leaving for education and training or government postings, but returning home eventually; the largest Nauruan community outside Nauru is in Melbourne, Australia. This demographic encouragement for population growth is unique amongst Pacific island countries, all of which are trying to reduce their rate of reproduction, not encourage a higher one. For Nauruans it is a feature of their pride in their community and their desire to maintain their social viability.

TOWARDS INDEPENDENCE

From 1949 to 1992 the Nauruan population has grown steadily in number with no further setbacks. Mining has continued with more and more growing land being lost, but more and more Nauruans have gained cash wealth in the process—presenting a strong double dilemma.

Cash is thus the major means of obtaining food. Apart from some fishing, some coconut toddy, and the vegetables the Chinese grow to serve in their restaurants, all other food is imported. In the 1950s and 1960s diets were considered satisfactory, even though high in imported carbohydrates, rice and flour and breakfast cereals (Kirk, 1957). Health reports to the United Nations mentioned no major nutritional concerns.

But Nauruans were still getting only a small proportion of the profits from phosphate at this time. And they were losing their lands (see Pollock, 1992b). They were also not in control of their own island, as BPC ran it as a United Nations Trust through Australian administration. And outsiders brought in to work phosphate almost outnumbered Nauruans. So 1968 was the date set for Independence, and also for taking over phosphate mining.

Another unsettling issue was the concern, mainly of Australians, to relocate the Nauruan population when phosphate ran out. Nauruans rejected any relocation plan. They had seen what had happened to the Banabans from Ocean Island and wanted to maintain the integrity of their own population.

Since Independence in 1968 and the purchase of their own phosphate mining facilities from the British Phosphate Commission for $A20 million, Nauruans have taken care of their own affairs. They have invested the profits from phosphate sold on the open market in the welfare of their people, and in other Pacific enterprises, such as Air Nauru and hotels, as well as in international banks, companies and real estate. In the 1970s they succeeded in stamping their Nauruan identity on the rest of the Pacific and the wider world. They have sought to present a positive image of wealth that assists the other much poorer Pacific island nations. Their leader, the late Hammer de Roburt, also reinforced this picture of Nauruan identity in the forefront of Pacific island affairs. Large body size may be considered in Pacific terms an appropriate manifestation of their status.

This positive picture of Nauruans controlling their own affairs was marred by the world-wide release in 1976 of a study reporting that the

Nauruan population had one of the highest rates of diabetes in the world. An epidemiological survey found that 25% of the adult Nauruan population was diagnosed as having maturity onset or non-insulin-dependent diabetes, and another 8% had high rates of glucose intolerance (Zimmet, 1979). The story of this small obese population was spread around the world as epidemiological phenomenon, and picked up by the popular press. The self-image of a newly emerging nation was thus scarred by the negative publicity about an unhealthy population.

Nauruans were characterized, along with a number of other Third World societies, as having a high incidence of diabetes, with strong negative connotations. Similar rates of prevalence were found in Australian Aborigines, Pima Indians and Mexican Americans. Neel (1962) has suggested that such populations may have a "diabetic genotype" that is unmasked by a change to a westernized lifestyle. Obesity, a high caloric western diet low in fibre and high in fat and sugar, together with reduced physical activity, are considered the major precipitating factors for the 20-plus age group(Zimmet, 1979:144). Labelling obesity as due to a genetic difference has not eased the negative publicity.

The slur of obesity was considered to be too harsh by the Nauruans themselves, as they had a different view of their body size. Large body size had been a key factor in the survival of their population, not a deleterious one. It was part of their positive identity.

MODERNIZATION

Obesity, and its association with diabetes, has become labelled a "disease of modernization," with the Nauruan population placed by epidemiologists at the forefront of this phenomenon. Zimmet explains this prevalence in the Pacific by locating these two diseases in the third stage of his framework of epidemiologic transition. Stage I was the Era of Pestilence and Famine brought by voyagers when death rates were high and little population growth occurred. Stage II was the Era of Receding Pandemics when infectious diseases were less destructive and Pacific island populations began to increase. Stage III, the Era of Degenerative and Man-made Diseases, such as diabetes and hypertension, affects mainly those populations that have adopted a western lifestyle. Such a lifestyle is a mark of modernization, as contrasted with those societies that continue to live in a more traditional lifestyle (Zimmet, 1979: 145).

There are several difficulties with this general argument about diabetes and obesity that are also espoused by other epidemiologists working in the Pacific (Prior, 1976; Baker, Hanna and Baker, 1986).

Firstly Zimmet's framework for epidemiologic transition in the Pacific is too limited. It does not go back in time in enough detail to consider cultural practices in place at the time Europeans arrived. Nor does it consider a very deep-seated value of food as a means of communication. In Rarotonga, Tahiti, Samoa, Tonga and Wallis we know that chiefs were at the centre of a food distribution network, and that they ate well when visitors recorded those events. We also have indications that at puberty women in Tahiti underwent fattening processes, particularly those associated with Arioi society, and that women in Futuna and Wallis were, and are still today, expected to eat well, not to work and to put on weight when they first move to live with their husband's family and before the birth of the first child, so that the mother-in-law cannot be charged with neglect by the birth mother (Pollock, 1987 field notes).

Secondly we must ask why did diabetes "suddenly" appear in these populations in the 1970s? Why did it not appear when the populations were obese at contact? Can the same standards of obesity and overweight be applied to all populations, or are we using inappropriate standards? The Japanese have decided they need a measure more appropriate to their own lifestyle (*see* papers in Baba and Zimmet, 1990). Closer consideration of demographic and historical events will help clarify modern-day epidemiological occurrences, but they must be taken in a broader framework.

Thirdly, modernization is a process. The term cannot be applied to contemporary populations by designating today's rural populations as "traditional" in contrast with urban populations which are considered "modern." In the Pacific the distinction between these two is very small because there is a great deal of flow between rural and urban areas. They are not isolated either in terms of resources, or of physical features. Both of these populations have been affected by modern ideology, they are on the receiving end of new values via radios, in some cases television and videos, and magazines, have relatives who have been overseas or lived in an urban centre. Both groups work, both reproduce and both eat. Is it that diabetes is "catching" in the sense that overeating is socially induced, that is, by the concept of the meal?

Using modernization as the theoretical hook for these epidemiological transition ideas does not clarify why diabetes appeared in the
1970s. Diabetes came to the fore in epidemiological studies in the
1970s as Neel's (1962) hypothesis was tested on a number of nonwes-
tern societies. But the association between obesity and diabetes was
(and still is) under question by some researchers, as are the standards
by which we assess overweight and obesity (see Baba and Zimmet,
1990; Introduction above). As populations in the modern world are
assessed also in terms of reported weights, BMIs (see Introduction),
hip/thigh ratios, and other standards, it is becoming clear that the
higher ranking weights need to be increased to fall more realistically
in line with current statistics, much the way Recommended Dietary
Intakes have been adjusted in the 1960s and 1970s.

If diabetes is a disease of modernization, and modernization is associated with urbanization, cash income and wage work and imported food, then why did Nauruans not develop diabetes in the
1920s and 1930s when they first experienced this lifestyle; why did it
wait to manifest itself until the 1970s? The answer lies in the interest in
diabetes in developing countries in the 1970s (and the money for research) aroused by Neel's work in South America that yielded the
"thrifty gene" hypothesis, and studies of Pima Indians in the U.S. Epidemiologists moved their focus of attention from infectious diseases
to these noninfectious or "man-made" diseases such as diabetes, hypertension and cardiovascular disease. Prior's work on these "new"
diseases as manifest in the Tokelau atoll project, Zimmet's diabetes research throughout the Pacific, and Baker and his colleagues' work on
Samoans in four locations have all used the concept of modernization
as the key concern (Prior, 1976; Zimmet, 1979; Baker, Hanna and
Baker, 1986).

Historical factors such as those raised here are important considerations because they can show a wide range of concerns impinging on
obesity, such as past fertility patterns and irregularities in the food
supply. Ethnographic data from earlier periods yields descriptions of
body size, and foods consumed, mainly subjective, but nevertheless
indicative of patterns to be explored further. Body image data within
its social context is sparse, particularly for early times, but nevertheless where available must be incorporated into considerations of obesity.

Not the least of the difficulties with the "obesity as a disease of modernization" viewpoint is the negative image it implies, and its
directedness, mainly at women. Nauruan women expressed their

concerns to me about the connotations of the labels when they identify themselves as from Nauru. They are proud of their identity, which has emerged out of a heritage in which biological and social events have been permeated by cultural practices. Their identity is slightly different from that of other Pacific Island people. Two major invasions, one by the members of the British Phosphate Commission (British, Australian and New Zealand), and a second by the Japanese during World War II, as well as American bombing, brought new ideologies and caused major disruption to local resources. They also took their physical toll on Nauruans, with new kinds of food, a period of regular food supply, broken in 1943–45 by two years of starvation, and then a steady growth of reliance on imported food (Pollock, 1991). But the price was the loss of their land, which was literally carried away to make others land-rich. With Independence cash flow has increased throughout the community, enabling more food and liquor and other consumables to be imported. And through the increased world network of communications they learn that they are at the forefront of a new era, that of Degenerative and Man-Made Diseases.

Thus we have argued here that modernization needs to be carefully rethought to incorporate cultural values associated with a group body image. In many societies the group is more important than the individual for setting values. Fattening processes are a part of ethnography that have not been widely considered for their implications for population growth, social status and health. Subjective measures need to be incorporated with objective ones sought by epidemiologists and human biologists. A more "rounded" picture of the social contexts of health issues should throw more light on societies such as Nauru. The associations between obesity and diabetes and other health concerns need to be more clearly established before a population's collective body image and positive identity is turned into a derogatory headline.

CONCLUSION

Fattening processes as part of the beauty concept in Nauru and other societies of the Pacific (see Pollock in press b) need to be considered in a broader framework than they have heretofore. Cultural, environmental and genetic factors must all be included as they affect one another, not as separate categories.

The process of fattening on Nauru was a strong manifestation of their cultural values. Upper-class women received cultural and physical support for their reproductive abilities. Tabus and cultural practices were part of the process that ensured the population survived metaphysically and physically. Together these cultural and genetic elements contributed significantly towards the continuity of the population despite the vagaries of climate and population size, and disruptive events such as mining and World War II. The celebrations recognizing a young girl had reached puberty indicate that at some time in the past it may have been fairly common for women not even to start to menstruate, either because of being undernourished due to the irregular food supply, or because of sterility due to disease.

Genes alone would not be sufficient to enable a young woman to put on weight in Nauru; she needed the special attention of her relatives to provide her with the food by redirecting the meagre resources in her direction. And those foods would not be redirected unless body size had positive connotations, such as beauty. Thus according to the supporting cultural practices the young, newly menstruating woman was singled out to join the small group of women on whom the burden of reproduction for the whole Nauruan community rested. And the whole community supported and commended the effort.

While the new values came in with mining, some of the old values persisted. Love of food and admiration of large body size are as much part of the new scene as they were of the old. What have changed are many of the material surroundings and negative values associated with large body size that have been superimposed on the society.

Further increase in the high rates of diabetes seems unlikely. Zimmet (1979) has already referred to the 1976 figures as an "epidemic." I have suggested elsewhere (Pollock, ms) that this may be due to those who were poorly nourished as children during World War II reaching the age of susceptibility to maturity-onset diabetes. Alternatively those figures may reflect a post-Independence affluence and thus high consumption. One piece of data we sorely need is a person-by-person household consumption survey at four different times during a year to give a comprehensive picture of the nutritional standing of Nauruans.

When phosphate mining finishes, changes in food consumption are likely. Nothing will grow locally unless vast amounts of topsoil are brought in to cover the area topside where pinnacles may be cut down; this is a very expensive proposal to the Nauru Rehabilitation Commission, and seems unlikely at this time. So all food will still be imported. But Nauruans are likely to restrain their spending because they will then be on a finite source of income. If soil is brought in, the Chinese may establish market gardens consisting of vegetables, as they have elsewhere in the Pacific. But proximity to the Equator and the periodic droughts will make this risky. I suspect that the traditional love of food by Nauruans will persist; it will just be more difficult to satisfy.

Reduced consumption may reduce the rates of diabetes. Or then again it may not. If diabetes has a genetic base, as some epidemiologists have argued, then the social contexts which accentuate its onset may be in the past, as argued above. In any case, monitoring diabetes rates and food consumption in Nauru will lead to clarification of our understanding of this disease.

By drawing together commentary on cultural practices, demographic processes and historical events, we have shown that on Nauru large body size was actively promoted in the past as a sign of beauty. So it cannot be considered "a disease of modernization." Large body size has been recorded for this society for over 100 years. It has not been produced only by the attributes of modernization, cited by epidemiologists and human biologists.

The inclusion of obesity as a noninfectious disease also requires further clarification. That diabetes, obesity's consort in the negative imagery, may be a recent disease in the Pacific, remains to be ascertained. That the two are weakening or limiting in some way for this population, and others in the Pacific and elsewhere also needs further proof—that is, does diabetes contribute directly to x numbers of deaths?

The connotations of the term obesity also need reconsideration. A range of different measurements is now used, all of which are applied to place some people's body weight over a standard and others under it. Obesity has negative associations in English that are now spreading to nations using English as a second language, but where large body size has a much more positive image.

Body image is an important concept at national as well as individual levels. Nauruans themselves are concerned about the negative aspects of their collective body image being spread around the world with no chance to defend themselves. They have not the communication technology to counter the world-wide impact of scientific papers that have presented the world with an overwhelmingly negative image of Nauru (fat = lazy, out of control, unintelligent, for example).

This chapter has shown that large body size has a strong positive cultural base that has been overlooked by those considering only the physical, biological and medical phenomena. The whole label of obesity needs to be rethought as a culturally sensitive term so that we can accept large body size positively without the necessity of associating it with disease factors. Beauty has many forms.

NOTES

Nancy J. Pollock gained her Ph.D, from the University of Hawaii. Her research interests have focussed on the sociocultural meanings of food with particular interest in Pacific societies. Her book tracing five hundred years of changing food habits in the Pacific, entitled *These Roots Remain* was published in 1992 (University of Hawaii Press). She is currently Senior Lecturer in the Department of Anthropology at Victoria University in Wellington, New Zealand.

REFERENCES

Baba, J., and P. Zimmet 1900. *World Data Book of Obesity*. Excerpta Medica, Elsevier.

Baker, P., J.M. Hanna and T.S. Baker (eds.) 1986. *The Changing Samoans*. Oxford University Press, New York.

Beaglehole, J.C. (ed.) 1962. *The Endeavour Journal of Sir Joseph Banks*. Angus and Robertson, Sydney.

Beller, A. 1977. *Fat and Thin. A natural history of obesity.* Farrar, Strauss and Giroux, New York.

Delaporte, Mrs. P. 1920. The men and women of old Nauru. *Mid Pacific* 19(20), 153–156.

Ellis, A.F. 1936. *Ocean Island and Naura*. Angus and Robertson, Sydney.

Ellis, A.F. 1950. Rehabilitation of Nauru and Ocean Islands, *New Zealand Journal of Agriculture* 80, 213–214.

Frisch, R., and J. McArthur 1974. Menstrual cycles: Fatness as a determinant of minimal weight for height necessary for their maintenance or onset. *Science*, **185**, 949–951.

Hambruch, P. 1914–15. *Nauru. Ergebnisse der Sudsee Expedition 1908–1910.* L. Friedriksen, Hamburg.

Houghton, P. 1991. The early human biology of the Pacific. *Journal of the Polynesian Society* 100(2), 167–196.

Kayser, P. 1917–18. Die Eingebornen von Nauru (Sudsee). *Anthropos* **12/13**, 313–337.

Kirk, Nancy 1957. *Dietary Survey of Nauru*. Commonwealth Department of Health, Canberra, Australia.

Kretzschmar, K.E. 1913. Nauru. *Cyclostyled*.

Mason, L. 1947. Marshall Islands Report. Coordinated Investigation into Micronesian anthropology (CIMA).

∨ McGarvey, S.T. 1991. Obesity in Samoans. *American Journal of Clinical Nutrition* **53**, 1586s–1594s.

Neel, J.V. 1962. Diabetes Mellitus: A thrifty genotype rendered detrimental by progress. *American Journal of Human Genetics* **14**, 353–362.

Pollock, N.J. 1985. The concept of food in a Pacific society. *Ecology of Food and Nutrition* **17**, 195–203.

Pollock, N.J. 1987. *Nauru Report*. Report to the Commission for the Rehabilitation of Nauru, Melbourne, Australia.

Pollock, N.J. 1991. Nauruans during World War II. In Geoff White (ed.), *Remembering the Pacific War*. Centre for Pacific Island Studies, University of Hawaii, Occasional Paper #36.

Pollock, N.J. 1992a. *These Roots Remain*. University of Hawaii Press.

Pollock, N.J. 1992b. *Land for Nauruans: Mining, money and misunderstandings*. Paper for Folk Law Conference, Wellington.

Pollock, N.J. in press a) World War II on Nauru, *ISLA*, Guam .

☞ Pollock, N.J. in press b) *Fat as a concept of beauty*. Pan Pacific Arts Association Conference Proceedings, April 1993, Adelaide.

Prior, Ian 1976. Nutritional problems in Pacific islanders. *Proceedings of the New Zealand Nutrition Society*.

Rallu, J.L. 1990. *Les Populations Oceaniennes aux XIXe et XXe sieécles*. Institut d'Études Demographiques, travaux et documents, Cahier No. 128, Paris.

Rhone, R.D. 1921. Nauru, the richest island in the South Seas. *National Geographic* **40**(60), 559–589.

Silverman, M. 1971. *Disconcerting Issue*. University of Chicago Press, Chicago.

Simpson, T.B. 1844. Pacific navigation and British seamen. *Nautical Magazine and Naval Chronicles* **13**, 99–103.

Stephen, E. 1936. Notes on Nauru. *Oceania* **7**(1), 34–63.

Underwood, J. 1989. Population history of Nauru, a cautionary tale. *Micronesia* **22**(1), 3–22.

Wedgwood, C. 1936. Report on research work in Nauru island, central Pacific. *Oceania* **6**(4), 359–391; **7**(1), 1–33.

Weeramantry, C. 1992. *Nauru. Environmental Damage under International Trusteeship*. Oxford University Press, Oxford.

Zimmet, P. 1979. Epidemiology of diabetes and its macrovascular manifestations in Pacific populations: The medical effects of social progress. *Diabetes Care* **2**(2), 144–153.

Zimmet, P., H. King, R. Taylor, L.R. Rape, B. Balkau and K. Thoma 1984. The natural history of impaired glucose tolerance in the Micronesian population of Nauru. *Diabetologia* **26**(1), 39–43.

6

Taste, Food Regimens and Fatness. A Study in Social Stratification

ANNEKE H. VAN OTTERLOO

INTRODUCTION

The growing incidence of overweight, fatness and obesity in recent decennia is a modern industrial phenomenon, which is attributed largely to overfeeding (de Boer and Deurenberg, 1987). This phenomenon stands in remarkable contrast to the widespread thinness and ill-health caused by malnutrition in pre-industrial and early industrial times. In the Netherlands for instance, G.J. Mulder, a well known physician active around 1850, complained of a series of illness and health problems relating to food habits of the so-called "peoples' class." These habits were part of lifestyles which were defined in the first place by deep poverty. The foodways of the rich were, however, criticised as well: overfeeding was as important a health-risk as undernourishment, although this problem was far less common (Mulder, 1847). Considering recent data on the unequal distribution of obesity among different socioeconomic strata (Baecke *et al.*, 1983), fatness seems to have trickled down from the top to the bottom of the social scale.

Then and now, fatness is only possible in a situation of affluence. Large quantities of food have been available to all strata of the population only relatively recently. The rise in importance of a new standard of beauty relating to body shape seems to be an accompanying phenomenon which is spreading downwards among social classes as well. Fat bodies are no longer seen as a sign of wealth and freedom from want, which in Mulder's time may probably still have been the case. To the contrary, fatness is considered a worry both from a physical and an aesthetic point of view. Heavy societal pressure to possess slim bodies for women as well as for men forces them to control their appetites. This development towards an ideal of moderation is an aspect of what Elias called "the civilising process" (Elias, 1978). This civilising of appetite (Mennell, 1985), and Bourdieu's notion of the classificatory character of taste (Bourdieu, 1986) are taken as a cue to the research reported here.

RESEARCH QUESTION AND METHODS

This study tried to throw some light on a few correlates of fatness anchoring in aspects of lifestyle. The research concentrates on differences in opinions and practices between families of the professional class and two types of working class, respectively. These have to do with taste, food choices and health, food regimens (especially those limiting or regulating much fat and sweet foods), body images and body management. All of these are supposed to belong to a complex of attitudes relating to body weight and to be, as a whole, part of peoples' lifestyles. An impressive way of approaching differences in matters of taste is proposed by Bourdieu. His concept of "habitus" (Bourdieu, 1986: 169–226) is used here to connect lifestyles with differences in sociostructural circumstances. Mothers of 6–12 year old children (15 from the professional class, 14 underclass mothers receiving state grants because of their or their husbands' lack of paid work, and 17 skilled working-class mothers) were chosen as respondents because as "gatekeepers" they should be considered the best informants about food preferences in the family.

The method of research was ethnographic. Semistructured interviews, lasting about two hours, were held with a total of 46 mothers, representing two distinct social strata. Respondents were encouraged to comment freely and to talk about their own feelings and experiences. All interviews were fully tape recorded and transcribed.[1] The sampling was done in cooperation with a regional agency of youth health care. Mothers coming to the agency for a check-up were asked to participate in the project. From those willing mothers a careful selection was made according to the 3 usual criteria of socioeconomic status: occupation, education and income. This procedure resulted in two groups of respondents representing families of relatively "high" and "low" socioeconomic status, but these were of unequal size. The most numerous group of working-class mothers was split further according to type of income: wages or social security grants. This seemed to be a relevant distribution as to food choices. Thus, 46 respondents finally were divided into three nearly equally distributed groups: 14 mothers belonging to "social class" IA (the category of "grant receivers"), 17 mothers belonging to IB (the category of "wage earners") and 15 mothers belonging to II (the category of "professionals") (Goudsblom, 1986).

SOCIAL DESIRABILITY AND SOCIAL CLASSIFICATION

In an interview situation participants try to present themselves to their partners of discussion as acceptably as possible. This is true for interviewers and interviewees alike. Especially among the working-class families in the sample, the researchers felt they were not seen as "one of us," and vice-versa. Although we had taken pains to assure the respondents beforehand we only wanted to know their opinions and practises and did not come for any supervision, we observed that the mothers (especially those from class I) felt the urge to present themselves as "competent mothers and housewives."

If a bias towards social desirability sometimes may have been a characteristic of the answers this does not mean they are less valuable. The behaviour respondents want to show is what they think is good and right in the interviewer's eyes. This is in most cases the behaviour they aspire to, but are not always able to realise. Because we wanted to know valued opinions and motivations for their reported behaviour, this is no serious drawback. In addition their answers were checked by asking about feelings and experiences as well. The impression of competency consists of four aspects (Goffman, 1959) called "Managing the impression."

The first was concealing the necessity to economise; most mothers were, however, very open in matters of price and economy; the second, exaggerating quantities of socially valued foods, for instance sort drinks because of their connotation of luxury and ease, and milk for health reasons; thirdly, underrating "socially despised" foods like sweets and cola drinks, at least from the point of view of competent mothers exerting prudent regimes over their families. Lastly, showing knowledge about vitamins in fresh vegetables and fruits and (less frequently) about the importance of variety in meals.

Working-class mothers showed competency, but presented attitudes (in the eyes of the interviewers) of resistance, indifference, insecurity, imitation and acceptance. These attitudes were less evident in the group of professional class respondents who wanted to be considered competent mothers. Communication between "them" and "us" was enacted on the same wave length, evidence of shared standards of middle-class behaviour (Bourdieu, 1986: 117).

TASTE, FOOD REGIMENS AND FOOD CHOICES

Preferences: Taste of Necessity and Taste of Luxury

An important purpose of the research consisted in groping for any indication of differences in taste among our respondents, compared to those found by Bourdieu in France (1986. chapters 3, 5, 7). This sociologist typifies working-class preferences as a "taste of necessity." This means that their preferences and choices in the field of cultural consumption are bound to their social class position. As far as the dinner table is concerned, this points to their preference for cooking and eating foods because of their "habitus" and their occupational and financial situation. This same position in society induces Bourdieu to speak of a "taste of luxury" in the case of the middle classes; these people have the opportunity to develop a more selective taste. Distinction is manifest in the importance attached to rules, forms, choices and qualities in food and eating as opposed to material necessity. French working-class families like "the good life": eating and good cooking is very important compared to other social activities. They prefer "cheap, fat and filling foods and large portions," also, meat and vegetables must be well-cooked. French middle classes prefer light, delicate and lean foods, also *crudités* (raw vegetables), which are more expensive although healthy.

In general, it turned out that comparable tendencies are discernible in the Dutch data. Attitudes, regimens and preferences of the mothers we interviewed differed in rather consistent ways between the social classes I (working class) and II (professional middle class), while differences between the subgroups IA and IB ("grant receivers" and "wage earners"), although present were much less conspicuous. As far as taste is concerned, working-class respondents reportedly liked foods which were similar in some respects to those preferred by their French counterparts. To the observers these were filling, fat, sweet and cheap. The preference for sweet is more of an English than a French taste.

A central element of what may indeed be aptly called a "taste of necessity" is the fondness for *meat*. Most families eat meat because Father wants to eat it. Pork is considered cheaper and softer (especially for the children) than beef. Bacon and chops are the preferred cuts, as they are not seen as fatty. Most mothers bake them well and do not use the fat. They do not like fat gravy either, and are horrified at the idea of eating "really fat" pieces of meat such as pork rind and pig tails, of which they remember their fathers and grandfathers were fond. One or two mothers do continue the tradition of eating crackling (baked fat) and sopping bread in the gravy.

Thus, working-class families in our sample are not particularly fond of fat meat: they eat pork rather than beef, not because it is more greasy (which mothers do not realise) but for its cheapness. Another reason to shun pork is the modern "chemical" way of breeding pigs. This dislike of fat is remarkable in view of the rise of fat-consumption since World War II. The difference between "observable" and "hidden" fat is relevant here. The strong preference for meat has to be understood in terms of its "filling" character, which is especially satisfying for those actually doing heavy manual work, or for those with a fond memory of what their fathers and grandfathers ate. Another reason is found in the aspect of luxury. Working-class families have only recently been able to afford to eat meat every day. Mothers remembered they often had meat only on Sundays as a child, which is similar to group IA ("grant receivers"), whose income does not permit them to eat meat every day: this is an important difference from group IB ("wage earners").

Another indispensable part of the hot meal belonging to the "taste of necessity" are fresh *vegetables*. These must be well-cooked in water and be prepared with a simple sauce and/or some spices. Raw vegetables are consumed only in summer; these mostly consist of green salad or cucumber, nothing else. Potatoes are eaten frequently, sometimes alternated with macaroni or spaghetti, while rice is eaten exclusively as *nasi* (Indonesian name for cooked rice), an Indonesian dish served with spices, meat and vegetables. Dessert if present always consists of ready-made (sweet) custards or sometimes yoghurt. Working-class families in our sample have a definite preference for white bread. Mothers admitted to having tried brown bread, "but they really do not like it" and husbands insisted on white bread to take to work. Most mothers offered both types, white and brown, which practically never means the full-grain quality bread. Here the mechanisms at work are the same as comparisons among meat, where white bread used to be a highly prized luxury food until less than a generation ago. Working-class mothers continue to buy white bread; moreover they cannot afford whole-grain bread, which is much more expensive.

Professional middle-class representatives among our respondents are conspicuous in their differences; they prefer a wide variety of different types of food. Middle-class mothers do not prepare meat every day, they replace meat with fish, cheese or eggs. Their choice of meat is beef rather than pork, although pork is eaten often. They buy less fatty, more expensive, smaller cuts of meat. Quality in these families refers to the choicest and most exclusive food, while in group I (A+B) it means something different, not rotten and good-looking. Vegetables (always fresh in group II as well) are more varied, exclusive and special; they are moreover eaten raw more often, mixed with herbs, fruits or other delicacies and eaten as a side dish. Potatoes are frequently prepared in different ways or replaced by pasta, rice, or grains. Desserts are more varied, too, and the preference for brown or whole-grain bread definitely dominates over white bread. White bread is consumed in its luxury forms, as baguettes or rolls. In conclusion, their preferences can be tentatively labelled as a "taste of distinction." The described differences in taste between the classes may contribute to the differences in body weight observed elsewhere, although it must be realised the data represent "verbal behaviour" only.

Food Regimens

All respondents, to repeat, try to present themselves as competent mothers. This includes methods of caring and training in matters of food as well, which is implied in Bourdieu's theory, but not elaborated on. Yet mothers in different classes follow different procedures. An important aspect of distinction is the degree of respect they have for the idiosyncratic preferences of their children and husbands. Likes and dislikes are traits one has to live with or which ought to be modelled. Working-class mothers appear to be more inclined to accept their children's and husband's tastes as given facts than middle-class mothers are. More than once they said, "we eat what we like so they have this right as well."

Yet there are boundaries to the freedom of the young; even in the more permissive working-class milieu stands the rule: children have to learn to eat everything. They must first taste a bit before they are allowed to dislike a certain food. The reasons for this are practical and "social" at the same time, allowing "don't like" means mothers will end up with several pots on the table instead of one. Moreover, refusals by children or husbands to eat are considered a bother to the orderly social event of the common meal in both social strata as well. As a "professional" mother expressed it: "In view of their future positions they have to get used to all possible dishes." At the same time this claim of mothers is more or less attenuated by making concessions to individual tastes in their families. "Finishing one's plate" seems an outdated rule for most children of our respondents, because parents think it is bad to urge food onto children. "Otherwise they are not allowed to leave the table" continues to be practised in some middle-class milieus only, but even here quantities are reduced when children don't feel like eating. Other adaptive techniques consist in spreading apple sauce over "the dishes they really dislike," changing the sequence, or offering alternatives.

The most problematic part of the meal for mothers and children is vegetables. Greens are seldom liked by the young without a thorough education by mothers considering them as indispensable foodstuffs in view of the vitamins therein (more of health arguments below). Meat is much less an obstacle: most children like it. The same is true for potatoes and for desserts. Children have to be taught to eat a proper meal and so mothers try, but with a different rigour according to class. This disciplinary task is also relevant where the likes of children are concerned. Here mothers do not deal with awful vegetables, but with delicious sweets, cookies, soft drinks and savoury snacks such as crunchy chips and french fries. All these delicacies present themselves to children's eyes conspicuously and abundantly. There is no need to inspire them; instead mothers need to set boundaries to their appetite. In this respect the influence of social class is obvious again, as we will see.

None of the mothers we met relaxes her rules for children in respect of eating sweet and savoury snacks, which they would generally prefer and tend to overeat.

The same is true for the extensive range of sweet sandwich-spreads available in the Netherlands. Working-class mothers' regimens in matters of "much, fat and sweet" are considerably more permissive than those of their middle-class counterparts. On the condition children eat something of their regular meals, "they can take what they like and how much they like," in some cases without asking permission first. But "finished is finished;" mothers buy cola drinks (the cheap varieties), sweets and other snacks only once a week. Respondents in group IA appear to be less restrictive than most of those in group IB, but in group I as a whole, regimens are much looser than in group II.

Middle class mothers (group II) submit their children to a lot more rules around sweets and snacks which are at the same time more complicated. Their basic attitude to the likes and dislikes of their children is educative; appetites must be adapted and moderated. In contrast to working-class mothers (group I), they conceive of tastes as qualities which are to be molded and modelled rather than to be met. A more strict approach to children's dislikes and a lot more claims of discipline as to their likes follow from this attitude. For their children this means fewer sweet sandwiches, soft drinks, sweets and snacks fewer times of the day or even of the week. In the afternoon when children come home from school, tea or juice is drunk instead of a cola drink (which is very much frowned upon) or one of the sweet dairy-based drinks. Quite a few mothers in group II are very critical of these inventions of the food industry: "too sweet, taste awful," while in families in group I they partly replace plain milk. The use of french-fried potatoes really discriminates between the classes: working-class mothers let children have their choice of this preferred snack (or meal) at least once a week, while most "professional" mothers say they offer this snack only once a fortnight or more.

At the same time a liberating deviation of these disciplines is enjoyed at special occasions. The weekends rather function as a safety valve in middle-class more than in working-class families. At these occasions, for instance, it is allowed to finish a complete box of chocolate grains (a spread for bread) for only one breakfast. An exclusive weekend connotation adheres to other treats and special delicacies as well, for instance pastry, desserts, drinks and snacks. It is remarkable that the range of such foods offered to children is smaller in working-class families, while the number of occasions is larger. In middle-class families the variety of sweets, treats and snacks is larger, but the number of occasions to enjoy them is kept smaller.

Reasons for Food-Choices: Tasty or Healthy

A recurrent theme in the interviews was the question: why? We discussed extensively the reasons mothers used to explain their choices in the field of food. All of them had definite rules and regimens in selecting, preparing and serving food, but what were their motives? In assessing their answers one must realise anew the element of social desirability which colours their answers. Besides, talking about one's reasons for behaviour always contains an aspect of legitimation *post facto*. Nevertheless we got a good impression of the differences in arguments used alongside the lines of social class.

The most conspicuous distinction between groups I and II is the overwhelming importance of the criteria "tasty" as a guide to food choices and regimens in the first-mentioned stratum. Working-class mothers, though, differ among themselves in combining "tasty" with other criteria, for instance "cheap," "easy to prepare" and "fit to spoil husband and children." All of these have to do with the specific social position of the mother in her family and of the family in society; we come back to this later. The other key motive in the discussions, "healthy," was not combined with "tasty"; it scored, besides, definitely second in rank, although reference to it was made frequently.[2] Middle-class mothers, in contrast, reverse the ranking order of "tasty" and "healthy," while admitting they account for both criteria.

BODY IMAGES AND BODY-MANAGEMENT

Body Images and Motivations

A most important topic of research concerns the feelings and attitudes of the body and body controls. The theme of "body discipline" (Turner, 1984) was introduced by asking respondents if they had ever had any problems with the weights of their children, their husbands or themselves. Questions of slimming and dieting are central in the lives of many modern western women. Mothers of primary school children are, in addition, constantly aware of the normal growth in length and weight of their children: for this process they are held responsible. Moreover they feel they are more or less in charge of their husband's weight, too. Therefore their views on body-shapes may be a revealing aspect of the aforementioned complex of attitudes and lifestyle concerning taste and eating. In this respect too, differences between the classes are the focus of our interest.

The pervading interest in, and trouble with body weight among our respondents is most striking. Only a few mothers said the subject did not interest them; most of the others admitted to having had a problem either with one of the family members or with their own bodies. Here too, interesting differences and similarities between the groups manifested themselves in the aspects we distinguished: body images or ideals of body shape, motivation (aesthetic, fear of social degradation, practical or health-related arguments) and body management (or body discipline); all of these differ from each other according to their reference to children, men and women.

About half of our working-class respondents said they have had feelings of anxiety about their children's weight, while only one professional mother said the same. Check ups with school physicians decreased these worries: their professional knowledge about body weights and growth patterns changed attitudes to semi-professional know-how communicated to us with astonishing ease by the mothers. The mothers of thin children preferred them to be fatter and vice-versa. Ideal body shapes of children for both classes exist somewhere between the extremes of fat and thin, but the motivations differ; mothers in group I mentioned reasons of aesthetics and derision, while those in group II touched on health reasons. Deviant body-weights of husbands are mentioned by one third of the mothers, about equally distributed over groups IA, IB and II. Most of these men are judged as being too fat, but there is a notable difference in the comments on this situation—working-class mothers say their husbands "are not hampered by their fatness at all," while their middle-class counterparts think they "do not feel fit" and explain their worries about this by pointing at possible health risks in the future. They feel very responsible for their husbands' bodies, which is not true for working-class mothers. Reasons of social derision in the case of fat men were not mentioned at all, while aesthetics plays a minor part: in this respect no differences between the classes exist.

Yet most of the troubles that respondents of both groups experienced with their own body weights, now or in the past, were that most of them preferred to be slimmer than they actually were, but for a few the reverse was true. Motives for the possession of slim bodies applying to women appeared to be more varied than those for men or children, "not being able to buy pretty clothes" (practical), "I'm so ashamed of myself" (social contempt), "I do not feel fit" (health) and "it is ugly" (aesthetic). The possession of a slim body is evidently a prescription for women which is independent of class. This is not true for men. In this respect differences between the sexes appear to be more important than those between the social strata. How deeply this ideal of feminine beauty is internalised can be illustrated by the next quote (group IA), "I am never ill, but it is just for your own self, isn't it? . . . yes and I don't need to do it for my man . . . he weighs 105 kilos himself so I don't have to slim for him." Another mother of the same group and in the same situation realised the existence of social pressure in these matters, "I am feeling fine but it is the opinion of others . . . other people think it is odd . . . they talk you into . . ." She prefers nevertheless to be much slimmer because she thinks appearances are important. A respondent (IB) said; "I am so ashamed of myself . . . unhealthy? People say so and perhaps it is true but the most important thing is it is ugly!"

Most respondents in both working-class categories explain their wish to slim with comparable motives. The most remarkable distinction from the comments in group II is the absence of references to health. The criterion of "feeling fine or not feeling fine" comes close, but it is of a short-term character. Fatness is not associated at all with possible health problems in the future. These are played down or even negated. The idea to prevent health problems is strange and requires a constraint from outside, "When your physician advises you to get your weight down you'll feel more urge to . . . if there is some compulsion. . . ."

The connection of fatness with health rather than with appearance and beauty in the first place for the group of middle-class mothers is a consistent trait, body weights have to be permanently watched, "I think it is important because I feel constrained to live healthier when slimming" and "I have to slim, not because of my physician's advice, but in my own opinion. For health reasons." Aesthetic motives are not absent of course, but they are always mixed up with health reasons, while arguments of shame are not mentioned.

Ideal body images do not differ very much among our respondents, at least for women and children. For men they do. Working-class mothers' opinions are much more easy or indifferent as to fat than are middle-class mothers' attitudes. Moreover, there is an obvious shift in motives and arguments for ideal slim-but-not-too-thin body shapes moving from working-class to middle-class groups; from beauty and shame to health. These body images may be a base for efforts at body

management and, more generally, be connected with food preferences (and regimes) or in Bourdieu's words (1986: 190):

> "Tastes in food also depend on the idea each class has of the body and of
> the effects food has on the body, that is, on its strength, health and
> beauty, and on the categories it uses to evaluate these effects, some of
> which may be important for one class and ignored by another, and
> which the different classes may rank in very different ways."

Efforts at Body Management

Measures taken by our respondents, if any, to achieve or maintain the
desired body weights of themselves and their families, were an important topic of discussion. While many mothers of thin children preferred them to be fatter, they accepted thinness, knowing they were
healthy. Only two of them actually tried to feed children extra bits
(pieces of sausage, hot porridge with cream) in spite of the opinion of
the school physician. As to fat husbands, respondents' reactions differed, working-class wives in our sample only felt like doing something about weight control in a few cases. They are generally easy on
their husbands and do not expect any incentives for their own efforts
to slim, either. Men seem to take some action by themselves only in the
case of pursuing sports such as football or body building. This last
type of discipline, centering around strength, involves a lot of dieting.
As several respondents explained to us, it is evidently a typical working-class ideal of the (male) body (Bourdieu, 1986: 210–211).

Middle class respondents, however, showed uneasiness about the
growing dimensions of their husband's belly. They are like Steffy, a
dentist's wife, who urges him to moderate his appetite ". . . but this is
very difficult. He eats what he likes and is fond of a good piece of
(sometimes fat) meat, baked eggs for lunch and even takes syrup and
sugar in his custard. Then I say, 'You should take yoghurt!'" But her
policy is a little ambivalent because she thinks it pitiful to him to for-
bid him what he likes. The word "pitiful" is used repeatedly by our
respondents in connection with the refusal of foods to husbands or
children for reasons of body weight.

Most efforts at controlling weights undertaken by our respondents,
however, concern their own bodies. The endeavours to slim appear
not to be dependent on social class, but successes in reaching that goal
are. Some women in group I such as Sonja, a bench-worker's wife,
said, "I keep slimming again and again, I reduce, but afterwards I im-

mediately gain weight." Others try a whole series of measures like Elly, married to a cleaner, who wants to get rid of her fat belly, ". . . keep-fit course, gymnastics, step-ups, dieting, eating regularly and having breakfast, abstaining from french fries . . . but not one kilogram is lost; (it) did not help at all." She has given up on her efforts completely, now denying the relationship between eating and fatness. Yet in this respect she is an exception; most respondents in group I know the causes perfectly, like Katja (IB), weighing 100 kg (220 lbs): "I've periods of gorging and then I can't leave anything in the cupboard . . . it is caused by eating too much, I am not a strong-natured person."

Gorging periods are mentioned by group II as well. Hortense is as obsessed with her repeated failure to control her appetite as is Katja, but there is one conspicuous difference, she does not appear fat at all! Nevertheless she says "I know that if I am not slimming I eat very poorly . . . treating my body very badly . . . very unhealthily . . . I simply cannot control myself. Extremely weak!" Her "wicked" behaviour consists of devouring complete packets of biscuits and liquorice and drinking bottles of cola. She appears to consider these acts as real sins against health. In this way she comes very near to Veronica (IB), a Jehova's Witness, who knows it is written in the Bible that gluttony is a sin.

Hortense's gorging obsession is an exception among our middle-class respondents. Willemijin, a scientist's wife, told an emotional story of an opposite problem which she recently overcame, her anorexia nervosa. While the majority of this group of mothers had problems controlling their body weight, they also confessed to knowing of the temptations and yielding, but in fact they all have their bodies under control, firstly for their health and lastly for beauty reasons. None of them is really fat either; their success in this respect forms a remarkable contrast to their working-class counterparts. Apparently they are propelled by internalised motives of health rather than by external appearances of social shame, which is more often the case in group I. This contrast fits Elias' (1982) notions on the differences in ways of control between the social strata, and is in accord with Bourdieu's contention "that the body is the most indisputable materialisation of class taste" (1986: 190).

THE DIFFERENCES WEIGHED: SOME CONCLUDING REMARKS

Although we did not gather data on fatness itself we think the material on food regimens and body controls presented here may be relevant for an interpretation of the social distribution of this phenomenon. It is striking that, even in our small sample, we only met fat-looking mothers in the working-class group while they were lacking in the other. The consistent differences in the complex of attitudes concerning eating and body weight we found to exist between both groups, representing "high" and "low" in social stratification, are evidently the more important results of this study. Taste, regimens and choices as to food on one side and body images and controls on the other are all part of a whole lifestyle comprising other attitudes (concerning health, for instance) and behaviour as well. Distinctions in lifestyle are largest between the working and the middle-class groups in our sample, yet even minor differentiations presented themselves within both groups of working-class mothers.

Several interrelated interpretations can be tentatively proposed for a resultant chain of distinctions between "high" and "low." To begin with the mothers themselves, most of them are full-time housewives and in the small social unit of the family they are dependent on husband and children for the approval of their work. An important part of their working existence consists of dealing with food and cooking. This is a rather traditional but no less a real situation. It is understandable that they like to please and not to obstruct the palates of members of their family. Food is one way of spoiling them a little because of its social functions of conviviality and delight. Mothers in comparable social positions will be subdued by the same social pressures, independently of class.

Class positions interfere in these pressures in the following way: Working-class mothers have less chances and possibilities to resist these pressures because of the more deprived situation in which they have to live. Bourdieu's concept of "habitus" (1986: 171) affords a clear view of the way in which these "life situations," conventionally named socioeconomic circumstances, influence "lifestyles." Habitus refers to the social backgrounds by which people act, perceive and appreciate aspects of material and immaterial culture, in this case food and body shapes. At the same time habitus influences their evaluation and classification of other peoples' practises and values. Both of these functions of habitus result in a hierarchy of tastes or lifestyles enacted by people belonging to a related stratification of class positions. In other words, mothers with a low level of education, a low occupational status (for their husbands and for themselves) and a low income are not "fit" to appreciate the importance of a distinguishing "healthy taste." Their position in and outside of the family is a very dependent one and they yield to the pressure of the appetites of husband and children and last of all themselves. This contributes to the often-observed hedonistic character of the lower-class culture.

Yet yielding to internal or external pressures concerning appetite is not a static phenomenon. The above-mentioned differences in regimens between mothers represent different social strata and are an aspect of the educational practises which are generally characteristic of their lifestyles. These differences in disciplining children are a consequence of the relative positions of dependency and interdependence of society at large. The stress on strictness and discipline is a typical middle-class trait which has a long history. It belongs to the "process of civilisation" in which, according to Elias (1982), mechanisms of controlling behaviour have changed and developed over centuries. This general evolution from a more external form of control by others into a more internalised form of self-control takes place at unequal pace for the different social strata. The "civilising of appetite" (Mennell, 1985: 20–40) is an aspect of this process. It refers to the growth of a more strict and stable form of disciplining of impulses for food and eating, and to an exchange of quality for quantity.

The emphasis on quality and refinement, be it gastronomic or for health, is only possible in life situations which permit a certain distance from necessity. Our society has only recently changed to a land of riches where tidbits and delicacies are available to everyone. Working-class families have only recently participated in affluence; this is a time to enjoy food and not to postpone the gratification of appetite in view of future health. It can be assumed their time to learn discipline and self-control has not yet been long enough, but eventually it will come. In this process social constraints will play an important part.

Fat food was liked in the past by Dutch society because of its taste and its nutritious qualities. Looking fat was also valued positively. Nowadays, however, fat food is feared because of its fattening qualities (not in the first place for taste, although *visible* fat is negatively valued). The fear of becoming fat has to do with reasons of health, beauty and social competition: a slim body is a source of high status.

NOTES

Annecke van Otterloo lectures in the Department of Sociology at the University of Amsterdam. She has done research on religion, life styles and eating habits. Her recent book is entitled: *Eating and Appetite in the Netherlands 1840–1990. A historical and sociological study.* Bert Bakker, Amsterdam, 1990.

1. The research was done by Anneke van Otterloo and Juul van Ogtrop, Department of Sociology and History, University of Amsterdam.
2. Conversations with mothers belonging in group IA about health and illness as a guideline in food choices produced comments such as "Why consider that? We all die in the end!" Such comments resemble an attitude of fatalism, found in a group of labouring-class British women (Pill, 1983), expressing a view of illness as something external and out of control.

REFERENCES

Baecke, J.A.M., J. Burema, J.E.R. Frijters, J.G.A.J. Hautvast and W.A.M. van der Wiel-Wetzels 1983. Obesity in young Dutch adults: I Socio-demographic variables and body mass index. *International Journal of Obesity* 7, 1–12.

Baecke, J.A.M., J. Burema, J.E.R. Frijters, J.G.A.J. Hautvast and W.A.M. van der Wiel-Wetzels 1983. Obesity in young Dutch adults: II Daily life style and body mass. *International Journal of Obesity* 7, 13–24.

Bourdieu, P. (1986). The habitus and the space of lifestyles. In *Distinction, A social critique of the judgement of taste*. Routledge and Kegan Paul, London/New York. pp. 169–226.

de Boer, J.O., and P. Deurenberg 1987. *Voeding en overgewicht*. Samson Stafleu, Alphen, Rijn, Brussels.

Elias, N. 1978. The history of manners. In *The Civilising Process. Sociogenetic and Psychogenetic Investigations*, Vol. 1. Basil Blackwell, Oxford.

Elias, N. 1982. State formation and civilisation. In *The Civilising Process*, Vol. 2. Basil Blackwell, Oxford.

Goffman, E. 1959. *The Presentation of Self in Everyday Life*. Doubleday Anchor, New York.

Goudsblom, J. 1986. On high and low in society and in sociology. A semantic approach to social stratification. *Sociologisch Tijdschrift* 13, (No. 1) 3–18.

Mennell, S. 1985. The civilising of appetite. In *All Manners of Food. Eating and taste in England and France from the Middle Ages to the present*. Basil Blackwell, Oxford. pp. 20–39.

Mulder, G. J. 1847. *De voeding in Nederland in verband tot den Volksgeest*. H.A. Kramer, Rotterdam.

Pill, R. 1983. An apple a day ... some reflections on working class mothers views on food and health. In Anne Murcott, (ed.), *The Sociology of Food and Eating. Essays on the sociological significance of food*. Gower House Groft, Aldershot England. pp. 117–128.

Turner, B.S. 1984. The disciplines. In *The Body and Society. Explorations in social theory*. Basil Blackwell, Oxford. pp. 157–176.

7

Vegetarianism and Fatness: An Undervalued Perception of the Body

LAURENCE OSSIPOW

INTRODUCTION: FATNESS AS SEEN BY VEGETARIANS

Vegetarians rarely show any excess weight. In today's western societies they are considered, and consider themselves as slim. Through the study of 116 articles published in the medical literature between 1980–1987, it appears that anthropometric figures are usually lower for vegetarians (and especially for their children) when compared to official norms (*see*, for example Van Staveren *et al.*, 1985; Fulton, Hutton and Stitt, 1980). Dwyer *et al.* (1980a,b), who carried out extensive research on vegetarians in the U.S., state that the growth curves obtained for vegetarian (school) children were from 0.5 to 1.0 kg and 1 to 2 cm smaller, depending on age, sex and diet, than were curves for a reference population of nonvegetarian children. In general, height is affected more than weight. Calculated curves for children fed macrobiotic diets are inferior to those obtained for other vegetarians. Measurements of females are more consistently affected than males and their diets reflect higher animal food avoidance. Finally, the caloric supply seems to be lower than commonly recommended norms, although the quantity of proteins appears to be sufficient. With different measurements from those relating weight to length (subscapular skinfolds, arm-muscle circumference) the same researchers point out in another study (Dwyer *et al.*, 1980b) that, while only a few of these children are overweight, quite a few are lean.

For Levin, Rattan and Gilat, (1986), the average weight of the Israeli vegetarians examined was significantly lower than that of the omnivores (60.8 kg versus 69.1 kg), even though the vegetarian diet supplied a significantly higher amount of calories than the non-vegetarian diet (3,030.5 versus 2,626.8 kcal/day).

Recent studies such as NIN (Canadian National Institute of Nutrition), 1990, recall that quantity, and also quality, of fat eaten affects weight. Thorogood *et al.* (1990) demonstrate for example, that health-conscious individuals have a low intake of saturated fat. Many researchers now consider that vegetarian food is close to new dietetic norms, even closer than omnivorous food.

Except for recent studies, the above-mentioned research should be considered cautiously for several reasons. First, although research has been carried out with a different attitude than that prevalent in the 1970s (which was often negative towards vegetarians), some of these studies are still tinged with a certain reserve towards the subject. This is due to prejudice rather than to "scientific distance," as revealed by the terms used by some researchers when referring to their informants and their diets. The latter is, for example, described as being a hobby, a fancy, or faddism. Second, from a methodological point of view, we can deplore the fact that this research is undertaken with rather small numbers of cases, of whom we rarely know the exact diet, or how long the adherents have been following it. For example, certain nutritionists mention vegetarianism when studying a diet partially made up of meat products (regular consumption of poultry and fish). In other respects, a good number of investigations deal with vegetarianism in general, starting with observations of various groups of Indians who migrated to Great Britain or to the U.S., and whose diet differs from western vegetarian practices. Moreover, research is rarely based on simultaneous analysis of food consumed and the beneficial or negative effects it can cause, as revealed by blood sample analyses. Nutrients supplied by the diets are frequently calculated from tables of food composition that are not suitable for vegetarians.[1] Finally, and what is most striking, the majority of the consulted studies takes the interaction of physical, sociological and psychological factors into little account.

In Geneva, 47.2% (from a sample of 22 women and 14 men) of persons examined by Paoliello (1987) approach an ideal weight (the theoretical optimal weight worked out according to the Lorentz formula). Forty-four and four–tenths percent are below these values, with an ideal weight below 20% of the ideal, and 5.6% exceed the desirable norm (23.1% above the ideal weight). A survey that I conducted in Geneva to complement the ethnological facts collected previously showed that the majority of vegetarians—for all types of diets usually followed for more than ten years—are close to standard ideal weight (see Table I). Five men (25% of the males) and eleven women (65% of the female population) are slightly below the theoretical ideal weight. Three men exceeded the norm. Children and teenagers (most of them brought up as vegetarian from birth) are often below ideal weight according to medical standards. We should keep in mind that only a small number of children and teenagers were examined (see Table II) without knowing the overall curve of their growth. These remarks are of concern for the girls especially.

The absence of stoutly built vegetarians is usually explained by referring to weight that is either identical to or inferior to that of the norms. Researchers have pointed to factors such as:

- deficiencies in intake of different nutrient elements (such as vitamin D) which could disturb weight and especially growth;

- a medium or lower caloric intake, although some researchers (as seen previously) notice a supply that is higher than that of omnivores;

- a lower consumption of saturated fats and alcohol;

- a diet with a richer fibre content, which could be either a cause of bad absorption (see remarks made by Levin, Ratten and Gilat, 1986), or a quick way to satiety (according to some dietitians);

- some nutritionists such as Freeland-Graves et al. (1986), collaborate with psychologists, looking for another type of explanation for the lower caloric intake of vegetarians. According to them, vegetarians control their weight because they have a great dietetic awareness.

TABLE I. Height and weight of 36 adults on vegetarian diets, Geneva

Sex[a]	Age (years)	Height (cm)	A Weight (kg)	B Ideal body weight[b] (kg)	Difference between A/B (kg)
1	22	176	65	69.5	−4.5
1	31	176	73	69.5	3.5
1	32	173	55	67.25	−12.25
1	34	172	68	66.5	1.5
1	34	173	65	67.25	−2.25
1	38	182	61	74	−13
1	39	158	67	56	11
1	41	160	63	57.5	5.5
1	42	175	68	68.75	−0.75
1	42	174	68	68	0
1	44	170	68	65	3
1	45	167	70	62.75	7.25
1	46	170	60	65	−5
1	50	176	65	69.5	−4.5
1	51	175	62	68.75	−6.75
1	52	182	63	74	−11
1	59	166	81	62	19
1	63	170	55	65	−10
1	68	182	76	74	2
2	20	160	44	56	−12
2	29	153	43	51.9	−8.8
2	29	169	52	61.4	−9.4
2	30	165	60	59	1
2	39	166	58	59.6	−1.6
2	39	165	48	59	−11
2	39	150	40	50	−10
2	41	160	49	56	−7
2	41	160	47	56	−9
2	44	163	52	57.8	−5.8
2	45	168	53	60.8	−7.8
2	46	168	57	60.8	−3.8
2	47	168	55	60.8	−5.8
2	49	165	46	59	−13
2	50	163	55	57.8	−2.8
2	51	161	55	56.6	−1.6
2	62	172	54	63.2	−9.2

[a]Key: 1 = male; 2 = female
[b]Lorentz' formula:
   Height(cm) − 100 − { [Height(cm) −150] / [4 for males, 2.5 for females]}

TABLE II. Height and weight of 17 children on vegetarian diets, Geneva

Sex[a]	Age (years)	Height (cm)	Ideal height (kg)	A Body weight (kg)	B Ideal body weight[b] (kg)	Difference between A/B (kg)
3	3.5	98	98	15	15	0
3	4	100	101	18	16	2
3	5	105	108	18	18	0
3	7	120	120	21	22	-1
3	8	125	125	22	24.5	-2.5
3	9	128	130	24	27.2	-2.3
3	10	131	136	28	30	-2
3	11	144	140	28	33	-5
3	17	172	171	60	61	-1
3	18	150	171	49	62	-13
3	18	185	172	69	62	7
4	3	93	93	13	13.8	-0.8
4	5	105	107	15.5	17.2	-1.7
4	7	120	118	24	21.2	2.8
4	10	135	135	30	30	0
4	11	142	140	34	33	1
4	15	160	159	44	53	9

[a]Key: 3 = boys; 4 = girls
[b]Ideal body height/weight compared with curves for reference population of nonvegetarian children (Sempe/Pedron, Paris, 1970).

VEGETARIAN DIETETICS

As an ethnologist, I will try to explore the question of weight in a wider context. I will also examine what slimmers (persons attempting to lose weight) and weight are associated with, and why stoutness is considered badly by the vegetarian informants I met. As with fieldwork carried out in a foreign culture, this ethnological approach to vegetarianism includes both immersion in and distance from the group under study, and their ideas about their own culture. It aspires to render the symbolic representation attached to food and to examine differences between belief and daily habits. However, it does not pretend to discuss positive and negative nutritional aspects from a dietetic and medical point of view. This analysis is based on representations drawn from more than fifty semi-directed interviews with vegetarians, living in Geneva and other French-speaking parts of Switzerland. Since 1983, I have also observed various activities: cooking classes, training courses, lectures, meetings and general assemblies of vegetarian or macrobiotic societies. Other sources of information were correspondence and informal contacts with the network of informants.

Ovolactovegetarianism, as defined by the interviewees and their literature, is a diet excluding all meat elements coming from dead animals, such as fat, stock and gravy, but it allows products from a living animal, such as eggs, milk, and honey. The main part of the diet is based on different cereals, and on leguminous plants, fruits and vegetables (about one-third cereals and leguminous plants to two-thirds fruits and vegetables). A great majority of vegetarians consume only a very small quantity of eggs and milk, which are generally ingredients rather than food in themselves. These vegetarians also prefer light "natural" cheese. *Vegans* never use animal products. *Raw food eaters* are usually vegans, eating raw products originating from plants. Nevertheless, there are some raw food eaters who also consume some raw meat products. They follow *instinctotherapy* developed in Switzerland and later in France. Their history will not be touched on in this article. A macrobiotic diet is a diet of Japanese origin, with elements borrowed from Chinese philosophy.[2] At present, except for macrobiotic informants, who cook two thirds of their food, vegetarians place great importance on raw food.

From "Light" to Cosmic Food

For vegetarians,[3] food not only represents a material element to be ingested to make the body function but it also serves to establish a physical and spiritual bond with Nature, and in a wider sense with the Cosmos (Dubisch, 1985). For some, these "places" are inhabited by a divine force, and for others by an energy spiritually superior to that of the human being. Most highly valued are elements which bind them to this idealised "nature," which they visualise as little domesticated: in this value system fruits, then wild or cultivated vegetables precede cereals, produced by agriculture (though from a quantitative point of view cereals come first in order of preference). Raw food eaters who are deeply in favour of a "natural nature," wish they could eat only "wild" plants or fruits.

Similarly, vegetarians classify their food either as "dead" or as "living" according to how far from or close to Nature they are perceived. Some foods are condemned as being unhealthy when "polluted" by pesticides, fertilisers and additives, or when grown under glass, out of the ground, on soil substitutes (rock fibres or peat) containing nutrients. Above all they are considered as denatured, deprived of the "vibrations" that would allow them to communicate with Nature. Products to be consumed should be seasonal as well.

According to these informants, meat—steak for example—is a typical example of a dead foodstuff, being necessarily produced by slaughter, and, at least in their opinion, it is frequently denatured either by hormones or other substances injected during fattening, by preservatives or by a lengthy period in cold storage. Meat is also discredited because, according to vegetarians, it would be preferable to consume vegetables or seeds directly rather than through the ingestion of an animal (see Figure 1). An exaggerated consumption of this type of "concentrated" food, typical of the so-called carnivores, leads away from Nature. Although often practised by vegetarians, cooking is another "denaturing" factor. As an example, they mention that vitamins are destroyed during cooking.

Vegetarians qualify their food as "light," being taken in small quantities, having a low lipid content, being a living foodstuff and often eaten raw. In this sense they compare it to "rich," "fat," "heavy," and "dead" food used by "carnivores" (omnivores as a matter of fact): "steak and fries" are a good example of such food. Vegetarian food is considered "light" because it is characterised by a fluid and rapid intestinal transit. As explained by numerous informants, a chymus stagnant in the intestines causes putrefaction and produces toxins. Therefore, they try to ease digestion from the very start, at the stage of ingestion, by chewing their food thoroughly.

One must have a clean body in order to be correctly connected with the natural world (Nature and Cosmos), with other people and with oneself. Thus the body should be quickly freed from any loss of energy from digestion. An informant explained: "When I used to eat lots of cheese, sausages and beer, my sensitivity to others was different. . . . Theoretically, a clean body allows another type of life in terms of contacts with others, and a better self-knowledge." Another stated that "a lighter diet brings a clear mind." Though all traces of food should disappear quickly from the body, some nutritious elements can be absorbed without any difficulty, vitamins for example.

There is a "double" perception of bodily functions which includes on the one hand, a *maximum elimination* (using purges such as enemas and fasts) and on the other *economy and conservation* (autoreabsorption of certain nutrients) which is a cyclic paradigm.

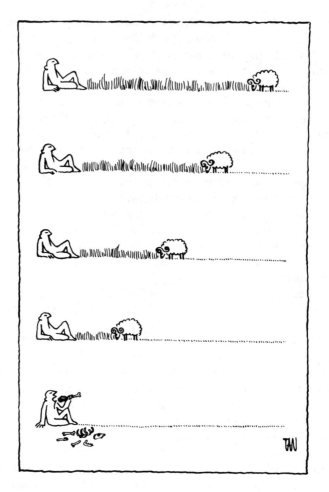

Figure 1. Carnivore: A consumer at the second degree?

Although not practised by all, one of the cures, which is fashionable at present in the vegetarian milieu, is urinotherapy (drinking one's own urine). This therapy is principally attributed to Ayurvedic medicine, which is of Indian origin. Its aim is auto-immunisation against certain illnesses, by the "re-injection" of eventual toxins in order to resist illness that could develop. It is also intended to recover certain vitamins or salts that would otherwise be eliminated. Drinking urine allows one to learn and appreciate everything that is produced by the

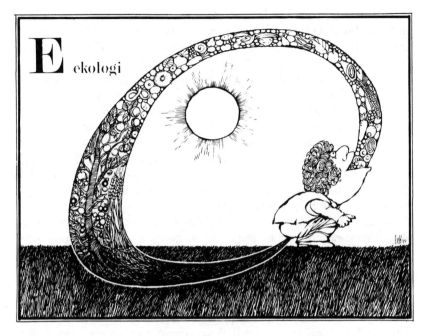

Figure 2. Food, Body and Cosmos: A perpetual cycle.

body. A doctor informant writes that, by tasting one's urine, the curist, "becomes more careful of his/her own way of eating. He/she feels more responsible for the state of his/her body, and becomes aware that he/she by ignorance and unawareness, created the troubles he/she is suffering from."

Another circle exists, which includes factors outside of the body. By returning human excrements to the "nourishing earth," natural compost will be produced with the help of water, air and sun, which will become a soil for growing food later eaten by vegetarians (*see* Figure 2).

Rarely do vegetarian women suffer permanently or occasionally from dysmenorrhea or amenorrhea. Nutritionists associate these states with a low calorie, low fat diet. Although some female informants perceive these disorders as pathological, others consider menstruation as useless for the proper functioning of the body. These women feel lighter and physically less affected by a phenomenon they cannot control. A male informant pointed out that amenorrhea prevents wasting a precious source of blood and iron.

The maximum absorption for a minor waste turns out to be symbolised in "breathernism," of which many raw food eaters dream. They imagine human beings who would function with perfect economy, living on water, then exclusively on air and solar light. In principle, this cosmic food has no toxins, as the Cosmos can only be perfect, and would require no elimination. The body would communicate directly with natural and/or divine forces. To illustrate their theory, raw food eaters mention numerous fasters about whom they have read in vegetarian or religiously oriented journals.

This concern for economy and profit can also be applied to a field that is more down to earth. According to these informants, it would be possible to feed the entire planet with cereals and sprouting seeds more efficiently than with meat (*see* Figure 3).

As far as sexuality is concerned, moderation seems to be the ideal. Sexuality is not forbidden, but it should be experienced as a relationship that favours emotional life as much as spiritual and physical exchange. Some (males) consider it preferable not to ejaculate as this is equivalent to a loss of energy.

Others feel that sport is a waste of energy, and it is to those who commit excesses and have to compensate. Sport seems particularly related to "carnivorism." Nevertheless, young vegetarians do go in for certain sports such as sailing, skiing (especially cross-country), walking and swimming, since these activities exemplify "controlled energy," suppleness, contact with Nature, and here again these activities seem to offer a feeling of lightness and fluidity (on this subject, *see also* Pociello, 1981). Sports or other activities should develop spiritual as much as physical qualities, of which yoga or meditation are often cited by informants.

Vegetarians speak of a body which "forms a whole with the soul." Yet they live it as divided into two parts. One part, the top (heart, soul, spirit, aura) which is the centre of the Immaterial, reflects the celestial Cosmos. But what appears to be too mental or intellectual is rejected for what is seen as sensitive and emotional. The bottom part, (intestines, stomach, sexual organs) is more likely to be tarnished, yet deserves attention, as it links us to the terrestrial part of the Cosmos.

"Relax," "listen to your body," "let yourself go," say vegetarians. This advice, very close to the paradoxical orders described by Bateson *et al.* (1981), does not reflect the entire reality of vegetarian behaviour. Indeed, everything seems to lead towards a permanent control of the body. Informants follow food and health rules to cure an illness, to be

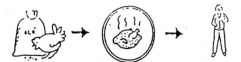

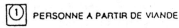

With the quantity
of cereals needed
to feed 1 person
with meat

AVEC LA QUANTITÉ DE CÉRÉALES OU'IL FAUT POUR NOURRIR

PERSONNE A PARTIR DE VIANDE

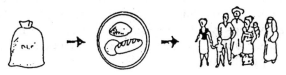

we can feed
7 persons with
bread

ON PEUT NOURRIR

PERSONNES A PARTIR DE PAIN

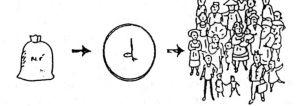

and more than
20 persons with
sprouting seeds

ET PLUS DE

PERSONNES A PARTIR DE GRAINES GERMÉES

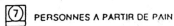

Figure 3. Benefits of eating naturally—meat versus grains. From Dr. Soliel (1985). *Graines germées et jeunes pousses* (Germinated grains and young sprouts). Edition Soliel, Imene-Bourg, (Geneva), Switzerland.

in good health, and not to grow unhealthy, but also to control their body and themselves. The body is the base on which every change is inscribed daily and in a concrete way. It is a "Being" to be fed from the Inside, by spiritual exercises or personal experiences, as well as from the Outside by a precise choice of food.

In order to understand vegetarians better, the body and food need to be representative of the world socially. According to the sociologist Pierre Bourdieu (1979), this care for the body, this ease in speaking about it and the acceptance of deferred pleasure (progress in food habits and spiritual attainment, for example) seem to be characteristic of the so-called upper and middle classes. Vegetarians do modify their way of life and their relationship to their group of origin in a relatively wide sense. They are usually recruited from non-manual workers, executives, managers and liberal professions. Many are teachers, professors and artists, or are working in medical or paramedical circles. For reasons which are too long to explain here (such as different value systems, for example), a worker or a member of the "lower" class is unlikely to become a vegetarian or share this style of life and way of thinking.

WEIGHT: AN INNER STATE OF MIND

The representations that vegetarians elaborate about the body and the world do not deal much with the question of body weight. Weight does not matter much, either as a mass or as a measurement. As seen previously and as underlined by Schwartz (1986) in several chapters about cures and diets fashionable at the end of the nineteenth century, it is the feeling of lightness that prevails. This feeling is above all an inner state of mind. But it can also be transmitted by the overall appearance that vegetarians reveal or try to reveal by a supple walk, calmness, simplicity and the comfort of their clothes, in natural fibres.

Self-assessment in terms of weight or stoutness is salient only when vegetarians are confronted by omnivores whom they try to convince of the value of their way of life. This also became an issue when I specifically questioned them about losing, gaining, or keeping their weight. Weight loss and stability are attributed to a "light" diet, with a high fibre content, composed mainly of fruits and vegetables, which are often eaten raw and with little preparation. Vegetarians insist on the well-balanced aspect of their diet explained by the particular way they combine foods, notably for proteins. The absence of nibbling (eating at moments other than those explicitly reserved for meals) and the distaste for sweets are often proudly noted. But, actually, regular observation reveals that they often nibble in between meals (fruits, nuts and biscuits) and that they consume desserts with pleasure. Those who considered themselves too skinny said they gained weight when they stopped eating stimulating foods, such as coffee and meat. Only in this case is a gain of weight acceptable. Vegetarians also associate a gain or excess of weight with the nonrespect of food and health rules. Thus, those who put on weight are guilty, as they endanger their own health.

"Pure Vegetarians" Versus "Plump Carnivores": A Question of Toxins

Fat people are usually "carnivores" less responsible than others. Vegetarians are not disgusted by omnivores who are fat because they look fat, but because, according to the informants, they present a dirty body that is heavily "poisoned" by meat and denatured products. One of the rare fat vegetarians I know spent his time relating his periodic fasts. His past as a "carnivorous" restaurant owner weighed on his conscience. He is allowed to be fat but has to explain that he is pure and cleared of his ex-greed. A Buddha or a guru can be plump without being suspected of impurity.

Following Mauss (1923) and Fischler's demonstration concerning "la symbolique du gros" (1987), we could also qualify this type of fat person as "good." In our system of values, they symbolically compensate their accumulation of food by returning something else to the vegetarian network. The fat vegetarian is devoted to investing money, energy and time in a vegetarian association, while the guru offers his knowledge. Conversely, vegetarians are particularly revolted by the "fat carnivore" who gets fat at the Third World's expense (see also Fischler, 1987: 267–270). The "fat carnivore" returns nothing, does not eliminate, and due to obesity, he/she is often ill and incurs more expenses, for example, medical, than he/she contributes.

Thus a light body is imagined as clean and preferably thin, for aesthetic reasons but not at all costs. In any case, vegetarians refuse to submit to the models of slimness frequently seen in the media at the moment.

Notions of slimness and obesity are connected to certain beliefs of the world,[4] which helps others to perceive who are vegetarians and those who are carnivores. This can be deduced from certain social behaviours which are appropriate for the particular diet and views about the body.

Because some practitioners of macrobiotics smoke, drink beer and sometimes eat fish, they are suspected by vegetarians (ovolactovegetarians, vegans and raw food eaters) of excess. They also feel that

TABLE III. Some concepts associated with slimness and fatness, as seen by Swiss vegetarians

	Slim	Fat
Food and body qualities	vegetarianism light fluid pure clean lively raw supple smoothness mild sweet, unrefined	carnivorism heavy, rich, greasy crystallised polluted dirty dead cooked stiff strength strong spicy, prepared
Food qualities and representations of nature	natural whole unrefined wild "natural" Nature vegetable and animal undomesticated animal "good instincts" Cosmos	denatured processed refined cultivated domesticated Nature animal domesticated animal world, massive breeding "low instincts" industrial world
Registers	elimination/ conservation	monopolising/ wasting

these macrobiotic informants lack vitality. Vegetarians assume this lack to be due to overcooked food. Adherents of a macrobiotic diet are not considered fat but as less "light" because they are less "lively." They are classified as being closer to carnivores.

Raw food eaters and vegans direct more or less the same reproaches to ovolactovegetarians, for their excess intake of dairy products and cooked food.

Macrobiotics adherents accuse vegetarians of being too skinny and ethereal, due to an alleged excessive consumption of vegetables and raw food. They consider an excess of *yin* as negative and connected with illness and, in particular, with cancer.

Omnivores, however, qualify vegetarians as "skinny," "peaked," "gloomy," and "droopy," and they associate this diet with a lack of strength and a passive nature. Nevertheless this image has begun to change. Ovolactovegetarianism, or a moderate vegetarianism is, rightly or wrongly, becoming seen as a "healthy" diet, which prevents various diseases, notably cardiovascular. These diets are associated with the contemporary wish for slimness.

Vegetarians are both delighted and disappointed with this growing popularity, while the sceptics consider this to be a chance for a "denatured recuperation." According to them, and as I have tried to present it, health, slimness and lower weight are not sufficient for improving the human being. For there is no possible lightness without Cosmic harmony and spiritual effort!

NOTES

Laurence Ossipov is an assistant (*Cheffe de travaux*) at l'Institut d'ethnologie of the University of Neuchatel in Switzerland. His doctoral research is on vegetarian and macrobiotic networks in the French-speaking part of Switzerland as well as among migrating peoples.

1. Except for Truesdell, Whitney and Acosta (1984).
2. Like *yin* and *yang*, two complementary principles or energies. For an approach to the history of raw food eaters and macrobiotic adherents, *see* Ossipow, 1989a. For a more thorough discussion of various types of food and the structure of observed meals *see* Ossipow, 1985; 1989b.
3. The following remarks apply to vegetarians as a whole. As revealed by various surveys, the representations described are principally of feminine origin, as women compose about two thirds of the adult vegetarian population. The questionnaire concerning weight is an exception.
4. See Table III. For a different but complementary outline refer to Dubisch, 1985.

REFERENCES

Bateson, G., R. Birdwhistell, E. Goffman, E.T. Hall, D. Jackson, A. Scheflen, S. Sigman and P. Watzlawick 1981. *La nouvelle communication.* Seuil (ed.). Paris. Texte recueillis et presentes par Y. Winkin; traduction de D. Bansard, A. Cardoen, M.C. Chiarieri, J.P. Simon et Y. Winkin.

Bourdieu, P. 1979. *La distinction. Critique sociale du jugement.* Minuit (ed.). Paris.

Dubisch, J. 1985. You are what you eat: Religious aspects of the health food movement. In A.C. Lehmann and J.E. Myers (eds.), *Magic, Witchcraft,* and Religion: An anthropological study of the supernatural. Mayfield, London; Palo Alto. pp. 69–77.

Dwyer, J.T., E.M. Andrew, I. Valadian, and R.B. Reed 1980a. Size, obesity and leanness in vegetarian preschool children. Journal of the American Dietetic Association 77(4), 434–439.

Dwyer, J.T., E.M. Andrew, C. Berkley, I. Valadian, and R.B. Reed 1980b. Growth in "new" vegetarian preschool children using the Jenss-Bayley curve-fitting technique. American Journal of Clinical Nutrition 37(5) 815–827.

Fischler, C. 1987. La symbolique du gros. Communications 46, 255–278.

Freeland-Graves, J.H., S.A. Greninger, G.R. Graves and R.K. Young 1986. Health practices, attitudes and beliefs of vegetarians and nonvegetarians. Journal of the American Dietetic Association 86(7), 913–918.

Fulton, J.R., C.W. Hutton and K.R. Stitt 1980. Preschool vegetarians: Dietary and anthropometric data. Journal of the American Dietetic Association 76(4), 360–365.

Lewin, A., J. Rattan and T. Gilat 1986. Energy intake and body weight in ovo-lacto vegetarians. Journal of Clinical Gastroenterology 8(4), 451–453.

Mauss, M. 1980 (1923). Essai sur le don—Forme et raison de l'échange dans les sociétés archaïques. In Sociologie et Anthropologie. PUF: Paris. pp. 144–273

National Institute of Nutrition (NIN) 1990. Risks and benefits of vegetarian diets. NIN Review 12, (supplement to report NIN 5(1), January 1990, Ottawa, Canada.

Ossipow, L. 1985. La cuisine du corps et de l'âme: l'apprentissage du végétarisme. In P. Centilivres et J.L. Christinat (eds.), Recherches et travaux de L'institut d'ethnologie 6, Institut d'ethnologie Neuchatel, 203–211.

Ossipow, L. 1989a. Le buffet crudivore: approche ethnologique de l'instincto-thérapie et de l'alimentation dite vivante. In Du sauvage, du vivant et du cru. Université de Bourgogne Editions universitaires de Dijon. Cahiers du stage, "Ethnologie de l'alimentation," organisé à Dijon par la direction régionale des affaires culturelles de Bourgogne 17–19, Novembre 1988.

Ossipow, L. 1989b. Le végétarisme: Vers un autre art de vivre? cerf/Fides, Paris. 125 pp. (Bref).

Paoliello, C. 1987. Etude sur les végétariens de Geneve et alentours. Ecole de diététique, Geneve (Travail de diplôme).

Pociello, C. 1981. La force, l'énergie, le grâce et les réflexes: le jeu complexe des dispositions culturelles et sportives. In Sports et société: Approche socio-culturelle des pratiques. Vigot, Paris. pp. 171–237.

Schwartz, H. 1986. Never Satisfied—A cultural history of diets, fantasies and fat. The Free Press, New York.

Thorogood, M., L. Roe, K. McPherson and J. Mann 1990. Dietary intake and plasma levels: Lessons from a study of the diet of health conscious groups. British Medical Journal 300, 1297–1301.

Truesdell, D.D., E.N. Whitney and P.B. Acosta 1984. Nutrients in vegetarian foods. *Journal of the American Dietetic Association* 84(1), 28–35.

Van Staveren, W.A., J.H. Dhuyvetter, A. Bons, M. Zeelen and J.G. Hautvast 1985. Food consumption and height/weight status of Dutch preschool children on alternative diets. *Journal of the American Dietetic Association* 85(12), 1579–1584.

II

PHYSICAL AND SOCIAL ASPECTS

8

Potential Advantages and Disadvantages of Human Obesity

NEVIN S. SCRIMSHAW and WILLIAM H. DIETZ

"Leave gormandizing: know the grave doth gape
For Thee thrice wider than for other men"
Shakespeare, Henry VIII.

INTRODUCTION

In any consideration of the relationship between diet and disease, it is appropriate to examine first the dietary conditions during the paleolithic period to which humans are genetically adapted. There has been no time for significant further genetic adaptation, either to the development of agriculture some 10,000 years ago or to the radical dietary changes of the past one-hundred years in industrialized societies. Judging by information on the diets of contemporary African Bushmen and Australian Aborigines who, until recently at least, were still living as hunters and gatherers, the paleolithic diet was one of great variety and relatively high in animal protein (Eaton, Shostak and Konner, 1988). The diets of contemporary aborigines in both tropical and subtropical regions are remarkably constant in amounts (Lee, 1968), but they must forage for food over a wider area, and expend

147

more energy to do so in unfavourable times. They also take advantage of less palatable foods.

Any animal eating periodic meals, including man, takes in food in excess of immediate physiological needs with every meal, and daily dietary energy intake seldom coincides exactly with daily energy expenditure. Despite daily and weekly fluctuations in energy balance, most individuals with ready access to food maintain a remarkably constant weight from week to week. However, in industrialized countries average weight for height gradually increases until age 60 and then declines. In these populations a substantial minority becomes overweight or obese.

Obesity in industrialized populations has no practical advantage and has some serious, adverse health consequences to be discussed later. The significance of simple overweight in such a population is more controversial, perhaps because differences in body composition confound the interpretation of the relationship with disease. For most developing countries obesity is rare, and weight for height decreases with age after early adulthood. However, there are some interesting exceptions that would be worth examining for their biological consequences, including obese South Sea island royalty and ritual obesity in some African tribes. Moreover, obesity is increasing in developing countries as more persons become relatively affluent and less physically active.

Almost all published articles and chapters focus on obesity as a health and social problem in contemporary industrialized societies without reference to its historical and global dimensions. This paper will concentrate on the broad geographical occurrence and biological significance of obesity.

During the paleolithic period the genetic potential for rapidly converting excess food to fat would have permitted the acquisition of valuable energy stores for lean periods. As described later, such stores, until they are exhausted, not only make up for a temporary shortage of dietary energy but also minimize the drain on lean body mass of amino acids necessary for protein synthesis when dietary protein sources are curtailed. It may be significant that the stone figures of Stone Age women found in Europe and Siberia from the Upper Paleolithic period were all fat, as if this were the ideal.

When contemporary hunters in Africa kill an animal too heavy to carry home, they may gorge themselves with several kilos of the meat before returning to their group with all that they can carry (Lee and DeVore, 1968). In temperate regions seasonal variations in the availability of foods of plant origin were even more pronounced (Brown and Konner, 1987). The ability to digest and absorb a large amount of food at one time is also advantageous to the Nestlik and other Central Arctic groups who have almost no vegetables in their diet and who depend on fauna whose numbers and distribution vary markedly (Balikci, 1968). The animal bones in archaeological excavations suggest that in Northern Europe large animals were even more important in the diet.

Unfortunately, the same inborn metabolic capacity to consume excess food and convert it efficiently to adipose tissue that may be advantageous to populations with limited and variable food supplies can be seriously disadvantageous to those whose food supplies are abundant and reliable, and whose energy requirements are reduced by sedentary life styles (Weiss, 1980). With abundant and reliable food supplies such a trait is conducive to obesity (Beller, 1987; O'Dea, 1988). In a few of these situations, such as among royalty in some Polynesian societies, positive social values are attached to what is elsewhere considered morbid obesity. Other examples are Sumo wrestlers in Japan and young male wrestlers in Polynesia (*see* Chapter 2; Beaglehole and Beaglehole, 1938). However, for most it is a social disadvantage. Regardless of the society, obesity is a health hazard (Bray, 1987).

Before exploring the consequences of overweight and obesity in humans it is necessary to define these terms. A social definition of obesity would be fatness beyond the socially accepted norms for a given society. Medically, obesity is defined as a body mass (wt in kg/ht in m^2) in excess of 27.8 in men and 27.3 in women (NIH Consensus Panel, 1985). These values approximate 120% of ideal weight for age and gender. Although the term "overweight" is in common use, no widely used criteria define the term. Therefore, we will use obesity in the following discussion as a dichotomous term that does not reflect the severity of the excess weight. The acceptable range has been determined mainly from U.S. life insurance statistics, despite some questions as to their bias, but more recently data from the U.S. National Center for Health Statistics have been used (Simopoulos, 1987).

The extensive literature on the relative value of various other anthropometic indices, including skinfold thicknesses, for appraising body composition, overweight and obesity is beyond the scope of this article. Although the use of different indices may affect the proportion of individuals judged obese and the strength of the correlations between obesity and the increased risk of various diseases, the differences are not pertinent for the present discussion.

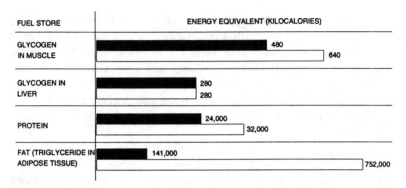

Figure 1. Energy stores in a normal adult (black bar) and obese adult (white bar). Each pair of bars is on a different scale. In obese persons the amount of fat, the main energy store is five to six times greater than in persons of normal weight.

FAT AS AN ENERGY STORE

Fat constitutes the principal energy reserve in the body. Among normal adults, only 1.0 kg or less of body weight is glycogen, the storage form of body glucose. Because glycogen is approximately 75% water, 1.0 kg of glycogen supplies 250 g of glucose with a caloric equivalent of approximately 800 kcals.

In the average 70 kg man, 15% of body weight (10.5 kg) is fat, whereas in the average 50 kg woman, 25% of body weight (12.5 kg) is fat. The caloric equivalent of fat-free mass is 1 kcal/g because approximately 75% of fat-free mass is water. Body fat has a caloric equivalent of 7.2 kcal/g. Therefore, men of normal weight store approximately 75,000 kcal and women approximately 90,000 kcal in fat. From these figures one can calculate the additional energy stores in varying degrees of overweight and obesity. Figure 1 shows energy stores in normal and obese adults.

Women have a greater amount of subcutaneous fat than men, which provides an added buffer for the stress of child-bearing. A fairly rapid increase in body fat is a normal feature of puberty in girls, whereas boys lose fat during the same period. There is some evidence that menarche requires a certain degree of adiposity (Frisch and Revelle, 1970), a convenient way of ensuring that women do not become pregnant for the first time until their bodies can nourish a fetus. It is noteworthy that fattening huts are common in Africa for adolescent girls of the elite (Brown and Konner, 1987) and among the Fellahin in

Egypt a fat woman is considered to have more room to bear the child and nourish her children (Ammar, 1954). Fat accumulates during pregnancy and is subsequently utilized as an energy source during the first six months of lactation.

MECHANISM OF ADAPTATION TO STARVATION

When food intake is grossly deficient or lacking, the body mobilizes its tissue reserves for survival. It must supply both energy for maintenance and amino acids for essential protein synthesis. Normally the principal fuel for the brain is glucose. A rapid drop in its continuous supply brings about confusion, coma and if prolonged, results in death.

The human brain requires between 100 and 145 grams of glucose (equivalent to about 400 to 600 kcalories) per day, but the body's main reserve of glycogen in the liver is considerably less than 100 g, and not all of it is available. Thus, the available glycogen stores in the liver are not even sufficient for the duration of the overnight fast between the evening meal and breakfast.

There is no net synthesis of glucose from fat. The glycerol of triglycerides from fatty tissue provides a source for glucose synthesis, but only about 16 grams per day. Therefore, glucose needs are met by the mobilization of amino acids from skeletal muscle. These are used for the synthesis of alanine that furnishes its carbon skeleton to the liver for the synthesis of pyruvate (Cahill, 1978). Pyruvate then serves as a major precursor for glucose synthesis in the liver. The remaining amino acids mobilized are used for necessary protein synthesis. Without this mechanism, lean body mass would be rapidly depleted, and the survival time of even obese starving individuals would be quite short.

Fortunately, an alternate mechanism provides substantial fuel for the brain as well as for skeletal and cardiac muscle, thereby greatly prolonging survival time in starvation. The blood of subjects who are starved, even briefly, shows an accumulation of ketone bodies, primarily acetoacetic and beta-hydroxybutyric acids that are derived from fat and that can serve as an energy substrate in place of glucose. Figure 2 compares brain energy sources after an overnight fast and after 5-6 weeks of fasting. Figure 3A shows the high uptake of glucose by major tissues after an overnight fast and Figure 3B shows the reduced uptake after 5 weeks of starvation. These adaptive responses do not completely eliminate the breakdown of body protein for gluconeogenesis but do reduce it to minimum levels.

Nevin S. Scrimshaw and William H. Dietz

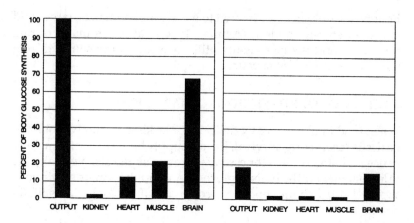

Figure 2. Under normal circumstances the energy required by the brain comes from glucose (bar at the left), but after five to six weeks of starvation other compounds furnish approximately 70% of the energy required.

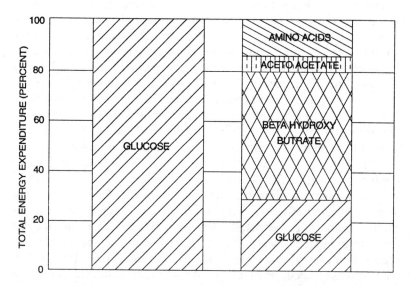

Figure 3. After five weeks of starvation (right) glucose synthesis is less than 20% of that after a normal overnight fast (left) and brain uptake has decreased proportionately. The relative decrease in glucose uptake by the heart and kidney is even greater.

These metabolic responses give the human body a remarkable capacity for surviving without food for long periods. The Irish revolutionary, Terence MacSwiney, survived for 74 days in 1928 before dying of starvation. The biblical fasting period of 40 days and 40 nights is well within the capability of a well-nourished adult. Obesity greatly prolongs this period, as has been repeatedly demonstrated during total fasting. For example, a 30 year old woman who ate no food for 236 days reduced her weight from 128 to 84 kg, and a 51 year old woman fasted for 249 days and reduced her weight from 128 to 95 kg. (Young and Scrimshaw, 1971). Neither of these women suffered adverse side effects that could be attributed to lack of food, nor have most other obese patients who fasted to lose weight.

A young child receiving a diet that is grossly inadequate in dietary energy can prolong survival for many months by the above mechanism, although the child becomes progressively more marasmic as body fat stores are utilized. After these stores are utilized, lean body mass must furnish amino acids for both essential protein synthesis and energy. At this point death ensues rapidly.

A child who develops kwashiorkor as a result of a diet that is deficient in dietary protein relative to energy dies in a matter of days unless a good source of protein is given promptly. A "sugar baby" form of kwashiorkor was formerly seen in Jamaica and some parts of Africa when a child received abundant calories from cassava but little protein. Such children appear blubbery. In marasmus, the mobilization of amino acids from skeletal muscle for gluconeogenesis results in their availability for protein synthesis. It is for this reason that biochemical and clinical signs of protein deficiency are not seen in marasmus or in starvation. However, in the case of kwashiorkor sufficient dietary energy is ingested to block the tissue breakdown that supplies amino acid precursors for the internal gluconeogenesis in marasmus (Scrimshaw and Behar, 1961). Glucocorticoid hormone plays a major role in mediating this response because it is catabolic for muscle tissue and anabolic for liver cells; plasma glucocorticoid levels remain low in kwashiorkor and relatively high in marasmus (Scrimshaw and Behar, 1961).

DISADVANTAGES OF FATNESS

Fat-free mass is greater in the obese because of both an increase in muscle mass to support the increased body mass and the greater nuclear mass of hypertrophied adipose tissue. Because fat-free mass is the principal determinant of basal metabolic rate and accounts for the largest fraction of total daily energy expenditure, obese individuals have an increased maintenance energy requirement. The amount of dietary energy intake that is utilized for weight gain, therefore, may be a very small part of the significantly higher food intake of the obese individual. Presumably, because food intake is greater, the obese individual is widely perceived as a social deviant in contemporary cultures.

Although, as we have seen, the temporary storage of excess calories as body fat constitutes a normal, and originally adaptive, physiologic response to the ingestion of excess calories, the prolonged accumulation of body fat was not a normal characteristic during the evolution of humankind. It is not surprising, therefore, that obesity is accompanied by a variety of adverse biological consequences that depend on age and circumstances. In contemporary societies there are also social consequences that bear more heavily on children.

Children and Adolescents

In children and adolescents, obesity has multiple effects on growth. The height for age and the bone age of overweight children are greater than in their non-obese counterparts, and obese girls have early menarche (Dietz and Schoeller, 1982).

Obesity can be a severe social handicap for a child. For example, when young U.S. children were presented with profiles of a variety of children with handicaps, they invariably listed the obese as the children that they least wanted as friends and ascribed a variety of negative social characteristics to them (Straffieri, 1967). These attitudes commonly evolve to discrimination and persecution by peers and frequent playground teasing and name-calling. The lack of oversized clothing for children is a visible example of the institutionalization of such discrimination. These experiences of obese children reflect the social reality. They are among the last chosen to play on teams, other children tease them, and they are self-conscious about their weight.

Despite the discrimination, the sense of self-worth of obese young children is similar to that of the nonobese, but by adolescence the social messages become internalized with the development of a negative self-image that may be life-long. In another study (Stunkard and Mendleson, 1967) adults who were obese as children, but of normal weight as adolescents, had a body image comparable to that of individuals who had never been obese, but adults who had been obese as adolescents had an extremely negative body image and feelings of low self-worth.

Obesity in the pediatric age group is related to the later development of cardiovascular risk, and hyperlipidemia is already found in as many as 20% of obese children. Total serum cholesterol is elevated; high-density lipoprotein cholesterol is low; and low-density lipoprotein cholesterol is increased. This pattern of cholesterol distribution poses a high risk for future cardiovascular disease.

Although noninsulin-dependent (type II) diabetes mellitus is rare in obese children, its precursors are common. Glucose tolerance is abnormal and the degree of hyperinsulinemia is directly related to the degree of body fatness. Finally, although hypertension occurs in approximately one percent of children, over half of those with persistent hypertension are obese. The increase in fat-free mass that accompanies obesity may play an etiologic role (Weinsier *et al.*, 1985).

Adults

In adults, the discrimination that begins in childhood persists but becomes more subtle with advancing age. Abundant anecdotal evidence suggests reduced job opportunities and promotion among the obese. Part of the higher prevalence of obesity among those in a low socioeconomic class may be causal (Gortmaker *et al.*, 1993). There is some tendency for obese women to be perceived as less desirable mates and therefore for them to marry downward in socioeconomic group.

In adults the medical complications of obesity also occur with a high prevalence. Obesity predisposes to gall stones, usually of the cholesterol type. Chronic obesity changes the center of gravity so that the lumbar curve of the vertebrae first becomes lordotic, followed by a compensatory thoracic kyphosis and eventually a cervical lordosis producing a forward position of the head. There is also an increased frequency of flat feet and of bilateral arthritis of the knees.

In the Pickwick Papers, Charles Dickens graphically described a condition in some very obese persons characterized by hypoventilation, somnolence, cyanosis, tachycardia, raised central venous pressure, cardiac dilatation, hepatomegaly, and peripheral edema. It now bears the medical eponym "Pickwickian Syndrome."

Obesity accounts for approximately 25% of adult diabetes in the populations of North America and Europe. It has a higher prevalence among some societies that have undergone rapid transition from a traditional to a sedentary life-style with high sugar intake. Examples are modern Alaskan natives and Eskimos, American Indians (Knowler *et al.*, 1981) and some Australian aborigines (O'Dea, 1988).

The only dietary factor consistently related to the prevalence of diabetes in these populations is total caloric intake (West, 1978; Wyllie-Rosett, 1985). Moreover, the association of diabetes with adiposity in adults is evident in comparisons among populations and persists in both inter- and intrapopulation analyses (West, 1978). The risk of diabetes is directly related to the distribution of body fat. Men and women with an increase in upper body fatness (android distribution) are at substantially greater risk for abnormal glucose tolerance and hyperinsulinemia than are individuals with lower extremity fatness (gynoid distribution) (Kissebah *et al.*, 1982).

Even in individuals within the range of normal weight, blood pressure is, in general, proportional to weight. About one-third of obese individuals are hypertensive, and blood pressure increases with the degree of obesity (Report of the Hypertension Task Force, 1979; Kotschen and Kotschen, 1985). Weight loss alone is often sufficient to lower blood pressure (Kotschen and Kotschen, 1985). When combined with exercise and a diet with less saturated fat, blood pressure returns to normal in most individuals.

Obesity is also associated with an increased risk of cardiovascular disease and sudden death that is proportional to the degree of obesity (Hubert and Castelli, 1985). The most dramatic risks are for the most obese. For example, among young adult males in excess of 200% of ideal body weight, the mortality over a seven-year period was eleven times the expected rate for age (Drenick *et al.*, 1964). The extent to which the increased risk is due to obesity *per se* is unknown. Certainly much of it is mediated by the effect of obesity on the intervening diseases of diabetes, hyperlipidemia, and hypertension (Marks, 1960).

Pregnant Women

Among obese pregnant women, the rate of complications during pregnancy, delivery and post-partum is significantly increased. At the time of delivery the frequency of dystocia (difficult child-birth) is greater, and the infant's risk of excessive birth weight, neonatal hypoglycemia, hypocalcemia and respiratory distress syndrome all increase. Following delivery, obese mothers have an increased prevalence of episiotomy infections, thrombophlebitis, and pulmonary embolus (Edwards *et al.*, 1985; Kliegman and Gross, 1985). They are also more likely to develop gestational diabetes mellitus.

Cancer

There is increasing evidence that diets that are high in saturated fat influence the occurrence of some forms of cancer (National Research Council, 1989). One of the best known studies reports a significant correlation between the dietary fat of different ethnic groups and their rates of breast cancer in Hawaii (Kolonel *et al.*, 1981). Moreover, the incidence of breast and colon cancer is low in Japanese in Japan consuming a traditional diet but much higher among ethnic Japanese living in California. The principal differences are in the total quantity of fat eaten and the amount of fat from meat and dairy products (Buell, 1973). Positive associations have been found between excess weight and cancers of the gallbladder, biliary duct, endometrium, ovary, breast and cervix in women, and cancers of the colon and prostate in men (Lew and Garfinkel, 1979). While much of the effect of diet on breast cancer may be mediated through fat consumption and not through calorie consumption, obesity may contribute an independent effect (Miller, 1985).

Infection

Overfed dogs were found to have lowered resistance to distemper virus (Newberne, 1973). In human subjects increased morbidity from infections (National Research Council, 1964; Pitkin, 1976) significantly decreased bactericidal capacity (Palmblad, Halberg and Rossner, 1977) and reduced glucose oxidation (Kjosen, Bassue and Myking, 1975) of leukocytes has been found in obese subjects compared with those of normal weight.

ADVANTAGES OF OVERWEIGHT

As already indicated, it seems likely that the ability to store fat had a significant advantage during the paleolithic period when the current genetic make-up of the human race was established. For certain populations even today there is a clear advantage to a moderate increase in adipose tissue. Eskimos are known to have more subcutaneous fat than is characteristic of normal inhabitants of more temperate regions. This is an advantage for the maintenance of body temperature under conditions of extreme cold.

It is well established that morbidity and mortality from tuberculosis is greater in individuals who are undernourished (Scrimshaw, Taylor and Gordon, 1968; McKeown, 1976). The lower mortality from tuberculosis in obese patients is probably due to the buffer that body fat provides against the catabolic losses that occur in persons with infection (Berry and Nash, 1955). Mayer (1959) suggests that this may explain the popular association of stoutness with health in the western world, a concept that still persists in many developing countries. Despite the potential benefit of increased body weight on the outcome of tuberculosis infections, few other positive consequences of excess body fat can be demonstrated in developing countries.

Today there are many situations in which seasonal food shortages result in a loss of weight which is then restored when food crops are available. In the Gambia, for example, not only do women lose weight during the hungry season, but there is also a seasonal decrease in birth weight associated with an increase in infant mortality (Prentice et al., 1983). Severe seasonal variation in the food supplies of agriculturalists as well as hunters and gatherers is well documented (Whiting, 1958; Hunter, 1967). In many of the groups observed the accumulation of some meagre fat stores during the harvest season is essential for maternal and infant survival. The massive adipose tissue distributed over the buttocks of some African groups, the so-called "Hottentot bustle," which appears to be genetically determined, may represent useful energy stores that interfere minimally with heat dissipation. However, none of these examples involves obesity, or even obvious overweight.

SUMMARY

In summary, the capacity to metabolize excess food and store its energy as fat would have been advantageous to humans during the Paleolithic period when the human genome was determined. Adipose tissue can serve as an energy source during periods of seasonal food shortages and between kills of large animals. Added body fat acquired during pregnancy provides part of the energy required for the first six months of lactation.

The adipose tissue of well nourished individuals of normal weight enables them to survive at least 30 days of starvation with no permanent harm. Some morbidly obese individuals have survived over 200 days with no significant side-effects attributable to lack of food. This phenomenon occurs despite the fact that glycogen stores as a source of glucose are sufficient for only a few hours. Such extended survival is possible because ketone bodies derived from fat replace glucose as an energy source for the brain and cardiac muscle.

For contemporary populations in industrialized countries with abundant access to food and a sedentary life style, the conversion of excess food to fat has no advantage and exposes the individual to serious health hazards. The latter include an increased risk of diabetes, hypertension, heart disease, orthopedic abnormalities and, in exceptional cases, Pickwickian Syndrome. Obese individuals frequently experience social discrimination, which is particularly severe in its lasting effects on the self-image of adolescents.

NOTES

Dr. Nevin Scrimshaw is a clinical and public health nutritionist who founded the Institute of Nutrition of Central America and Panama (INCAP). He is Professor Emeritus of Massachusetts Institute of Technology where he headed the Department of Nutrition and Food Science. He continues to direct activities of the Food and Nutrition Programme for Human and Social Development for the United Nations University, Tokyo. In 1991 he was awarded the World Food Prize Laureate for his extensive work and publications in the field of nutritional deprivation. He is currently located at the Center for Population and Development Studies of the Harvard School of Public Health.

Dr. William Dietz is Associate Professor of Pediatrics at Tufts University School of Medicine and Director of Clinical Nutrition at the New England Medical Center, Boston. His undergraduate degree is from Wesleyan University, his M.D. is from the University of Pennsylvania, and he has a Ph.D. in nutritional biochemistry from Massachusetts Institute of Technology.

REFERENCES

Ammar, H. 1954. *Growing up in an Egyptian village.* Routledge and Kegan Paul, London

Balikci, A. 1968. The Nestlik Eskimos: Adaptive processes. In R.B. Lee and I. DeVore (eds.) *Man the Hunter.* Aldine, Chicago. Chapter 8, pp. 78–82

Beaglehole, E., and P. Beaglehole 1938. *Ethnology of Pukapuka.* Bernice P. Bishop Museum, Honolulu, HI.

Beller, A.S. 1987. *Fat and Thin: A Natural History of Obesity.* Farrar, Straus and Giroux, New York.

160   Nevin S. Scrimshaw and William H. Dietz

Berry, W.T.C., and F.A. Nash 1955. Studies in the aetiology of pulmonary tuberculosis. *Tubercle* **36**, 164–174.

Bray, G.A. 1987. Overweight is risking fate: Definition, classification, prevalence, and risks. In R. J. Wurtman and J.J. Wurtman (eds.), *Human Obesity. Annals of the New York Academy of Sciences* **499**, 14–28.

Buell, P.J. (1973). Changing incidence of breast cancer in Japanese-American women. *Journal of the National Cancer Institute* **51**, 1479–1483.

Brown, J.B., and M. Konner 1987. An anthropological perspective on obesity. In R.J. Wurtman and J.J. Wurtman (eds.), *Human Obesity. Annals of the New York Academy of Sciences* **499**, 29–46.

Cahill, G.F. 1978. Physiology of acute starvation in man. *Ecology of Food and Nutrition* **6**, 221–230.

Dietz, W.H., and D.A. Schoeller 1982. Optimal dietary therapy for obese adolescents: Comparison of protein plus glucose and protein plus fat, *Journal of Pediatrics* **100**, 638–644.

Drenick, E.J., M. E. Swendseid, W.H. Blahd and S.G. Tuttle 1964. Prolonged starvation as treatment for severe obesity. *Journal of the American Medical Association* **187**, 100–105.

Eaton, S.B., M. Shostak, and M. Konner 1988. *The Paleolithic Prescription*. Harper and Row, New York.

Edwards, L.E., W.F Dickes, I.R. Alton and E.Y. Hakenson, 1985. Pregnancy in the massively obese: Course, outcome, and obesity prognosis of the infant. *Obstetrics and Gynecology* **66**, 299–306.

Frisch, R.E., and R. Revelle 1970. Height and weight at menarche and a hypothesis of critical body weights and adolescent weights. *Science* **169**, 397–399.

Gortmaker, S.L., A. Must, J.M. Perrin, A.M. Sobol and W.H. Dietz 1993. Social and economic consequences of obesity. *New England Journal of Medicine* **329**, 1008–1012.

Hubert, H.B., and W.P. Castelli 1985. Obesity as a predictor of a coronary heart disease. In R.T. Frankle, J. Dwyer, L. Moragne, and A. Owen (eds.), *Dietary Treatment and Prevention of Obesity*. John Libbey, London. pp. 125–136.

Hunter, J. N. 1967. Seasonal hunger in a part of the west African savanna: A survey of body weights in Nangodi, north-east Ghana. *Transactions Institute of British Geography* **41**, 167–185.

Kissebah, A.H., N. Vydelingum, R. Murray, D.J. Evans, A.J. Harz, R.K. Kalkhoff and P.W. Adams 1982. Relation of body fat distribution to metabolic complications of obesity. *Journal of Clinical Endocrinology and Metabolism* **54**, 254–260.

Kjosen, B., H.H. Bassue, and O. Myking 1975. The glucose oxidation in isolated leukocytes from female patients suffering from overweight or anorexia nervosa. *Scandinavian Journal of Clinical Laboratory Investigation* **35**, 447–454.

Kliegman, R.M. and T. Gross 1985. Perinatal problems of the obese mother and her infant. *Obstetrics and Gynecology* 66, 299–306.

Knowler, W.C., D.J. Pettitt, P.J. Savage and P.H. Bennett 1981. Diabetes incidence in Pima Indians: Contribution of obesity and parental diabetes. *American Journal of Epidemiology* 113, 144–156.

Kolonel, L. N., J.H. Hankin, J. Lee, S.Y. Chu, A.M.Y. Nomura and M.W. Hinds 1981. Nutrient intakes in relation to cancer incidence in Hawaii. *British Journal of Cancer* 44, 332–339.

Kotschen, J.M., and T.A. Kotschen 1985. Obesity and hypertension. In R.T. Frankle, J. Dwyer, L. Moragne, and A. Owen (eds.), *Dietary Treatment and Prevention of Obesity*. John Libbey, London. pp. 137–146.

Lee, R.B., and I. DeVore (eds.) 1968. *Man the Hunter*. Atherton, Chicago, IL.

Lee, R.B. 1968. What hunters do for a living, or how to make out on scarce resources. In R.B. Lee, and I. DeVore (eds.), *Man the Hunter*. Atherton, Chicago, IL. Chapter 4, pp. 30–48.

Lew, E.A., and L. Garfinkle 1979. Variations in mortality by weight among 750,000 men and women. *Journal of Chronic Disease* 32,563–576.

Marks H.H. 1969. Influence of obesity morbidity and mortality. *Bulletin of the New York Academy of Medicine* 36, 296–312.

Mayer, J. 1959. Obesity: Etiology and pathogenesis, *Postgraduate Medicine* 25, 100–105.

McKeown, T. 1976. *The Modern Rise of Population*. Academic Press, New York/San Francisco.

Miller, A.B. 1985. Obesity and cancer. In R.T. Frankle, J. Dwyer, L. Moragne, and A. Owen (eds.), *Dietary Treatment and Prevention of Obesity*. John Libbey, London. pp. 1555–1566.

National Institutes of Health 1985. Consensus development panel on the health implications of obesity. *Annals of Internal Medicine* 103, 977–1077.

National Research Council 1964. Postoperative wound infections. *Annals of Surgery* 160: Suppl. 2.

National Research Council 1989. *Diet and Health: Implications for reducing chronic disease risk*. National Academy Press, Washington, D.C. pp. 768.

Newberne, P.M. 1973. The influence of nutrition response to infectious disease. *Advances in Veterinary Science and Comparative Medicine* 17, 265–289.

O'Dea K. 1988. The hunter-gatherer lifestyle of Australian Aborigines: Implications for health. In *Current Problems in Nutrition, Pharmacology and Toxicology*. John Libbey, London/Paris. pp. 26–36.

Palmblad, J., D. Hallberg, and S. Rossner 1977. In *Malnutrition and Host Defense*. Karolinska Institute, Stockholm. pp. VI–1—VI–16.

Pitkin, R.M. 1976. Abdominal hysterectomy in obese women. *Surgical and Gynecological Obstetrics* 142, 532–536.

Prentice, A.M., M. Watkinson, R.G. Whitehead, W.H. Lamb and T.J. Cole, 1983. Prenatal dietary supplementation of African women and birth weight. *Lancet* I, 489–492.

Report of the Hypertension Task Force. 1979. Vol. 9. Washington, D.C. NIH Publication No. 79-163:59-77, U.S. Dept. Health, Education and Welfare.

Scrimshaw, N.S., and M. Behar 1961. Protein malnutrition in young children. *Science* **133**, 2039–47.

Scrimshaw, N.S., C.E. Taylor and J.E. Gordon 1968. *Interactions of Nutrition and Infection*. WHO Monograph Series No. 57, Geneva. pp. 329.

Simopoulos, A.P. 1987. Characteristics of obesity: An overview. In R.J. Wurtman and J.J. Wurtman (eds.), *Human Obesity*. New York, *Annals New York Academy of Sciences* **499**, 4–13.

Staffieri, J.R. 1967. A study of social stereotype of body image in children. *Journal of Personal and Social Psychology* **7**, 101–104.

Stunkard, A.J., and M. Mendleson 1967. Obesity and the body image: I. Characteristics of disturbances in the body image of some obese persons. *American Journal of Psychiatry* **123**, 1296–1300.

Weinsier, R.L., D.J. Norris, I.R. Berch, R.S. Bernstein, J. Wong, M-U Yan, R.N. Pierson, Jr. and T.B. Van Itallie, 1985. Obesity and hypertension. *Hypertension* **7**, pp. 578–95.

Weiss, B. 1980. Nutrition adaptation and cultural maladaptation, An evolutionary view. In N.W. Jerome, R.F. Kandel and G.H. Pelto, (eds.), *Nutritional Anthropology*. Redgrave, Pleasantville, New York. pp. 147–179.

West, K.N. 1978. *Epidemiology of Diabetes and Its Vascular Lesions*. Elsevier/North-Holland, New York, pp. 579.

Whiting, M. G. 1958. *A Cross-Cultural Nutrition Survey*. Doctoral thesis, Harvard School of Public Health, Cambridge, MA.

Wyllie-Rosett, J. 1985. Obesity in the etiology and treatment of type II diabetes. In R.T. Frankle, J. Dwyer, L. Moragne and A. Owen (eds.), *Dietary Treatment and Prevention of Obesity*. John Libbey, London. pp. 147–154.

Young, V.R., and N.S. Scrimshaw 1971. The physiology of starvation. *Scientific American* **225** (No. 4), 14–21.

9

Obesity and Physical Fitness: An Age-Dependent Functional and Social Handicap

JANA PARIZKOVA

INTRODUCTION

Body fatness is a continuing phenomenon, and except for some clear-cut morbidity situations, it has always been difficult to agree on the cut-off points on a world-wide basis. From this it follows that up to now we have had difficulty in assessing the prevalence of obesity in children, adults and people of advanced age. It has also been difficult to compare the prevalence of obesity in different parts of the world. At a meeting of the Regional Office of the World Health Organisation in Warsaw, 1987 (WHO, 1988), this problem was discussed. In the resulting report, entitled "Measuring obesity," it was suggested that obesity in adults should be established at a level of a body mass index (BMI) of 30 or higher (WHO, 1988): a BMI higher than 25 means the initiation of overweight. For children and adolescents the values for classifying obesity have not been fully agreed upon, as BMI varies significantly depending on various stages of growth. Special growth grids were established by Rolland-Cachera *et al.* (1982), showing that the critical values of BMI for the classification of obesity also differ according to age.

Obesity is more correctly defined as an excessive accumulation of fat related to muscle and all other tissues of the body. However, the measurement of fat is not so easy as the evaluation of BMI, even if we use simple methods such as the measurement of skinfolds by calipers. In adult males the reference value of depot fat is 14% and up to 25% in females (Brozek *et al.*, 1987). But again a general consensus has not been reached. BMI correlates significantly with the amount of depot fat (kg) assessed by densitometry (Parizkova 1977; Parizkova, Markova and Weissova, 1988), with a value for males r = 0.901, and for females r = 0.927, p < 0.001. A special problem is the relationship of obesity to functional capacity and physical fitness which varies according to age.

Excess fat deposited in the body of a small child is generally considered an advantage, and not a drawback, as it might be later on in life. This advantage follows from the protective effect of deposits of fat in regard to various diseases, mostly of the respiratory and gastrointestinal systems, at early stages of life. Not very long ago, when health care and hygiene were at a lower level, fatter children had a better chance of surviving infectious diseases than thin children. The old masters painted angels and children who, by today's standards, would be judged obese, but who then may have had a greater chance of survival, as may be the case in developing countries today.

Such a view has changed recently in the industrially developed countries and also in the affluent social strata in developing countries. There has been evidence of the changed metabolic situation manifested, for example, by a pathological level of various blood lipids connected in some cases with childhood obesity. This situation can mean, for such an individual, an adverse prognosis as regards the development of cardiovascular diseases in adulthood or in advanced age, for example (Parizkova *et al.*, 1986a,b). In a group of preschool children (n = 54) a significant correlation was found between the percentage of body fat and the level of triglycerides (r = 0.494, p < 0.01) as well as that of cholesterol (r = 0.448, p < 0.01; Parizkova, Markova and Weissova, 1988).

In Czechoslovakia, the prevalence of obesity in preschool age children is very low, namely 2 to 3% when using as criteria the 97th percentile of body proportion, that is, BMI of about 18–19 (which corresponds approximately to the similar percentile in the growth grid of Rolland-Cachera et al., 1982), and also to growth grids based on longitudinal measurement of Czech children (Prokopec and Bellisle, 1993)

METHODS

A follow-up study was performed on 2,587 boys and 2,505 girls in Czechoslovakia five months before they entered primary school. These children had an average age of 6.4 years, 5 months before entering primary school. The level of functional capacity and physical fitness was tested in three subgroups of these children—lean (up to 3rd percentile), normal (25th–75th percentile) and obese children (above 97th percentile)—as measured by body proportion, in which BMI and circumference measures varied accordingly (Figure 1).

RESULTS

Motor development differed much less than somatic characteristics—only the results in the standing broad jump were significantly greater in lean and normal boys as compared to obese boys, and in lean girls as compared to obese girls (Figure 2). The performance in the 20 m dash and skill tests such as throwing a cricket ball and forward roll did not differ according to body proportion and BMI. Findings show that as regards motor abilities overweight small children are not so handicapped as their older peers. The evaluation of performance of the modified step test characterising cardiorespiratory efficiency also does not show significantly worse results in the overweight than in the normal preschool children (Parizkova et al., 1983).

In school age children the prevalence of obesity is at least doubled, exceeding the value of BMI 20 and 25–30% depot fat in the body, evaluated by means of densitometry, and/or skinfold thickness measurement and the calculation of the percentage of depot fat with the help of regression equations and nomographs derived for our population of children (Parizkova, 1961a,b, 1977). Some authors evaluated it as 10–15% of our childhood population. Any handicap from the burden of excess fat during dynamic play and exercise becomes much more apparent; many functional parameters deteriorate in these as compared to normal children. The measurements of the aerobic pow-

SOMATIC INDICES IN NORMAL ☐, ASTHENIC ▨ AND OBESE ◺ PRESCHOOL CHILDREN

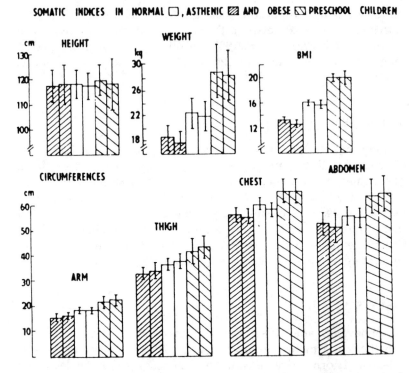

Figure 1. Somatic indices (height, weight, BMI, and arm, thigh, chest and abdominal circumferences) in normal, asthenic and obese Czech preschool children.

er characterising functional capacity and efficiency of the cardiorespiratory system, assessed by the measurements of oxygen uptake during a maximal work load on a treadmill (Sprynarova and Parizkova, 1965) or on a bicycle ergometer, revealed significantly worse results in the growing obese subjects, and the same applies to the comparison of the obese and normal children as regards the results of step test, vital capacity, performance in running, jumping and the like (Parizkova and Hainer, 1989).

Such reduced functional capacity results, moreover, in adverse psychological consequences—inferiority complexes causing, for example, increased aggressive behaviour in obese youngsters. On the other hand, some obese children compensate in other spheres and become

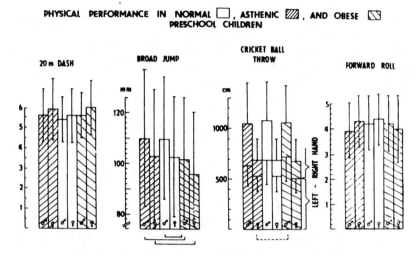

Figure 2. Selected physical performance by normal. asthenic and obese Czech preschool children.

very good pupils at school, or dominate in other activities in which excess weight does not interfere.

The problem of obesity becomes very serious at puberty. This is especially noticeable in industrially developed countries, where during recent decades both feminine and masculine models are presented as very thin. Moreover, stars of cinema, theatre, sports, and pop music are not only lean, but are also presented as physically fit. Fashion has a sporty character for most age groups. All this results in a distressing position for an obese adolescent who has to face up to the negative attitudes of colleagues at school or even in the family. Clumsiness, unattractiveness to the opposite sex, are serious problems at this age. The deterioration of functional capacity and physical fitness described above is even more pronounced during dynamic performance, of which dance is one example. Only muscle strength, which correlates with total and lean body mass, may be higher, but often, due to physical inactivity and avoidance of exercise, the muscles may not be well developed. Excessive strain during physical activity due to the burden of excess fat in the obese individual further reduces time spent on exercise and total energy output.

In obese adolescent boys and girls the study revealed not only excess development of fat, but also that the amount of lean body mass was higher when compared with normal adolescents of the same age and height. In obese boys there was another change in body physique—the measure of bi-iliocristal breadth (the distance between iliac crests at the point which gives the maximum diameter) was significantly higher than in normal boys even when this diameter was corrected to allow for the thickness of subcutaneous fat (Parizkova, 1977). During more advanced stages of obesity secondary pathological, metabolic, body posture and joint changes may appear which are correctable only with difficulty. Primary endocrine disturbances causing obesity are rare during the growth period. Obesity is most often the result of absolute or relative overeating and hypokinesia (diminished motion).

Regulation of energy imbalance can thus be a very good remedy especially for obese adolescents in whom the establishment of an intensive exercise regime is easier than later on in life. For such a purpose, special summer camps, or whole-year institutional treatment where obese children and adolescents are admitted for necessary periods, are especially suitable. Weight reduction treatment by monitored diet and attractive, sufficiently intensive exercise is thus facilitated under conditions of collective life among other obese pupils. This applies also to the correction of adverse dietary and motor habits.

Such summer camps have been especially popular in Czechoslovakia: obese children and adolescents who voluntarily participated for seven weeks in these camps felt at ease there, as they were all equally handicapped. The care of the children was on a high level, as medical doctors and physical education instructors supervised the daily regimen of the children. A monitored diet of 1,700 kcal (7.1 mJ) per day along with regular, adequate exercise was introduced. Before entering and after leaving the camp, children were tested in the psychological laboratory of our Research Institute for Physical Education (body composition measured by densitometry, aerobic power, motor testing, and the like) and also interviewed by a psychologist. Further tests concerning the level of physical performance in selected sport disciplines were performed at the beginning and at the end of the camp, that is, before and after the reduction of weight and excess fat.

Often, children who to begin with were not able to achieve, for example, the 50 m run, or to swim at all, succeeded in undergoing these tests at the end of the summer camp. There was an effort to create a competitive but cheerful atmosphere. The greatest stress was on exercise, as too great a reduction of food intake resulted in reduced development in height (Parizkova, 1977). When children felt too tired after

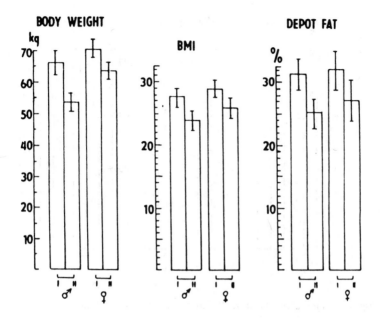

Figure 3. Posttreatment measures of body weight, BMI and depot fat in obese Czech preschool children.

an all-day exercise program, they, however, never refused to participate in a dancing party!

Results of a seven-week treatment in a summer camp for obese boys and girls aged 12 to 13 years are shown in Figure 3. Even when body weight, BMI and the percentage of depot fat did not decrease to normal values, the improvement was significant. The same applied to the efficiency of the cardiorespiratory system—oxygen intake during a standard work load on a veloergometer related to total body mass in both boys and girls, and to lean body mass in boys only. Vital capacity increased significantly after reduction treatment in both sexes (Figures 3 and 4; Parizkova 1977, 1993). Performance in running, jumping, swimming, throwing, muscle strength and results of skill tests also improved considerably. After this treatment and reduction of excess fat, children and adolescents felt more confident, and many of them continued in exercise and controlled eating even under home conditions without regular control. Thus they were able to preserve the positive results of treatment and were also able to establish better contacts

Jana Parizkova

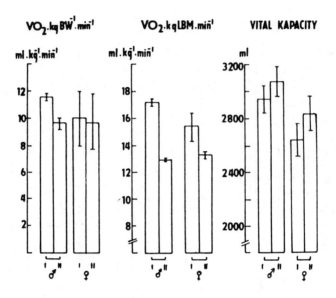

Figure 4. Vital capacity of posttreatment obese Czech preschool children.

with other normal children. On the other hand, some children returned home and reverted back to their old habits and thus regained weight. Their developmental curve of weight and fatness oscillated due to changes in physical activity and dietary regimens for several years (Parizkova, 1977, 1982, 1993, Parizkova *et al.*, 1993).

This experience indicates the usefulness of organising such summer camps for all obese children. In more advanced cases treatment in special year-round institutions with normal schooling would be desirable. Bulgaria had very good experience in this type of treatment (Tupuzov, 1986).

DISCUSSION

In adults, when life patterns are already established, the impact of obesity varies markedly. It also depends on whether obesity has developed in adulthood, or whether it has lasted since childhood. In most cases obesity is again a handicap, especially in some professions, and for women. When trying to find a marriage partner the choice and availability of a desirable mate is difficult for the obese. Fertility may

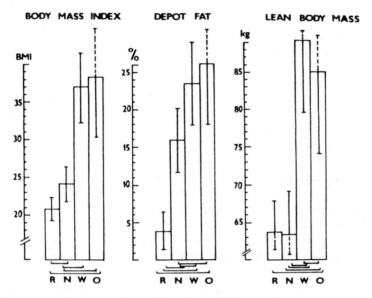

Figure 5. Body mass index, depot fat and lean body mass in runners, normal-weight individuals, weight lifters and obese adults.

also be reduced in obese women; massive obesity of the mother may have an adverse impact on the offspring.

Obesity which develops after several pregnancies is not judged or criticised as severely as in a young single woman. The same applies to a settled man with a successful professional career. In some professions obesity does not interfere, especially when the work is nonphysical. In any case, the level of functional capacity and physical fitness are reduced, which concerns mostly dynamic, aerobic performance.

In the industrially developed countries workers in furnaces, slaughterhouses, transport and brick-kiln jobs, for example, where great muscle force is still required, are mostly robust and muscular, but sometimes also obese. In competitive sport, heavy athletes such as weight-lifters and wrestlers have a body weight, BMI and the percentage of depot fat significantly higher when compared to athletes of dynamic sports disciplines (runners), but also when compared with subjects in the normal population. Weight-lifters have very similar BMI and percentage of depot fat to obese subjects treated in special clinics for the obese, the only difference being that the absolute amount of lean body mass is higher (Figure 5). The most excessive values of depot fat have been found in Japanese Sumo wrestlers who are still the most popular athletes in that country (see Chapter 2). However, the health of these adored and rich athletes may be poor—prediabetic changes have been proved in Sumo wrestlers with the highest body weight, and this can be corrected only after they reduce weight (Kuzuya et al., 1975). If weight and fatness are not reduced, such athletes suffer not only from diabetes, but also from atherosclerosis and other cardiovascular diseases, and die early.

In adulthood, the reduction of excess weight becomes a great problem; in serious cases clinical treatment of at least four weeks is necessary (Hainer et al., 1986). As in children, primary endocrine disturbance is also rarely found in adults. Chronic imbalance between energy intake and output is responsible for excess deposition of fat. This imbalance, however, can be corrected by reduced energy intake though a substantial increase in energy output is difficult due to various secondary pathological changes in the cardiorespiratory system. However, clinical treatment involves physical exercises adapted for such purposes. These exercises do not decrease obesity unless they are combined with a reducing diet.

Reduction of weight in adults is accompanied by changes in the percentage of fat (decrease of skinfolds, circumferences, BMI; waist-hip ratio mostly remains the same). This runs parallel with further positive changes such as a decrease in systolic and diastolic blood pressure, level of cholesterol, triglycerides and so forth (Hainer et al., 1991, 1992). Patients still remain overweight after four weeks of such a treatment but an estimate of body composition from skinfold measures indicates some loss of lean body mass. Along with these positive changes a decrease in basal metabolic rate appears; the nitrogen balance is usually negative only at the beginning of the treatment in the clinic (Parizkova and Hainer, 1989). This type of treatment, along with psychological and behavioural interventions, improved the situation for the obese substantially, but many of the patients, as do obese children, deteriorate again under home conditions. In spite of the fact that it is always possible to improve the situation of obese adults, prevention started as early as possible remains the most important strategy for overweight control. Sooner or later the excess deposits of fat not only decrease functional capacity and overall physical fitness, but they result in pathological consequences attacking many systems and organs of the human body.

Age changes in body weight indicate a decrease of body weight in more advanced age, especially in men. This could result either from reduced body weight in old individuals or could reflect hig rates associated with obesity, or both. Nevertheless, quite a n obese individuals survive until very old age, and many n even underweight individuals die much sooner without a_r varent clinical problems. In some populations living to an extremely old age as for example in the Caucasian mountains, even overweight subjects can survive for a long time. This did not seem true for old, long-living populations, for example, in the Andes, and it is very rare in industrialized countries. (Fong, 1983). Long survival of the obese who stay in good health and have a good level of physical fitness relative to their age has remained a great problem for obesity researchers, as it is generally accepted that overweight diminishes the life span. But from a social point of view, obesity in advanced age, as in children, is more acceptable than in adolescents.

(CONCLUSION)

Extensive measurements in most industrialised countries have shown that obesity for all ages persists as a serious problem not only from the point of view of health, functional capacity and physical fitness, but also from the social and cultural aspects. Changes in social attitudes resulting from public relations and modifications of cultural and aesthetic criteria seem to have made the situation of most obese individuals difficult. Quite often incipient obesity, especially during adolescence, results in frustration leading to development of bulimia, inertia and hypokinesia, which can lead to further increases in body weight and fatness. Analysis of this serious health and social problem, and sensitive handling of the obese individuals, especially during the most important and prolific periods of life, can improve the situation. The development of an adequate and individualised programme of nutritional and physical activity may secure an optimal energy balance and turnover especially when started early in life.

NOTES

Jana Parizkova, M.D., Ph.D., S.Sc., is based at the Biomedical Centre, Faculty of Physical Education, Charles University, Prague, Czech Republic.

REFERENCES

Brozek J., J. Parizkova, J. Mendez and H.L. Barkett 1987. The evaluation of body surface, body volume and body composition in human biology research. *Anthropologie XXV*, Vol. 3, pp. 235–259.

Fong, M.S. 1983. Demographic perspectives of aging. *Bibliotheca Nutritio et Dieta*, 33, 168–173 (Krager, Basel).

Hainer, V., M. Kunesova, V. Stich, J. Parizkova, A. Zak, V. Wernishova, P. Kozich, P. Hrabak, and L. Dedicova 1989. Very low energy formula diet in the treatment of obesity. *International Journal of Obesity*, 13 (Suppl. 2): 185–188.

Hainer, V., M. Kunesova, V. Stich, J. Parizkova and A. Zak 1991. Long-term follow-up of obese patients treated initially by very-low-calorie diet (VLCD). *International Journal of Obesity*, 15 (Suppl. 1): 1.

Hainer, V., V. Stich, M. Kunesova, J. Parizkova, A. Zak, V. Wernischova and P. Hrabak 1992. Effect of 4-week treatment of obesity by very-low-calorie diet on anthropometric, metabolic and hormonal indexes. *American Journal of Clinical Nutrition* 56, 281S–282S.

Kuzuya T., Y. Akanuma and K. Koseka 1975. Carbohydrate metabolism in obesity with special reference to the relationship of glucose intolerance and insulin hyperresponse. In Abstracts, Symposia and Free Communications. Xth International Congress of Nutrition, Kyoto, Japan. pp. 21.

Parizkova, J. 1961a. Age trends in fatness in normal and obese children. *Journal of Applied Physiology*, 16, 173–174.

Parizkova, J. 1961b. Total body fat and skinfold thickness in children. *Metabolism*, 10, 794–802.

Parizkova, J. 1977. *Body Fat and Physical Fitness*. Martinus Nijhoff B.V. Medical Division, The Hague.

Parizkova, J. 1982. Physical training in weight reduction of obese adolescents. *Annals of Clinical Research* 14, Suppl. 34:63–68.

Parizkova, J. 1989. Age related changes in dietary intake related to work output, physical fitness and body composition. *American Journal of Clinical Nutrition*, Suppl. 49(5), 962–967.

Parizkova, J. 1993. Obesity and its treatment by diet and exercise. In A. Simopoulos (ed.), Nutrition and fitness in health and disease. *World Review of Nutrition and Dietetics*, 72, 78–91. Karger, Basel.

Parizkova J., A. Adamec, J. Berdychova, J. Cermak, J. Horna and Z. Teply 1983. *Growth, Fitness and Nutrition in Preschool Children*. Universitas Carolina, Prague.

Parizkova, J. and V. Hainer 1989. Exercise therapy in growing and adult obese. In J.S. Torg, R.P. Walsh and R.J. Shepard (eds.), *Current Therapy in Sports Medicine*. B.C. Decker, Toronto, Canada. pp. 22–26.

Parizkova, J., V. Hainer, V. Stich, M. Kunesova and M. Ksantini 1993. Physiological capabilities of obese individuals and implications for exercise. In

M. Wahlquist and A.P. Hills (eds.), *Exercise and Obesity.* Gordon & Smith Co. Ltd., London.

Parizkova, J., E. Mackova, J. Mackova and M. Skopkova 1986a. Blood lipids as related to food efficiency in preschool children. *Journal of Pediatric Gastroenterogy and Nutrition,* **5,** 295.

Parizkova, J., E. Mackova, J. Kabela, J. Mackova and M. Skopkova 1986b. Body composition, food intake, cardiorespiratory fitness, blood lipids and psychological development in highly active and inactive preschool children. *Human Biology* **58,** 261–273.

Parizkova, J., E. Mackova and M. Weissova 1988. Dietary intake, body fat and blood lipids in preschool children. Cs. Gastroenterologie. In *Proc. 26th Conference of GEN (Group of European Nutritionists),* Prague. March 28–29.

Rolland-Cachera, M.F., M. Sempe, M. Guillud-Bataille, E. Patos, F. Pequinot Guggenbuhl and V. Fautrad 1982. Adiposity indices in children. *American Journal of Clinical Nutrition* **36,** 178–184

Sprynarova, S., and J. Parizkova 1965. Changes in the aerobic capacity and body composition in obese boys after reduction. *Journal of Applied Physiology* **20,** 934–937.

Tupuzov I.V. 1986. Model of prophylaxis and rehabilitation of child and adolescent obesity. In *Proceeding of National Scientific Conference of the Academy of Medicine, NIGH,* Sofia and BMI Pleven, pp. 60. (In Bulgarian).

WHO 1988. Measuring obesity classification and description of anthropometric data. Report on a WHO Consultation on the Epidemiology of Obesity. Warsaw, 21–23 Oct. 1987. Nutrition Unit, Regional Office WHO, Copenhagen.

——10——

Obesity and Overweight in Polish Men and Women: Social Determinants

JADWIGA CHARZEWSKA

INTRODUCTION

The effect of social environment on the prevalence of obesity has been revealed in populations at various levels of economic development. The correlations between obesity and socioeconomic status are described in detail in industrialised countries, such as the U.S. (Garn *et al.*, 1977; Lowenstein, 1976; Stunkard, 1978), United Kingdom and several other European and non-European countries (Goldbourt and Medalie, 1974; Khosla and Lowe, 1967; Kittel *et al.*, 1978; Silverstone, Gordon and Stunkard, 1969).

Essentially, in these countries the prevalence of obesity is inversely proportional to the socioeconomic status of the studied population groups, that is, the higher the social status the lower the prevalence of obesity. A different correlation has been described in countries with low national income such as the countries of South America and Puerto Rico (Stunkard, 1978; West, 1973).

The presence of different correlations in various population strata

177

and absence from the literature of a full agreement on observations concerning the prevalence of obesity in various social classes are due in a great degree to lack of an international, uniform criterion for diagnosis of obesity. In the nomenclature of the WHO Terminology Circular (1973), containing suggestions for a uniform nutritional terminology at an international level, separate definitions of obesity and overweight are given. According to this terminology, obesity is "excessive accumulation of fat" while overweight is "body weight above the normal range accepted for a given sex, age and body height in a population regarded as healthy."

Both these definitions, although completely correct, are so vague as to become arbitrary. This had led to a lack of uniformity in views presented in the literature. The situation is further complicated by the variety of methods used to determine obesity and overweight, and the tendency for oversimplification. In practice, the definitions of obesity and overweight are often used as alternatives to one another since these terms are usually regarded as synonymous.

None of the international organisations has indicated which method used for obesity determination is the most appropriate and so should be accepted as a standard. As yet, no generally agreed-upon definitions are available, apart from the above-mentioned ones. "Obesity" and "overweight" are understood by nearly every author slightly differently, although obesity has become a separate disease category.

The definition of obesity given above states that it is excessive accumulation of fat. Now the question arises, what is excessive accumulation and what amount of fat in the organism is harmful enough for human health to decrease the fitness of the organism?

Then, who is obese? We know that some amount of fatty tissue as a reserve tissue is justified both physiologically and from the standpoint of evolution. Through the greatest time span of our history, man was a gatherer and hunter. As estimated by Lee and Devore (among others, 1968), over 90% of all people who have been living on earth were gatherers and hunters, only 6% were farmers, and the remainder lived in societies at various levels of industrialisation. Thus, for the greatest part of our history, humans depended on the ability to win food through physical activity requiring a high energy expenditure. However, the availability of food was irregular, and periods of food shortage occurred frequently. The availability of fat reserves stored in adipose tissue made possible the use of this energy reserve during periods of increased requirements, for example, in hunger, disease and pregnancy. Thus, a reserve of fat was an advantage for people living an active way of life.

During our history of 40 thousand years *Homo sapiens'* physical structure has changed little, but formidable changes have occurred in the sociocultural life of this species, requiring adaptation to a less active way of life.

It may be assumed, in the light of high and increasing incidence of metabolic diseases, that a considerable proportion of human beings have not yet reached a sufficient degree of adaptation to the new conditions of life limiting physical activity. Thus it seems that the definition of obesity as a condition in which "excessive accumulation of fat" leads to decreased fitness of the body and health impairment would be most appropriate. However, establishing the upper range above which obesity could be determined quantitatively is a difficult and complex problem.

As yet, the cut-off points for the values of "obesity" and "overweight" have been arbitrarily set. Relatively more accurate definitions could be accepted only after extensive processing of sufficiently reliable empirical data which are unfortunately lacking.

Scant data in the world literature on these problems, and lack of information on the prevalence of obesity in various social groups in the Polish population, was the reason this study was undertaken.

METHOD AND SAMPLE

The analysed group of men was a random sample of 10% of men aged between 20–59 years, working in 14 institutions in Warsaw. The study was an integral part of the Polish Trial on Multifactorial Prevention of Ischemic Heart Disease.

In the years 1976–1979 a group of 2,343 men aged 20–59 years were randomly chosen and 1,808 were examined. The response rate was 77.2%. In the case of the second sample, 100 Polish women born in 1948 were randomly selected for the Multicenter Study on fat distribution in Europe under the auspices of the Agriculture University in the Netherlands, where 92 were examined. The response rate was 92%.

Two of the three methods generally accepted in the literature were chosen for evaluating obesity and overweight. Obesity was defined as follows: total body fat equal to 30% or more of body weight in males and 35% in females. Body fat was determined by the Durnin and Wormersley (1974) method, being the most common. It considers age and sex, and is relatively easy for use in most field investigations as it takes four skinfold measurements, at triceps, biceps, subscapular and iliac-crest. The Holtain caliper was used for these measures.

However, since even this method is too complex technically for certain field conditions, overweight was also determined with use of body height and weight measurements, using the definition that overweight is recognised when the value of the BMI index is equal to 29% or more in males and 26% or more in females. The BMI index is body mass in kg divided by body height in m^2.

Nevertheless, it should be added that although criteria of obesity and overweight were arbitrary, they fell within the 75th percentile of the total body fat or BMI in the Warsaw population. (Charzewska, Figurska and Wagrowska, 1981)

RESULTS AND DISCUSSION

In the light of criteria used, the prevalence of obesity in the whole male population of Warsaw was 14% and that of overweight was 18%. The difference between both criteria of the evaluation was small (Table I).

However, the relationship between obesity and overweight was quite different in the groups of young and older men (*see* Figure 1). The proportion of men with overweight increased particularly between the third and fourth decades of life, from 6% to 20%; after that age the curve forms a near plateau.

A period of the most intense rise in the proportion of obese men was noted at a later age than previously observed overweight increase, that is, between the 5th and 6th decades, when the relationships of obesity and overweight with age were different (Figure 1).

A fact worth stressing was that in a group of women aged 38 years, the difference between the proportions of obese women and women with overweight was much smaller than in men, being about 3% (*see* Figure 1).

Another question which may be asked is whether the difference between obesity and overweight is a reflection of age difference on the one hand or socioeconomic features on the other.

The social features analysed in this study were connected with the "style of life" of the social classes, a factor that might be a cause of greater prevalence of obesity in certain population groups. These features included: educational level, mean net income per capita per

TABLE I.   The prevalence of Obesity[a] and Overweight[b] in Warsaw

| | Age groups (years) | | |
	Younger 20–39	Older 40–59	Total 20–59
	%		
Obesity			
Males	3	24	14
Females	26	—	—
Overweight			
Males	11	23	18
Females	22	—	—

[a]Total body fat ≥ 30% in males and ≥ 35% in females.
[b]BMI ≥ 29% in males and ≥ 26% in females.

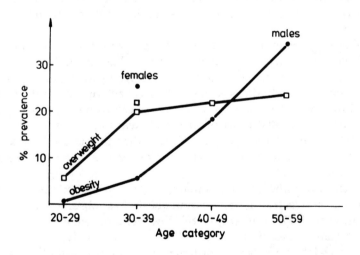

Figure 1.   The percent of prevalence of obesity by sex and age category, by criteria: total body fat ≥ 30% in males, ≥ 35% in females and overweight by critieria: BMI ≥ 29 in males, ≥ 26 in females.

family, degree of physical activity during occupational work and leisure time, and cigarette smoking. The degree of correlation between
social characteristics in the Warsaw group of males is shown in Table
II. It is evident that obesity was correlated with most social features
(Figure 2).

This part of the analysis of data is presented for the group of older
men, aged 40 years or older, since, as shown in Table I, both obesity
and overweight were present in a small proportion of younger men,
and thus their relation to social features was less evident.

Obesity was more frequent in men with a high educational level
than in those with lower levels. It was also more frequent in white collar workers than in those doing manual work, and in men with the
highest per capita income compared to those with lower income. The
highest proportion of obesity was found in men with low physical activity during occupational work, and nonsmokers were more frequently obese than smokers.

Those results generally confirmed the trends seen in U.S. males
(Garn et al., 1977; Stunkard, 1978). These researchers also observed a
positive relationship between affluence and the prevalence of obesity.
However, Stunkard (1978) suggested that obesity is also present in
less privileged groups.

For Warsaw women, it seemed that social features determined the
prevalence of obesity to a much greater degree than in men (see Figure 3).

Obesity was more prevalent in women with higher educational
levels than in those with lower educational levels, in divorced and
married women than in unmarried women and among multiparous
women than in childless women. Physical activity was not a factor
that differentiated the proportions of obese women, probably because the physical activity of all women was low. The effect of cigarette smoking on obesity was different than that in men, since the
proportion of obese women who smoked was higher than for nonsmokers.

Some other studies suggest that a very consistent but inverse relationship between social classes and obesity was observed in women
(Garn et al., 1977; Stunkard, 1978). However, a different pattern of results was obtained when the social features were analysed in relation
to overweight diagnosed according to the criteria of the Body Mass Index (see Figure 4).

The data indicate that smoking was the most important factor in
the prevalence of overweight, which was more prevalent among

TABLE II.   The Kendall rank correlation/*tau*, between social determinants in obesity study of Warsaw males, 1976–1979.

	1	2	3	4	5	6	7
1. Education	1.000	0.629*	0.420*	-0.479*	0.056*	0.005	-0.098*
2. Position		1.000	0.630*	-0.497*	0.067*	0.015	-0.072*
3. Occupation			1.000	-.0389*	0.087*	-0.021	-0.074
4. Physical activity, occupational				1.000	-0.056*	0.028	0.128*
5. Physical activity, in leisure time					1.000	0.044	-0.066*
6. Smoking in smokers						1.000	1.000
7. Smoking in population							1.000

*$p < 0.05$

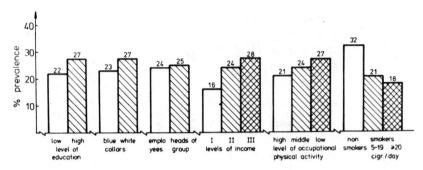

Figure 2. The percent prevalence of obesity by social determinants in Warsaw males aged 40–59 years.

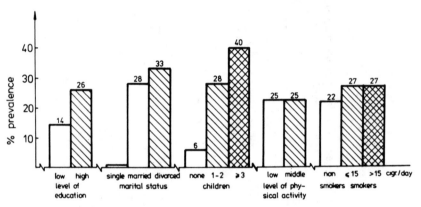

Figure 3. The prevalence of obesity by social determinants in Warsaw females aged 38 years.

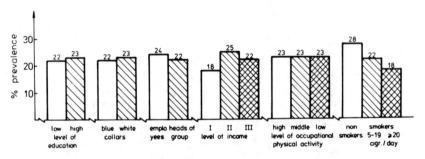

Figure 4. The percent prevalence of overweight by social determinants in Warsaw males aged 40–59 years.

nonsmokers than those smokers smoking over 20 cigarettes daily. Overweight was frequent in the group of men with a higher per capita income compared to the group with a lower per capita income. In industrialised countries results of studies on the relationship between social classes and overweight in terms of high relative body mass in men are rather conflicting. In Chicago (Garn *et al.*, 1977) and Birmingham (Khosla and Lowe, 1967), high relative body mass in males shows a tendency towards an inverse relationship, in contrast to Israel (Goldbourt and Medalie, 1974), Belgium (Kittel *et al.*, 1978), and to a lesser extent in Warsaw males.

Different trends in the relationship between social class and the prevalence of obesity and overweight are probably due, in part, to the variety of definitions and methods for assessing obesity and overweight. More studies are needed in order to explain the observed difference in the relationship between social and cultural factors and the prevalence of obesity.

CONCLUSION

The results obtained in this study made possible the following conclusions: in the Polish population, social features had an influence on the prevalence of obesity and overweight, but the influence on obesity was greater than for overweight.

The effect of some features on obesity was different between women and men. This should be kept in mind when data from various populations and countries are compared, since in most cases these data are not comparable, as obesity and overweight are not equivalent.

It is worth adding, finally, that although the aim of this study, as well as other similar studies of this type, was to estimate the social determinants of obesity, obvious implications for health are evident. Limiting obesity prevalence is an important part of prevention programmes for many diseases.

The outline of any prophylatic programme for obesity control must be based on a good knowledge of its social determinants for establishing which social groups are particularly prone to obesity development. However, since populations differ in levels of civilisation, urbanisation and culture, social determinants of obesity may be, and probably are, quite different.

NOTES

Jadwiga Charzewska received her Ph.D. and Ph.D. habilitatus from Jagiellonian University in Cracow. She works at the National Food and Nutrition Institute in Warsaw. Her interests include anthropology, nutrition and epidemiology. She is currently working on the effects of changes in socioeconomic conditions on the food intake and nutritional status (including the frequency of obesity) of children, adults and old people in Poland during the last ten years.

REFERENCES

Charzewska, J., K. Figurska, and H. Wagrowska 1981. The characteristics of the overweight and obesity indices. Part I. The use of the Quetelet index and other anthropometric patterns in interpopulational comparisons. *Przeg. Lek.* **38**, 277–282.

Durnin, J.V.G.A., and J. Wormersley 1974. Body fat assessed from total body density and its estimation from skinfold thickness: Measurements on 481 men and women aged from 16 to 72 years. *British Journal of Nutrition* **32**, 77–97.

Garn, S.M., S.M. Bailey, P.E. Cole and I.T.T. Higgins 1977. Level of education, level of income and level of fatness in adults. *American Journal of Clinical Nutrition* **30**, 721–725.

Goldbourt, U., and J.H. Medalie 1974. Weight-height indices. *British Journal of Preventive and Social Medicare* **28**, 116–126.

Khosla, T., and C.R. Lowe 1967. Indices of obesity derived from body weight and height. *British Journal of Preventive and Social Medicine* **21**, 122.

Kittel, F., R.M. Rustin, M. Dramamix, G.De. Backer and M. Kornitzer 1978. Psycho-social-biological correlates of moderate overweight in an industrial population. *Journal of Psychosomatic Research* **22**, 145–158.

Lee, R.B., and I. Devore 1968. Problems in the study of hunters and gatherers. In R.B. Lee and I. Devore (eds.), *Man the Hunter*. Aldine, Chicago. pp. 3–12.

Lowenstein, F.W. 1976. Preliminary clinical and anthropometric findings from the First Health and Nutrition Examination Survey U.S.A., 1971–1972. *American Journal of Clinical Nutrition* **29**, 918–927.

Silverstrone, J.T., R.P. Gordon and A.J. Stunkard 1969. Social factors in obesity in London. *Practitioner* **202**, 682–685.

Stunkard, A.J. 1978. Obesity and the social environment: Current status, future prospects. *Annals of the New York Academy of Sciences* **300**, 298–320.

West, K.M. 1973. Epidemiology of adiposity in regulation of the adipose tissue mass. Proceedings of the IV International Meeting of Endocrinology, Marseilles. *Excerpta Medica*, pp. 202–207.

World Health Organization, 1973. Food and nutrition terminology, Terminology Circular No. 27, Geneva.

11

Educational Attainment, Stress Hormones, Body Fat and Health: A Sociocultural Neuroendocrine Pathway?

DONNA L. LEONETTI, WILFRED Y. FUJIMOTO,
PATRICIA W. WAHL, GEOFFREY A. HARRISON,
and DAVID A. JENNER

INTRODUCTION

A full understanding of body composition and its relationship to health must ultimately come from an understanding of humans as *biocultural* beings: as products of the interrelationships among biological and sociocultural factors. Using data on adiposity, glucose tolerance, the catecholamines or "stress hormones," and educational attainment (as an index for sociocultural factors), this paper explores a set of such interrelationships in a sample of Japanese-American men. An hypothesis is then proposed that sociocultural factors and associated catecholamine secretory responses help regulate body fat distribution, which has implications for health, as seen here in glucose tolerance.

Obesity has long been known to be related to glucose intolerance. With the work of Vague (1956) and more recently, others (Evans et al., 1984; Feldman, Sender and Siegelaub, 1969; Haffner et al., 1986; Hartz et al., 1983; Kissebah et al., 1982; Mueller et al., 1984; Ohlson et al., 1985; Shuman et al., 1986; Stern and Haffner, 1986; Szathmary and Holt, 1983), the issue of body fat distribution rather than total adiposity as more critical to glucose tolerance has been actively pursued. Upper body obesity or android obesity (Vague et al., 1985), a high waist-to-hip ratio (Kissebah et al., 1982), and, more recently, intra-abdominal fat deposition (Sparrow et al., 1986; Newell-Morris et al., 1989) have been found to have strong associations with glucose intolerance.

The neuroendocrine system, as one of its functions, translates the individual's perceptions and emotions, as socially and culturally conditioned, into physiologic responses (Frankenhauser, 1975; Henry, 1982). The catecholamines, adrenaline and noradrenaline (or epinephrine and norepinephrine), are secreted from the adrenal medulla (primarily adrenaline) and sympathetic nerve fibres (noradrenaline only), and result from sympathetic nervous system activity. These hormones are involved in what is commonly thought of as "fight or flight" arousal or the "effort" response. As part of this response the catecholamines stimulate lipolysis, the breakdown of triglycerides stored in deposits of body fat for energy use (Pinter et al., 1967). Furthermore, specific fat deposits appear to be differentially sensitive to this lipolytic effect (Östman et al., 1979); in particular, intra-abdominal or visceral fat may be more sensitive to the lipolytic effects of adrenaline than is subcutaneous fat (LaFontan, Dang-Tran and Berlan, 1979). This differential sensitivity could, therefore, affect fat distribution, especially accumulations of intra-abdominal fat known to be associated with disease states (Sparrow et al., 1986; Newell-Morris et al., 1989).

Catecholamine production during daily living should reflect arousal and effort as individuals meet day-to-day challenges armed with training determined by their sociocultural world. This paper will focus on the educational attainment and associated characteristics of middle-aged and elderly Japanese-American men in relation to measures of catecholamines, body fat and blood glucose (Figure 1).

The study subjects are of the Nisei generation (American-born sons of immigrants from Japan). As children, the Nisei lived in homes

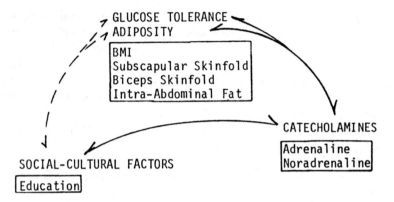

Figure 1. Diagram of interrelationships examined.

dominated by the Japanese cultural traditions of their parents and were economically and socially dependent on an immigrant community culturally rooted in a traditional Japanese agrarian past (Miyamoto, 1984). The predominant cultural orientation was toward hard work, educational achievement and socioeconomic mobility. A common educational goal was a college degree, which was achieved by about a third of the total Nisei generation. The formal education of the Japanese-American subjects took place in American schools and colleges and formed a most basic contribution to their exposure to and acculturation into American life. Besides serving as an indicator of lifestyle and health habits (Lambert *et al.*, 1982), educational attainment also represents achievement within American culture and society for Japanese-American men. Therefore, it can be viewed as a tool for coping with the American environment, understanding it and interacting with it in an accomplished manner. As a group the Nisei can be characterized as modern, urbanized, well-educated, and solidly in the socioeconomic middle class of the United States.

METHODS

Study subjects are from an estimated population of 1,542 Nisei male residents of King County, Washington, who were born between 1910 and 1939. The recruitment and selection of subjects have been previously described in detail (Fujimoto *et al.*, 1987a). Briefly, men with a self-reported history of diabetes or high blood or urine sugar as well as men with no such history were recruited in order to assure a broad spectrum of glucose tolerance levels in the sample. For the total sample, 229 men were enrolled in the study and were found to be representative of the Nisei men in King County with regard to age distribution, residential neighborhoods, and prefectures of origin in Japan of their parents (Fujimoto et al., 1987a), and to educational attainment (Leonetti, Fujimoto and Wahl, 1989).

The data analyzed in the present paper come from a subsample consisting of 124 Nisei men with a mean ($\pm$ SEM) age of 61.0 ($\pm$ 0.5) years. They include 54 men with normal glucose tolerance (NGT), 41 men with impaired glucose tolerance (IGT) and 29 men with noninsulin-dependent diabetes mellitus (NIDDM). No significant difference in age is found among the groups (Table I). These men remain from the larger sample of 229 men (Table I) after exclusion of those with missing values (n=7) and those taking a variety of medications that can potentially affect levels of catecholamines (decongestants, n=16, diuretics, n=54, adrenergic-blockers, n=42, and alpha-methyldopa, n=3). Men with diabetes using insulin (n=10) were also excluded. Some cases were excluded for more than one reason. As a result of these exclusions, the findings presented reflect the picture for those with less severe glucose intolerance (that is, not using insulin) and/or cardiovascular disease (for which many of the above drugs had been prescribed) or those with neither of these health conditions. However, the 105 subjects excluded do not differ significantly by age, educational attainment, residential distribution, or parental prefectural origin in Japan from the retained subjects.

All subjects participated in a 75-g oral glucose tolerance test (OGTT) which, along with individual medical histories, established the diagnostic categories using WHO criteria (World Health Organization Expert Committee on Diabetes Mellitus, 1980). This test provided the fasting and two-hour glucose levels. In a follow-up examination at approximately 30 months (range 28 to 34 months) of 92 (97%) of the nondiabetics (NGT, n=53; and IGT, n=39), a repeat OGTT identified 6 men who had newly developed diabetes.

Body fat measures presented here were chosen as representative of overall adiposity and of various deposition sites, that is, limb, subcutaneous truncal, and intra-abdominal areas. Weight was measured to the nearest hundredth kg on a calibrated balance scale with subjects clothed only in underpants and socks. Body mass index or BMI (kg/m^2), a measure of weight for height, was calculated. Skinfold thickness at the subscapula and biceps sites was measured to the near-

TABLE I. Sample numbers and age ($\bar{X} \pm$ SEM) by glucose tolerance categories (WHO criteria), Japanese-American men living in King County, Washington

	Total sample	Present sample	Age[a] (present sample)
Normal glucose tolerance, *NGT*	n = 79	n = 54 (68.4% retained)	60.7 ± 0.8
Impaired glucose tolerance, *IGT*	n = 72	n = 41 (56.9% retained)	60.5 ± 0.9
Non-insulin dependent diabetes mellitus, *NIDDM*	n = 78	n = 29 (37.2% retained)	62.4 ± 1.1

[a]Not significant by one-way analysis of variance.

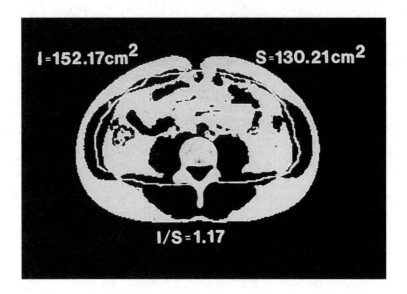

Figure 2. Computed tomography (CT) scan at the level of the umbilicus (top). White areas are fat and white line separates intra-abdominal fat from subcutaneous fat. Intra-abdominal fat equals 152.17 cm^2 in this individual.

est millimeter with Lange calipers (Tanner, Hiernaux and Jarman, 1981). A single (10 mm) computed tomography (CT) scan (GE 8800 Scanner) was taken of the abdomen at the level of the umbilicus (Shuman et al., 1986). Subjects underwent CT scans of the abdominal region without prior dietary or other intervention. A single scan has been previously shown to be representative of abdominal fatness (Borkan et al., 1982; Tokunga et al., 1983). Figure 2 shows a cross-section of the abdomen as produced by the CT scan with the fat shown in white. The fat area inside the abdominal cavity (see white line), was measured (cm^2).

Catecholamines were measured as the amounts excreted in the urine over a 24-hour collection period as previously described (Jenner et al., 1987). The urine collections were made during a day of usual activity and appear to represent the usual range of sympathetic nervous system activity experienced under free-living conditions (Jenner et al., 1987). The data on the catecholamines as measured by urinary excretion levels, of course, cannot take into account any alterations of blood levels through catecholamine metabolism and clearance. These measurements, therefore, may be somewhat imprecise as a reflection of catecholamine secretion. They do, however, provide the only noninvasive way to measure usual daily sympathetic nervous system responses.

The educational attainment variable has five levels: high school, technical school, some college, college degree, advanced degree. It is also dichotomized with respect to college education (some or none). Age is also statistically controlled because activity levels and the demands of working may decrease at older ages, particularly with retirement. Furthermore, age provides an adjustment for educational levels which were lower for the older Nisei than for the younger Nisei due to changing opportunities in their youth.

Educational attainment is also viewed in relation to other variables which reflect aspects of socioeconomic status and social life as follows: type of occupation (non-professional, professional); level of household income (less than $40,000/year, over $40,000/year); employment status (full-time, part-time, retired); marital status (ever married, never married); educational attainment of spouse (college, no college); having Caucasian or other non-Japanese friends (versus Japanese friends only); having friends from work (versus no friends from work), having average contact of over twice a month with each friend (versus less contact); going out usually as a couple if married (versus not usually going out as a couple), usually going out to restaurants or bars to which other Nisei go (versus not usually going to these places).

Two sample t-tests and one-way analysis of variance are used in comparisons of groups. Comparisons controlling for other variables use analysis of covariance. Where distributions of the data are skewed, nonparametric Mann-Whitney and Kruskal-Wallis tests of significance are substituted. Pearson zero-order or Spearman rank-order correlations are used, depending on distributions of the data. Chi-square tests of significance are applied to contingency tables. Multiple regression analysis of intra-abdominal fat is used to test for the effect of each variable given the effects of other variables in the model.

RESULTS AND DISCUSSION

The results presented in Table II show 24-hour adrenaline excretion to be inversely and significantly related to the amount of intra-abdomi-

Donna L. Leonetti et al.

TABLE II. Correlations of measures of adiposity with the catecholamines,, Japanese-American men living in King County, Washington

| | BMI (kg/m²) | Intra-abdominal fat (cm²) | Subscapular skinfold (mm) | Biceps skinfold (mm) | BMI Components | |
					Weight (kg)	Height (cm)
Adrenaline (μg/24h)	-0.07	-0.21*	-0.01	-0.08	0.02	0.12
Noradrenaline (μg/24h)	0.26**	0.07	0.13	0.05	0.33***	0.21*

Spearman rank correlations: *$p<0.05$, **$p<0.01$, ***$p<0.001$.

nal fat in the sample of Japanese-American (Nisei) men. Noradrenaline is positively and significantly related to body mass index, BMI, as
well as to both weight and height. This latter set of relationships suggests noradrenaline is more related to body size than to adiposity.
Subscapular and biceps skinfolds are not related to either catecholamine.

A number of other studies have found an inverse relationship between adrenaline and body fat (Young and Macdonald, 1992). Intra-
abdominal fat, in particular, has been shown to be particularly
sensitive to the lipolytic effects of adrenaline in an experimental setting (LaFontan, Dang-Tran and Berlan, 1979). However, the present
research is the first to show any association between adrenaline and
intra-abdominal fat within the context of ordinary daily living of a
sample of men representative of a population group.

The association of less educational attainment with more intra-abdominal fat is also observed (Table III). When intra-abdominal fat is
adjusted for BMI and age, the difference between those men with and
without college education is even more evident. BMI differences,
when adjusted for age, are nonsignificant by educational attainment.
Subscapular and biceps fat both reflect the results for BMI.

Much research has shown obesity to increase with lower socioeconomic class in the modern western nations (Stunkard, 1977), and
educational achievement is one important component of socioeconomic class. In this sample, although education is not related to BMI,
the finding of an inverse association with intra-abdominal fat is consistent with that reported by Björntorp (1988) in male subjects of an
association of low levels of education with high waist-to-hip ratios.
Waist-to-hip ratios are known to be correlated with CT measurements
of intra-abdominal fat (Ashwell, Cole and Dixon, 1985).

The further significant association of educational attainment with
levels of adrenaline but not noradrenaline is present (Table IV). In a
similar study of catecholamine excretion in the population of urban
Oxford in Great Britain on persons following their usual daily round
of activities, one sample of persons in professional and managerial occupations composed largely of persons with higher levels of education had distinctly higher levels of adrenaline than another sample in
manual occupations (Jenner et al., 1980, 1987). Thus, there may be differential levels of mental stimulation by occupational category or
associated life style that are reflected in these data.

In multiple regression analysis of intra-abdominal fat, BMI, adrenaline, education (as dichotomized), and age are entered (Table V). BMI

TABLE III. Measures of adiposity ($\bar{X} \pm$ SEM): BMI (also adjusted for age), intra-abdominal fat (also adjusted for BMI and age), subscapular skinfold, and biceps skinfold by educational attainment categories, Japanese-American men living in King County, Washington

Education (n)	BMI (kg/cm²)	BMI (age-adjusted)	Intra-abdominal fat (cm²)	Intra-abdominal fat (BMI adjusted)	Intra-abdominal fat (BMI and age/adjusted)	Subscapular skinfold (mm)	Biceps skinfold (mm)
High school (34)	24.1±0.5	24.9	110.1±9.6	123.0	121.8	15.7±0.9	6.06±0.43
Technical school (19)	26.4±0.5	26.6	129.9±10.9	118.1	117.8	19.6±1.2	8.26±0.94
Some college (24)	25.0±0.6	25.1	85.8±9.6	90.1	89.3	18.5±1.5	6.58±0.72
College degree (35)	24.9±0.4	24.7	101.8±8.0	106.4	106.7	18.0±0.8	6.34±0.42
Advanced degree (12)	26.3±1.0	25.4	88.6±13.0	78.6	80.1	18.5±2.6	7.83±1.19
F	2.71	1.59	2.53	4.31	3.38	1.54	2.00
P	0.033	NS	0.044	0.003	0.012	NS	0.099
No college (53)	24.9±0.4	25.4	117.2±7.3	118.2	117.3	17.1±0.8	6.8±0.5
College (71)	25.5±0.3	24.7	94.2±5.6	93.2	94.6	18.2±0.8	6.7±0.4
t-test: p	NS	NS	0.012	0.001	0.005	NS	NS

TABLE IV. Measures of catecholamine ($\bar{X} \pm$ SEM) by educational attainment categories, Japanese-American men living in King County, Washington

Education (n)	Adrenaline (μg/24h)	Noradrenaline (μg/24h)
High school (34)	7.6 ± 0.9	57.4 ± 3.8
Technical school (19)	6.8 ± 0.9	55.9 ± 4.5
Some college (24)	8.1 ± 0.7	61.3 ± 3.2
College degree (35)	8.4 ± 0.8	55.4 ± 2.7
Advanced degree (12)	9.7 ± 1.0	63.4 ± 4.7
Kruskal-Wallis: p	0.095	0.34
No college (53)	7.3 ± 0.6	56.9 ± 2.9
College (71)	8.5 ± 0.5	58.7 ± 1.9
Mann-Whitney: p	0.02	NS

is entered to account for that portion of intra-abdominal fat which may simply be a function of overall body fat. The inverse relationships of adrenaline and education to intra-abdominal fat are significant and indicate that each has an independent relationship to intra-abdominal fat with all the variables entered. Moreover, in step-

TABLE V. Standardized regression coefficients and p-values from regression of intra-abdominal fat, Japanese-American men living in King County, Washington

	β	p
BMI (kg/cm^2)	0.57	0.0001
Adrenaline (1n μg/24h)	–0.17	0.02
Education (college = 1, no college = 0)	–0.22	0.006
Age (years)	0.02	NS

wise regression of intra-abdominal fat, it is also evident that the entry of education decreases the p-value (from $p=0.005$ to $p=0.02$) and the standardized regression coefficient of adrenaline, indicating that education appears to account for a portion of the adrenaline-fat relationship. Given the lipolytic effect of adrenaline to which intra-abdominal fat is particularly sensitive, these associations present the basis for an hypothesis that day-to-day adrenaline secretion represents one potential mechanism through lipolysis by which intra-abdominal fat deposits may be regulated. Furthermore, since adrenaline secretion is sensitive to the interaction of an organism with its social and cultural environment, a possible neuroendocrine pathway from the environment to body fat distribution of the individual can also be hypothesized.

Fat deposition in the intra-abdominal region has relevance for disease states, particularly for diabetes and cardiovascular disease (Sparrow *et al.*, 1986; Newell-Morris *et al.*, 1989; Bergstrom *et al.*, 1990; Björntorp, 1990). The hypothesis presented above, therefore, potentially links body fat distribution and these disease states with sociocultural environmental factors via a neuroendocrine (sympathetic-adrenal-medullary) pathway. Björntorp (1991) has recently proposed a similar role for another neuroendrocrine (pituitary-adrenal-cortical) pathway. Indeed, it would not be surprising to find integrated effects of these two pathways once they are more fully understood.

In the present sample, significantly less adrenaline is found for those with NIDDM compared with those with NGT and IGT (Table VI). Noradrenaline, on the other hand, shows no significant differences. Spearman rank-order correlation coefficients are -0.191 ($p=0.034$) between adrenaline and fasting serum glucose and -0.265 ($p=0.003$) between adrenaline and two-hour serum glucose. The correlations of fasting and two-hour serum glucose with noradrenaline are not significant.

With respect to glucose tolerance, differences by educational attainment (Table VII) are also significant. The men with no college education are again distinguishable from those with a college education, showing higher amounts of fasting glucose and two-hour glucose than the more well-educated. There is also a clear and significant ($p < 0.003$) gradient in educational achievement by diagnostic group, with 74.1% of NGT men, 48.8% of IGT men, and 37.9% of NIDDM men having college experience.

In our previous research on the total sample of 229 Japanese-American men, BMI was related only in a marginally statistically significant

TABLE VI. Measures of catecholamines ($\bar{X} \pm$ SEM) by glucose tolerance diagnostic categories, Japanese-American men living in King County, Washington

	NGT	IGT	NIDDM	
	(n = 54)	(n = 41)	(n = 29)	p^a
Adrenaline ($\mu g/24h$)	8.6 ± 0.6	8.4 ± 0.8	6.4 ± 0.7	0.02
Noradrenaline ($\mu g/24h$)	57.7 ± 2.1	61.1 ± 3.0	53.9 ± 4.0	NS

[a]*Analysis of variance (Kruskal-Wallis)

TABLE VII. Measures of catecholamines ($\bar{X} \pm$ SEM) by educational attainment categories, Japanese-American men living in King County, Washington

Education (n)	Fasting glucose (mg/dl)	2-hr glucose (mg/dl)
High school (34)	121.6 ± 7.1	189.3 ± 17.1
Technical school (19)	131.3 ± 10.7	227.6 ± 24.8
Some college (24)	117.0 ± 9.8	176.6 ± 21.4
College degree (35)	109.1 ± 3.7	161.2 ± 11.3
Advanced degree (12)	98.2 ± 1.8	131.8 ± 10.1
Kruskal-Wallis: p	0.017	0.024
No college (53)	125.1 ± 5.9	203.1 ± 14.2
College (71)	109.9 ± 3.8	161.4 ± 9.4
Mann-Whitney: p	0.004	0.005

way to abnormal glucose tolerance. However, measures of site-specific fat—subscapular and biceps skinfold thicknesses, and intra-abdominal fat as determined by a computed tomography (CT) scan—were highly significantly related to abnormal glucose tolerance (Newell-Morris *et al.*, 1989).

Within this subsample, measures of adiposity are not strongly related to glucose tolerance, with no significant differences shown by diagnostic status for BMI, intra-abdominal fat, subscapular skinfold and biceps skinfold. Spearman rank-order correlation coefficients for fasting and two-hour serum glucose and measures of adiposity are either marginally significant or nonsignificant. In the present restricted sample, the effect of the exclusion of 105 of the subjects from the total sample, including the subjects with the most advanced diabetes and cardiovascular disease, was to truncate variability in the measurements of adiposity previously found to be associated with glucose tolerance in the full study.

However, in the present sample, high levels of intra-abdominal fat and low levels of adrenaline appear to be associated prospectively with worsening to diabetes. For the 6 men found to have newly developed NIDDM at 30 months follow-up, at the time of the initial examination their mean ($\pm$ SEM) intra-abdominal fat had been 147.9 ($\pm$ 18.8) cm^2 (versus 100.2 $\pm$ 5.5 for the 86 men remaining non-diabetic, Mann-Whitney $p=0.036$). Their adrenaline had been 4.44 ($\pm$ 1.12) μg/24 hr (versus 8.96 $\pm$ 0.5, Mann-Whitney $p=0.008$). These values were among the highest for intra-abdominal fat and the lowest for adrenaline levels. Only one of the six men had any college education. In previous studies we have also found the amount of intra-abdominal fat to be a significant predictor of subsequent development of diabetes in Japanese-American men (Bergstrom et al., 1990).

Associations between lower adrenaline and higher levels of fasting and two-hour serum glucose as seen in these subjects have not been previously reported.[1] In fact, a role for high (due to stress) rather than low adrenaline levels in the etiology of diabetes has been proposed (Surwit and Feinglos, 1988). However, no data have yet been presented that directly show this proposed relationship (Surwit, Schneider and Feinglos, 1992).

An estimate of the prevalence of NIDDM at about 20% among Nisei men ages 45 to 74 years indicates that this population may have four times the rate of diabetes reported for men in Japan and two times that reported for U.S. Caucasian men of the same ages (Fujimoto et al., 1987a). It thus appears that the high rate of diabetes in this population, as in other populations experiencing rapid westernization (Bennett, 1983; Taylor and Zimmet, 1983), may represent an historically recent rise in disease in response to the challenge of living within a changing social and cultural world. It may be that in facing that challenge some Nisei men were not well prepared, for any number of reasons often beyond their control, due to lack of social, financial and educational resources. The associations observed in the present study between glucose intolerance and lower levels of educational attainment are not

TABLE VIII.   Percent with economic and social characteristics by educational attainment categories, Japanese-American men living in King County, Washington

	No college	College	
	(n = 53)	(n = 71)	p^a
Professional occupation	1.9	54.9	0.0001
Income >$40,000/yr	30.2	54.9	0.01
Employment status part-time	15.1	2.8	0.02
Never married	11.3	4.2	0.2
Spouse with college education	14.9	35.3	0.02
(n=men ever married	(n = 47)	n = 68)	
Caucasian friends	18.9	47.9	0.002
Friends from work	26.4	42.3	0.1
Contact frequency $\geq$ 24/yr	69.8	52.1	0.037
Go out as couple	45.3	67.6	0.005
Goes to Nisei restaurants/bars	39.6	23.9	0.09

[a]Chi-square test

unique. In studies in the United States (Drury, Danchik and Harris, 1985) and Israel (Medalie et al., 1978), higher educational level has been found to be related inversely to glucose intolerance.

To gain a somewhat expanded understanding of how education reflects aspects of Nisei life we have examined characteristics of Nisei economic and social life as related to educational attainment (Table VIII). Higher achievement is associated with a better income, a high status occupation, and a spouse with high achievement. Lower achievement is reflected in never marrying and working part-time. For those with more education, more friendships with members of the majority population and people at work indicate open, but not overly dependent (less contact) friend relationships. Couple entertainment may indicate a tendency to have a close, American-style marital relationship which features companionship. For those with less education, going to Nisei-frequented establishments may reflect retreating behavior for the larger American society and possibly some insecurity in feelings about it. These data, although sketchy, help us infer some emotional aspects of Nisei lives and thereby to gain some insight into the relationship between adrenaline and education.

In addition, we can identify a profile characteristic of the above findings in two examples among our Japanese-American subjects (Table IX): never married men (n=9) and post-retirement, part-time employed men (n=10). These two small groups appear to be somewhat out of the economic and sociocultural mainstream of the population. They are never-married men who lack the basic life achievement of marriage and post-retirement, part-time employed men of marriage and post-retirement, part-time employed men who appear to lack the necessary financial or emotional resources to fully retire, yet also lack the vigor to sustain full-time employment. Both small groups show a strong tendency to have less education than other Nisei men, lower adrenaline levels (especially the part-time employed men), larger areas of intra-abdominal fat, and a tendency to have abnormal glucose tolerance (either IGT or NIDDM). Although numbers are small and statistical tests of significance therefore have little meaning (and are not presented), the total profiles are distinctive.

The results presented suggest that day-to-day levels of adrenaline may play an intermediary role in the distribution of fat in the body. Data such as these on adrenaline, gathered within the context of daily life rather than in experimental investigations, are very rare. Although adrenaline secretion is commonly thought of as being associated with stressful situations and experimental data indicate high levels of adrenaline might be potentially harmful to health (Henry, 1982), our data suggest that during ordinary daily living moderately higher levels of adrenaline may represent an adaptive condition expressed physiologically in adipose tissue regulation.

Perhaps, as with so many aspects of life, too much is a bad thing but too little is also not good. Rather than an indicator of stress, moderately higher day-to-day adrenaline levels may reflect a busy, confident, active lifestyle associated with and promoted by educational achievement. It has been demonstrated experimentally that persons who have higher excretion levels of urinary adrenaline out-perform those with lower excretion levels with respect to speed, accuracy and endurance (Frankenhauser, 1971). Also, persons who respond to mental work with decreased adrenaline output are less efficient than those with increased output (Johansson and Frankenhauser, 1973). Furthermore, psychological traits of those who have a stronger adrenaline response include greater "ego strength" (Roessler, Burch and Mefferd,

TABLE IX. Profile of educational attainment, adrenaline, intra-abdominal fat and glucose tolerance for never married versus ever married men and for part-time employed versus full-time employed men and retired men, Japanese-American men living in King County, Washington

	No college education	Adrenaline (μg/24h)	Intra-abdominal fat (cm^2)	Abnormal glucose tolerance (IGT or NIDDM)
Never married (n = 9)	6 of 9 (66.7%)	7.0 ± 1.6	123.9 ± 9.8	8 of 9 (88.9%)
Ever married (n = 115)	47 of 115 (40.9%)	8.1 ± 0.4	102.5 ± 4.8	62 of 115 (53.9%)
Part-time employed (n = 10)	8 of 10 (80%)	5.5 ± 0.7	133.0 ± 14.3	8 of 10 (80%)
Full-time employed (n = 79)	27 of 79 (34.2%)	8.3 ± 0.4	104.3 ± 6.0	45 of 79 (57.0%)
Retired (n = 35)	18 of 35 (51.4%)	8.2 ± 0.9	95.2 ± 7.5	17 of 35 (48.6%)

1967) and fewer depressive tendencies (Frankenhauser and Patkai, 1965). Indeed, decreased adrenaline response in stressful situations appears to indicate generally poor adjustment (Johansson and Frankenhauser, 1973). Finally, in relation to fat deposition, recent research indicates high waist-to-hip ratios are associated with various psychosomatic and psychiatric manifestations (Björntorp, 1988).

Less educational attainment may be an indicator of less successful coping by the individual leading to reduced adrenaline responsiveness. Alternatively, persons with initially low adrenaline responsiveness may have achieved less education. Positive correlations between school grades and adrenaline excretion have been found in children (Johansson, Frankenhauser and Magnusson, 1973; Lambert et al., 1969). If so, the entire developmental period would be included in this framework for understanding body composition and its relationship to the pathogenesis of diabetes (Leonetti, Fujimoto and Wahl, 1989). Since the relationship of educational attainment to intra-abdominal fat carries an additional significant effect independent of adrenaline on intra-abdominal fat, other functional pathways between educational attainment and intra-abdominal fat may also be present, for example, through dietary and other health-related habits influenced by educational level (Leonetti et al., 1991).

Of course, educational attainment could also affect catecholamine levels and intra-abdominal fat deposition in functionally independent ways. Further longitudinal research may elucidate the various possibilities. The results of the present research are based primarily on cross-sectional epidemiological data and as such they can only provide patterns that suggest directions for further research. It is, therefore, obvious that a complete understanding of the phenomena addressed here must take into account many more variables in order to confirm or reinterpret these results and to place them within the complex phenomena of which they are but one part.

ACKNOWLEDGMENTS

We gratefully acknowledge the statistical assistance of Jane Shofer. Cynthia Hendrix made all of the anthropometric measurements under the direction of L. Newell-Morris. W.P. Shuman provided the CT data. We are particularly grateful to the King County Japanese-American community for the support and cooperation they have given this study.

This research was supported by USPHS Grant DK-31170 from the National Institutes of Health and by facilities and services of the Diabetes Endocrinology Research Center (DK-17047), the Clinical Nutrition Research Unit (DK35816) and the University Hospital General Clinical Research Center (RR37).

NOTES

Donna Leonetti is Associate Professor of Anthropology, University of Washington, Seattle, Washington. She is Project Director for the Japanese American Community Diabetes Study, the Nisei Aging Project and the Study of Japanese American Kinship and Demography. Her research has been focused on Japanese Americans and biological and cultural aspects of their adaptation as a migrant population in the United States.

Wilfred Y. Fujimoto is Professor of Medicine in the Division of Metabolism, Endocrinology and Nutrition at the University of Washington, and Associate Program Director of the Clinical Research Center, University of Washington Medical Center, Seattle, Washington. He has been Principal Investigator of the Japanese American Community Diabetes Study and his major research focus is pathogenesis of diabetes mellitus and obesity.

Patricia W. Wahl is Professor of Biostatistics and Associate Dean of the School of Public Health and Community Medicine, University of Washington, Seattle. She is Co-director of the Coordinating Center for the Cardiovascular Health Study in Older Adults. Her research interests are in the application of statistical methodology to cardiovascular disease, diabetes and kidney disease.

G. Ainsworth Harrison is Professor of Biological Anthropology in Oxford University. His research areas are aspects of adaptation, growth and stress.

David Jenner is a faculty member of the Department of Medicine, School of Medicine, University of Western Australia, Perth, Western Australia. His research on interpopulation comparisons of catecholamine excretions began at the Department of Biological Anthropology, University of Oxford, in collaboration with Professor G. A. Harrison.

1. It is conceivable that the lower levels of adrenaline associated with diabetes could be the result of autonomic neuropathy, a complication of diabetes which would tend to reduce levels of catecholamine secretion. The fact that adrenaline but not noradrenaline is significantly lower in men with diabetes makes this explanation somewhat unlikely. Furthermore, our previous research on autonomic neuropathy in relation to glucose tolerance shows no significant differences among the three diagnostic categories for measures of autonomic neuropathy (Fujimoto *et al.*, 1987b).

206 Donna L. Leonetti et al.

REFERENCES

Ashwell, M., T.J. Cole and A.K. Dixon 1985. Obesity: New insight into the anthropometric classification of fat distribution shown by computed tomography. *British Medical Journal* 290, 1692–1694.

Bennett, P.H. 1983. Diabetes in developing countries and unusual populations. In J. Mann, K. Pyorala, and A. Teuscher (eds.), *Diabetes in Epidemiological Perspective*. Churchill Livingston, London. pp. 43–57.

Bergstrom, R.W., L.L. Newell-Morris, D.L. Leonetti, W.P. Shuman, P.W. Wahl and W.Y. Fujimoto 1990. Association of elevated fasting C-peptide level and increased intra-abdominal fat distribution with development of NIDDM in Japanese-American men. *Diabetes* 39, 104–111.

Björntorp, P. 1988. Possible mechanism relating fat distribution and metabolism. In C. Bouchard and F.E. Johnston (eds.), *Fat Distribution during Growth and Later Health Outcomes*. Alan R. Liss, Inc., New York. pp. 175–192.

Björntorp, P. 1990. "Portal" adipose tissue as a generator of risk factors for cardiovascular disease and diabetes. *Arteriosclerosis* 10, 493–496.

Björntorp, P. 1991. Hypothesis. Visceral fat accumulation: The missing link between psychosocial factors and cardiovascular disease? *Journal of Internal Medicine* 230: 195–201.

Borkan, G.A., S.G. Grezof, A.H. Robbins, D.E. Hults, C.K. Silbert and J.E. Silbert 1982. Assessment of abdominal fat content by computed tomography. *American Journal of Clinical Nutrition* 36, 172–177.

Drury, T.F., K.M. Danchik and M.I. Harris 1985. Sociodemographic characteristics of adult diabetes. In National Diabetes Data Group: Diabetes in America: Diabetes Data Compiled 1984. U.S. Department of Health and Human Service, PHS, NIH, National Institute of Arthritis, Diabetes, and Digestive and Kidney Diseases. NIH: Publication No. 85–1468, pp. VII-1-VII-37, Washington, D.C.

Evans, D.J., R.G. Hoffman, R.K. Kalkhoff and A.H. Kissebah 1984. Relationship of body fat topography to insulin sensitivity and metabolic profiles in premenopausal women. *Metabolism* 33, 68–75.

Feldman, R., A.J. Sender and A.B. Siegelaub 1969. Difference in diabetic and nondiabetic fat distribution patterns by skinfold measurements. *Diabetes* 18, 478–486.

Frankenhauser, M. 1971. Behaviour and circulating catecholamines. *Brain Research* 31, 241–262.

Frankenhauser, M. 1975. Experimental approaches to the study of catecholamines and emotion. In L. Levi (ed.), *Emotions—Their parameters and measurement*. Raven Press, New York. pp. 209–234.

Frankenhauser, M., and P. Patkai 1965. Interindividual differences in catecholamine excretion during stress. *Scandinavian Journal of Psychology* 6, 117–123.

Fujimoto, W.Y., D.L. Leonetti, J.L. Kinyoun, L. Newell-Morris, W.P. Shuman, W.C. Stolov and P.W. Wahl 1987a. Prevalence of diabetes mellitus and impaired glucose tolerance among second-generation Japanese-American men. *Diabetes* **36**, 721–729.

Fujimoto, W.Y., D.L. Leonetti, J.L. Kinyoun, W.P. Shuman, W.C. Stolov and P.W. Wahl 1987b. Prevalence of complications among second-generation Japanese-American men with diabetes, impaired glucose tolerance, or normal glucose tolerance. *Diabetes* **36**, 730–739.

Haffner, S.M., M.P. Stern, H.P. Hazuda, M. Rosenthal, J.A. Knapp and R.M. Malina 1986. Role of obesity and fat distribution in non-insulin-dependent diabetes mellitus in Mexican Americans and non-Hispanic whites. *Diabetes Care* **9**, 153–161.

Hartz, A.J., D.C. Rupley, R.D. Kalkhoff and A.A. Rimm 1983. Relationship of obesity to diabetes: Influence of obesity level and body fat distribution. *Preventive Medicine* **12**, 351–357.

Henry, J.P. 1982. The relation of social to biological processes in disease. *Social Science and Medicine* **16**, 369–380.

Jenner, D.A., V. Reynolds and G.A. Harrison 1980. Catecholamine excretion rates and occupation. *Ergonomics* **23**, 237–246.

Jenner, D.A., G.A. Harrison, I.A.M. Prior, D.L. Leonetti, W.J. Fujimoto and M. Kabuto 1987. Inter-population comparisons of catecholamine excretion. *Annals of Human Biology* **14**, 1–9.

Johansson, G., and M. Frankenhauser 1973. Temporal factors in sympatho-adrenomedullary activity following acute behaviour activation. *Journal of Biological Psychology* **1**, 67–77.

Johansson, G., M. Frankenhauser and D. Magnusson 1973. Catecholamine output in school children as related to performance and adjustment. *Scandinavian Journal of Psychology* **14**, 20–28.

Kissebah, A.H., N. Vydelingum, E. Murray, D.J. Evans, A.J. Hartz, R.D. Kalkoff and P.W. Adams 1982. Relationship of body fat distribution to metabolic complications of obesity. *Journal of Clinical Endocrinology and Metabolism* **54**, 254–260.

LaFontan, M., L. Dang-Tran and M. Berlan 1979. Alpha-adrenergic antilypolytic effect of adrenaline in human fat cells of the thigh: Comparison with adrenaline responsiveness of different fat deposits. *European Journal of Clinical Investigation* **9**, 261–266.

Lambert, C.A., D.R. Netherton, L.J. Finison, J.N. Hyde and S.J. Spaight 1982. Risk factors and life style: A statewide health interview survey. *New England Journal of Medicine* **306**, 1048–1051.

Lambert, W.W., G. Johansson, M. Frankenhauser and I. Klackenberg-Larsson 1969. Catecholamine excretion in young children and their parents as related to behaviour. *Scandinavian Journal of Psychology* **10**, 306–318.

Leonetti, D.L., W.Y. Fujimoto and P.W. Wahl 1989. Early life background and the development of non-insulin dependent diabetes mellitus (NIDDM). *American Journal of Physical Anthropology* **79**, 345–355.

208 Donna L. Leonetti et al.

Leonetti, D.L., R.W. Bergstrom, W.P. Shuman, P.W. Wahl, D.A. Jenner, G.A. Harrison and W.Y. Fujimoto 1991. Urinary catecholamines, plasma insulin and environmental factors in relation to body fat distribution. *International Journal of Obesity* 15, 345–357.

Medalie, J.H., J.B. Herman, U. Goldbourt and C.M. Papier 1978. Variations in incidence of diabetes among 10,000 adult Israeli males and the factors related to their development. In R. Levine and R. Luft (eds.), *Advances in Metabolic Disorders*, Vol. 9. Academic Press, New York. pp. 93–110.

Miyamoto, S.F. 1984. *Social Solidarity among Japanese in Seattle*. University of Washington Press, Seattle.

Mueller, W.H., S.K. Joos, C.L. Hanis, A.N. Zavaleta, J. Eichner and W.J. Schull 1984. The diabetes alert study: Growth, fatness and fat patterning, adolescence through adulthood in Mexican Americans. *American Journal of Physical Anthropology* 64, 389–399.

Newell-Morris, L.L., R.P. Treder, W.P. Shuman and W.Y. Fujimoto 1989. Fatness, fat distribution and glucose tolerance in second-generation Japanese American (Nisei) men. *American Journal of Clinical Nutrition* 50, 9–18.

Ohlson, L.O., B. Larsson, K. Svardsuss, L. Welin, H. Eriksson, L. Wilhelmsen, P. Björntorp and G. Tibblin 1985. The influence of body fat distribution on the incidence of diabetes mellitus. 13.5 years of follow-up of the participants in the study of men born in 1913. *Diabetes* 34, 1055–1058.

Östman, J., P. Arner, P. Engfeldt and L. Kager 1979. Regional differences in the control of lypolysis in human adipose tissue. *Metabolism* 28(No. 12), 1198–1205.

Pinter, E.J., G. Peterfy, J.M. Cleghorn, CJ. Pattee and H. Wetzel 1967. The influence of emotional stress on fat mobilisation: The role of endogenous catecholamines and the adrenergic receptors. *American Journal of Medical Sciences* 254, 634–651.

Roessler, R., N.R. Burch and R.B. Mefferd, Jr. 1967. Personality correlates of catecholamine excretion under stress. *Journal of Psychosomatic Research* 11, 181–185.

Shuman, W.P., L.L. Newell-Morris, D.L. Leonetti, P.W. Wahl, V.M. Moceri, A.A. Moss and W.Y. Fujimoto 1986. Abnormal body fat distribution detected by computed tomography in diabetic men. *Investigative Radiology* 21, 483–487.

Sparrow, D., G.A. Borkan, S.G. Gerzof, C. Wisniewski and C.K. Silbert 1986. Relationship of fat distribution to glucose tolerance. Results of computed tomography in male participants of the normative aging study. *Diabetes* 35, 411–415.

Stern, M.P., and S.M. Haffner 1986. Body fat distribution and hyperinsulinemia as risk factors for diabetes and cardiovascular disease. *Arteriosclerosis* 6, 123–130.

Stunkard, A.J. 1977. Obesity and the social environment: Current status, future prospects. *Annals of the New York Academy of Sciences* 300, 298–320.

Surwit, R.S., and M.N. Feinglos 1988. Stress and autonomic nervous system in type II diabetes: A hypothesis. *Diabetes Care* **11**, 83–85.

Surwit, R.S., M.S. Schneider and M.N. Feinglos 1992. Stress and diabetes. *Diabetes Care* **15**, 1413–1422.

Szathmary, E.J., and N. Holt 1983. Hyperglycemia in Dogrib Indians of the Northwest territories, Canada: Association with age and a centripetal distribution of body fat. *Human Biology* **55**, 493–515.

Tanner, J.M., J. Hiernaux and S. Jarman 1981. Growth and physique studies. In J.S. Weiner and J.A. Lourie (eds.), *Practical Human Biology.* Academic Press, London. pp. 8–16.

Taylor, R., and P. Zimmet 1983. Migrant studies in diabetes epidemiology. In J. Mann, K. Pyorala and A. Teuscher, (eds.), *Diabetes in Epidemiological Perspective.* Churchill Livingstone, London. pp. 58–77.

Tokunaga K., Y. Matsuzawa, K. Ishikawa and S. Tarui 1983. A novel technique for the determination of body fat by computed tomography. *International Journal of Obesity* **7**, 437–445.

Vague, J. 1956. The degree of masculine differentiation of obesities. *American Journal of Clinical Nutrition* **4**, 20–34.

Vague J., P.H. Vague, J.M. Meignen, J. Jubelin and M. Tramoni 1985. Android and gynoid obesities. Past and present. In J. Vague, P. Björntorp, B. Guy-Grand, M. Rebuffe-Scrive and P. Vague (eds.), *Metabolic Complications of Human Obesities.* Excerpta Medica, Amsterdam. pp. 1–12.

World Health Organization Expert Committee on Diabetes Mellitus 1980. Second Report. Technical Report Series 646. WHO, Geneva.

Young, J.B., and I.A. Macdonald 1992. Sympathoadrenal activity in human obesity: Heterogeneity of findings since 1980. *International Journal of Obesity* **16**, 959–967.

III

SOCIAL PHENOMENA ASSOCIATED WITH OBESITY

──12──

Changing Food Consumption and Body Images among Malays

CHRISTINE S. WILSON

INTRODUCTION

For the last two decades the diet, health and socioeconomic life of villagers in a *kampung* on the East Coast of the Malay Peninsula have been a focus of study for me, in which techniques of nutritional and anthropological research have been used. Formerly rural, remote and dependent on sea fishing for subsistence, this community has experienced marked socioeconomic change since the late 1970's due to exploitation of offshore oil in the South China Sea, that has altered the resource base, food choices and activity patterns, all of which influence body size and health.

This paper outlines initial findings on factors that contribute to obesity, and effects on them of dramatic changes recently experienced, particularly intensification of modernization, as observed 16 years after the first study was conducted.

METHODS

The research was conducted in 1968–9, 1970–1 and 1984. Data were collected using participant observation, open-ended and structured interviews, modifications of standard dietary survey techniques (Wilson 1970,1974) and, in the first two study periods, clinical examinations performed by physician colleagues. Corroborative medical and nutritional information was provided by local and national authorities throughout the research.

Household demographics, socioeconomic status, expenditures and food-sharing practices were determined by a combination of two complete censuses, one in 1968–9, the other in 1984, and daily inquiries of samples of households regarding income expenditures and numbers of persons participating in meals and other pertinent activities. Because of time constraints the data collected in 1984 were obtained chiefly by structured interviews on appropriate subsamples, except for the census-socioeconomic survey, which was done on every household.

RESULTS

Initial Studies

Twenty years ago about 5% of adults 16 years of age and above—14 males and 14 females—had body weights for height that would be termed obese, 20% or more above the "ideal" body weight given in life insurance figures (Briggs and Calloway, 1984). A like number was moderately overweight, and about the same number were marginally lean. Overweight was more prevalent in middle-aged women than in young adults, women busy with child-rearing and housekeeping under primitive conditions and men doing hard physical labour. (At 90.7kg (200 lbs) one woman in her 40s was nearly twice her "ideal" weight, 181.4% of "standard.") The majority of people 50 years and older were thin and there was a tendency to leanness in preschool and school-aged children.

Of 28 village children aged 6 months to 4 years (44% of the eligible toddler population) measured in a medical nutrition survey in 1969, only two had published "standard" weights (Jelliffe, 1966); 3 were about 90% of standard. The rest had lower weights that resembled those of Malaysian Army dependent children used for comparison (Wilson, 1970). In length/height the village children tended to resemble the Army dependents, both populations being below the Harvard (Stuart-Meredith) standards (see Weech, 1954). Records of height and weight measurements on 141 school children aged 6 through 11 years showed a population shorter and leaner than U.S. children of the same ages. The Malay children were at approximately the 10th percentile for both measures in each sex. Differences in weight from the U.S. sample were more pronounced than those for height. Indirect measures of body fatness in the toddler group (triceps skinfolds and midarm circumference) indicated very low arm fatness and relatively large muscle mass (significantly greater than that of the Malay child groups used for comparison), indicating a lean, well-muscled beginning to body development (Wilson, 1970).

Quantitative observations of meal and snacking practises and examination of household food procurement and consumption patterns indicated average caloric and protein intakes from the usual rice-plus-fish diet were adequate to maintain the body size of these relatively small, slight villagers (Wilson, 1970). A variety of social and economic mechanisms, including food sharing among kin and neighbours and shopkeeper credit extended to fishermen during winter storms, assured that food was distributed equitably, although meals might sometimes be low in some nutrients. The village social structure was egalitarian, and incomes reported were low and generally similar within a fairly narrow range. Few families had income and assets greater than the norm. Financial uncertainty of the principal economic base, fishing, and the socially institutionalised requirement for equal treatment of everybody minimised differences and overt envy but not an admiration of comfort and monetary good fortune. Although those classed as obese or overweight were not only the relatively more affluent, and there were thin people among the better-off, villagers valued a certain degree of overweight as evidence of financial ease or health. "Gemuk molek" they would say, Plump is pretty. Conversely, "kurus hudus"—thin is ugly. Although Malays used to fear the evil eye would affect a child praised by an outsider for fatness and healthiness (Skeat, 1900) and used roundabout terms to protect it, by the 1960s a fat, overfed baby was a source of pride, pointedly an example of health and the parents' ability to feed it well. Since protein-energy malnutrition was not uncommon in rural parts of Malaysia into the latter half of this century, and still is seen in some pockets of poverty (Chong et al., 1984), this attitude is understandable.

The approving attitude toward overweight applied also to non-Malays. When the investigator gained weight from many cups of very sweet coffee or tea taken in exchange for information and help, people remarked, "*Datang disini, menjadi gemuk-molek!*" You came here and got fat (plump)—it's attractive!

My housekeeper-friend Fatimah indicated the break-up of a first marriage and unhappy second one made her become thin. Only after return to her parents' roof, to some measure of peace (and ample food), did she resume the marginal obesity she considered her appropriate body size. Besides symbolising beauty and wealth, fat also indicated content, a life without strain. Indeed, "*makan, makan!*"—*eat,eat!* was urged on guests as the ultimate good a host could offer.

Extreme overweight was a source of ridicule and amusement. The woman who weighed 200 pounds was a frequent butt of jokes, some originated by herself. The title of her nickname, *Me' Gemuk* (Fatty), suggested she had been given the name early in life, since *Me'* is a common title for young girls prior to marriage, but other villagers indicated she had become grossly obese after age 40, despite continual hard work. Both village midwives were heavy, and approaching their 60s. Both were also hard-working. One admitted she sometimes wore a man's *sarong* (tube-shaped garment worn waist-down) because they were bigger than those made for women. She was one of the more affluent community members. Her colleague, though married to a famous *bomoh* (traditional medicine man) was, like *Me' Gemuk*, in more modest circumstances. Thus body size did not always reflect wealth.

Despite a substantial number of thin people in all age groups and food intakes that were sometimes marginally low, there were no overt signs of nutritional deficiencies in this *kampung* in 1968–9. Tuberculosis, upper respiratory illness, skin infections, intestinal parasites and lousiness were the chief health problems noted. "High blood" (hypertension) or more rarely heart problems were sometimes mentioned but other obesity-related health-impaired conditions were not reported, except that *kencing manis*—sweet urine, diabetes—was known but no one would admit to being affected. An indigenous treatment for diabetes was consumption of the bitter bean-like seeds of the *petai (Parkia speciosa)* or the related *jiring (Pithecolobium lobatum*: Wilson, 1985a). Both beans were said to be good treatment for obesity.

First Follow-up Study

Two subsequent research visits to this village (the second too brief to collect detailed data) showed only gradual changes in economic status and eating practises. A 1970–1 study of household economics and subsistence for several weeks during two seasons in 31 households indicated costs and incomes had risen about 10% in the intervening two years (Wilson, 1980). Body sizes and attitudes toward them were similar to those found in the earlier period. Two dozen adults were weighed before and after the fasting month of Ramadan,[1] during which all eating is done during the hours of darkness and extra amounts of sweet foods are consumed. Adult males, who worked less during these 29 days, tended to put on weight. Women, who put extra effort into housework and cooking special fast-breaking delicacies, remained the same size or lost weight, despite greater expenditures reported for food, especially high calorie items such as sugar, oil and condensed milk.

The food resources of villagers had expanded toward greater availability of commercial foodstuffs, including bread, rolls, sweet and plain biscuits and carbonated drinks, but the bulk of eating remained the traditional pattern of two rice meals a day with fish and vegetables fried or curried, and a snack, sometimes sweet, at breakfast and one or two other times during the day (Wilson, 1975). After mid-1969 about 20% of households raised up to a third of their annual consumption of rice in the village, or on land bought or leased elsewhere in the State. This productivity helped account for an increase of about 25% in average kcalories obtained from rice over earlier figures (Wilson, 1985b,1986a). Reported sugar and oil consumption remained about the same as values found in 1968–9.

Though western-type professional health care was sought for serious injuries, malaria and complications of pregnancy, and commercial tonics and patent medications were more widely used (for example, penicillin, available without a prescription, and "shots" for any perceived alteration of self-defined health), the majority of health disorders were defined in traditional ways. Correct recognition of a number of medical disorders was followed by nonscientific folk epidemiology as to their causation, but there was growing awareness that diabetes, obesity and hypertension were public health problems that could be alleviated or countered by cosmopolitan health treatment, although only a few cases were mentioned, and seldom with the degree of concern that would be assigned to them by westerners (Wilson, 1985a).

Second Follow-up Study

In 1984 the effects on village life and health of the sudden influx of outside monies into the region from offshore oil production that had begun about five years earlier was examined (Wilson, 1985b). They were many and notable. The numbers of dwellings, stable in earlier visits at 115, had increased to 171. The population had grown two-thirds to 960 individuals, mainly by internal biological growth. Whereas previously most adults were preliterate, and primary education was as far as most children were schooled, more than a quarter (255) of villagers in 1984 had had secondary schooling, and 21 had post-secondary training including some persons with university degrees.

Incomes had increased greatly in absolute terms, with considerable inequities in purchasing power and consumable property. Electricity in over 90% of homes (compared to 20% in 1968–69) had permitted introduction of the great common educator: Nearly two thirds of households had television sets, more than half of them in colour. Electricity had altered women's household and food-getting practises, and their physical activity. More than a third of households owned electric refrigerators, used to keep uncooked fresh food as well as leftovers. Similar numbers owned an electric rice cooker, blender, or both. Nine women had electric coconut graters. The meal pattern of rice with fish and coconut milk-based curries was not much changed, but methods of preparation were. Formerly coconuts were hand-grated and spices were pounded in a stone mortar, while home-raised rice was hulled by pounding the grains in a large mortar. These exertions were now supplanted by modern appliances, or ready-made purchasable ingredients. A village "factory" machine-ground curry spices for local and export sale, further removing the need for home pounding.

Whereas meals were formerly cooked over wood fires, most cooking was now done on kerosene- or gas-fueled stoves or cooking rings. Search for fuel and chopping it into suitable size had previously been one of women's daily chores. Another daily household task was the trip or trips to one of 49 village wells for water for food preparation and washing up. In 1984 75 households had their own well and, despite the considerable cost of installation, 62 householders had government-supplied water piped outside or within the house. Only 28 households now shared another's well. Thus by this decade a lot of vigorous and heavy work had been lifted from women's backs and arms, including laundry and sweeping. Half a dozen women had clothes-washing machines and a few owned vacuum cleaners.

Activities were reduced for both sexes and all ages. Automobiles, vans, or lorries, owned or rented, numbered 58 in 1984, contrasting with 3 or 4 in 1968–9. They were used as they sometimes are in developed locales to go half a mile down the highway to the new restaurant instead of walking or bicycling there. Bought hire-purchase, new or second-hand, the outlay these vehicles represent is further indication of greater availability of financial resources to many villagers. Although there were nearly twice as many bicycles (102) as motorcycles or motorscooters in 1984, the latter had largely replaced cycling, a former source of energy expenditure, for travel beyond the village.

Types of occupation had proliferated, many representing less active work than formerly. The number of fishermen were the same as 15 years before, 85 to 90, but the percent of men involved in fishing had declined from 70 to 44. Since nearly all boats were motorised, effort required in fishing was reduced. Almost half of other jobs held were clerical, teaching, driving, or some other semi-sedentary occupation. About one quarter of those of working age were unemployed or on welfare. There was no agricultural activity.

Because all food except fish for fishermen's families was purchased, amounts bought by 90% of households as reported in the census were converted to kcalories consumed per person per day by all persons over 18 months of age, and compared with similar data collected earlier. The amount of energy represented by rice had declined to half that consumed in 1970–1, nearly offset by an increase in kcalories from visible sugar, used chiefly in drinks and cooking at home, and an 83% increase in kcalories from fat, for a total per capita intake from these three foodstuffs alone of 1,341 kcalories (5,610 kJoules, Wilson, 1986a).

Further caloric sources, contributions of which have yet to be calculated, were flour, coconut milk used in curries, sweetened condensed milk, and snacks that included rolls with sweetened margarine, commercial cake, bread, sweet and plain biscuits, and other sources of invisible fat and sugar, noodles, packaged and tinned sweetened or soft drinks, ice cream, candies, potato crisps (chips), and a host of locally made snack items, variations of traditional foods that were calorically more dense than earlier counterparts. A common one, made locally as cottage industries, was dried fish chips, *kerupok*, reconstituted by frying in oil. Another popular breakfast or snack food was *nasi lemak*, "fat rice," boiled in coconut milk and served with a spicy fish or meat curry, taken several times a week. Such sweet rich foods were formerly reserved for special occasions and ceremonies.

Three additional sources of calories were introduced during 1984, two restaurants and a weekly night market. Men formerly took breakfast and snacks in coffee shops near home or work. The shops remained sources of quick calories, but the restaurants provided a new phenomenon, meals away from home midday and evening as well as breakfast. One did a brisk take-out business in the mornings of sweet or rich foods. Its meals included fried curried *mee* (Chinese noodles), or fried rice with shrimp. The other restaurant had a sophisticated menu of Thai and Malay food, curried, fried, or grilled. Besides fresh produce and household goods, the weekly market sold snack foods providing the buyer a second supper of calorie-dense foods such as fried curry puffs, fried *mee*, sweet rice cooked *lemak* (in coconut milk), and fish fried in batter. Since most of these foods were prepared at home by village women, the preponderance of fried items helps explain the increase in household oil consumption over earlier figures.

Three meals were still taken daily, but "lunch" or a bread meal was sometimes eaten at midday. Mothers cooked packaged noodles for children as morning or afternoon snacks, and complained that older children snacked on things from packets, *ringan*, light stuff.

Estimates of present day calorie intakes indicate that the traditional Malay snacking pattern substituting richer current items has more than compensated for the decrease in rice consumption, formerly the "bulk of consumption" (Wilson, 1985c). The two main meals—rice, fish and coconut-based curries—have not changed, but components have. Meat and chicken substitute for fish as new mobility makes larger markets and shops in the capital 12 miles away more accessible. Current diets are richer, calorically more dense than those to which adult villagers were accustomed in their youth. Higher caloric intakes and decreased physical activity probably explain a notable increase in numbers of overweight among the now middle-aged who were slim young people in 1968–9.

In 1984 the numbers of adult woman who were visibly overweight for height had more than tripled to 45 (21.7%). At least 15 men were similarly over desirable body weight. However, there was a new attitude toward it. A health questionnaire administered to a quarter of households produced reports of diabetes, headache, dizziness, heart and lung problems, hypertension, chest pain and kidney disturbances. One woman in her 60s had just died of diabetes, hypertension and kidney failure. Since the end of this follow-up study a man in his 50s was treated in hospital for a heart attack and returned safely home.

Willingness to seek cosmopolitan medical treatment is new (Wilson, 1986b). Though only two cases, these suggest others are at risk of consequences of "high blood," diabetes and obesity, understandable cause for increased anxiety in the community. Villagers' current perception that body size is related to these problems may be due to acceptance of health education by government professionals, but *kampung* people also seem to have reasoned it pragmatically for themselves. Cholesterol is not yet mentioned in the *kampung*; it may be before long. The principal cooking fat is red palm oil, produced in the country in quantity since the 1970s. Imported vegetable oils, available longer, are now less often used. Palm oil is relatively low in polyunsaturated fatty acids, and almost as high in saturated fat as coconut oil, the traditional cooking fat. Prudent diets for obesity and cardiac problems reverse the ratio of these types of fatty acids. (Recent studies suggest that palm oil is less cholesterogenic than other saturated diet fats, and unlike them does not induce thrombosis in experimental animals (Anonymous, 1988). (The factors involved require elucidation through further research).

DISCUSSION AND CONCLUSIONS

An increase in concern about overweight among younger people in this community may be due to awareness of what outsiders value. Television advertising uses slim young people in statusful activities. A 26-year-old housewife with secondary education, reared in an urban community before marrying into the *kampung*, embarrassedly requested permission to ask a personal question—not about money or family, but, how did I keep my figure trim? Did I eat differently to control my weight? Exercise? Her question was unusual for the community, but she may influence the attitudes of others. Exercise as a means towards body fitness was a new concept in this part of Malaysia. My friend Fatimah, now married to a successful businessman who prefers cosmopolitan-trained physicians, showed me a child's jump rope she had bought to help lower her now perceived too great body weight.

Fatimah and her husband visit the *kampung* frequently, passing on advice to receptive relatives and neighbours with interests beyond the village. The questions and concerns elicited in the 1984 study seem to be the beginnings of a change in health attitudes and behaviours in this village, needed because of major recent changes in diet and activity, from earlier bursts of intense effort and a diet relatively low in fats and calories to a more sedentary lifestyle with increased intakes of fats and easily assimilated carbohydrates, and increased deposits of body fat. Beginnings of modernised behaviours are partly responsible for these body changes. People who used to walk to a neighbour's or relative's to socialise and snack now sit at home, watching afternoon programs on *Talivisen Malaysia*.

There may be a genetic component to this trend toward fatness among Malays, a predisposition to become obese. They are the parent people of the Polynesians, some of whom are notably overweight (Bindon and Baker, 1985; *see* also Chapter 13.) I do not know of research on this aspect of obesity among Malays, but in earlier study periods I noted familial tendencies to stoutness, now blurred by others' increasing girth and pudginess.

Bindon has commented (1988) that eating taro, their essential starchy food, to Samoans will make one strong and, if thin, is prescribed as a curative. A common Samoan idea these days is that eating too much of it will make you fat. These people, too, now associate fatness with awareness of the relation between obesity and heart disease or diabetes (Bindon, 1988: 73). Lewis, working among the Micronesian peoples of Kiribati (1988: 89 ff) notes that urban residents now rely heavily on imported foods, particularly refined carbohydrates and fat. Most of these imports satisfy increased desire rather than supporting increased population (Lewis, 1988: 93). Rice and sugar consumption per person quadrupled between 1950 and 1977. Most of these Pacific populations earlier relied on a traditional type of diet, now much changed.

Since this Malaysian research was conducted other workers (Yassin and Terry, 1990, 1991) have reported dietary patterns and anthropometric characteristics of rural elderly women 55 years of age and above in the State of Negri Sembilan, in the western part of the country. This population, too, reported high use of rice, cooking oil, sugar and wheat-flour products (Yassin and Terry, 1990: 218). Both underweight and obesity were prevalent, and waist-hip ratios indicated excess body fat was preferentially deposited in the abdominal region, a finding associated elsewhere with increased risk for diabetes, hypertension and heart disease. Younger women in the sample were significantly taller and heavier, with a higher prevalence of excess body fat and more body muscle than older women (1991: 116).

These people (Wilson, 1985a,1985b)are changing their attitude toward body size to the western view that bigger is not necessarily better, as they become more aware of compromises in health that obesity can cause. It will be of interest to see what form their solution to this problem will take, and how it helps them deal with oncoming health problems.

Acknowledgments

The research reported here was supported by National Institutes of Health Grant AI–10051 to the Department of Epidemiology and International Health, University of California, San Francisco, through the U.C. International Center for Medical Research (UC–ICMR) at the Institute for Medical Research, Kuala Lumpar, Malaysia, and National Institutes of Health Grants GM–35,001–3 and AM–19152 to the investigator.

Special thanks are due to the Division of Human Nutrition, Institute for Medical Research, and its Director, Dr. Y.H. Chong, and the State of Terengganu Health Department, for continuing research support and advice throughout these studies.

The courtesy of 'Che Ismail b Mohd, Headmaster, Marang Primary School, in making available data on school child growth, is gratefully acknowledged, as are the clinical and research contributions of Dr. D.A. Mckay of the ICMR and Dr. J.C. White, University of Malaya School of Medicine, to these studies.

NOTES

Christine S. Wilson is a nutritionist-anthropologist and Editor of *Ecology of Food and Nutrition*. Her research has included ethnographic study of diet, nutrition and health in the culture and environment of Malay fishing people and urban Mexican Americans, composition of indigenous foods, effective methods for determining nutrient intakes, and effects of economic change on food behaviors and health. She has a bachelor's degree from Brown University and a doctorate from the University of California, Berkeley.

1. The official religion of Malaysia is Islam.

REFERENCES

Anonymous (1988). New findings on palm oil. *Nutrition Reviews* 45, 205–207.

Bindon, J.R. 1988. Taro or rice, plantation or market: Dietary choice in American Samoa. *Food and Foodways* 3, 59–78.

Bindon, J.R., and P.T. Baker 1985. Modernisation and obesity among Samoans. *Annals of Human Biology,*12(1),67–76.

Briggs, G.M., and D.H. Calloway 1984. *Nutrition and Physical Fitness*, 11th ed. Holt,Rhinehart and Winston, New York. pp. 160–164.

Chong, Y.H., E.S. Tee, T.K.W. Ng, M. Kandiah, R.H. Hussein, P.H. Teo and S.M. Shahid. 1984. *Status of community nutrition in Poverty kampungs*. Bulletin No. 22, Institute for Medical Research, Division of Human Nutrition, Kuala Lumpur, Malaysia.

Jelliffe, D.B. (1966). *The Assessment of the Nutritional Status of the Community*. World Health Organisation Monograph Series No. 53. World Health Organisation, Geneva, Switzerland.

Lewis, D.E., Jr. 1988. Gustatory subversion and the evolution of nutritional dependency in Kiribati. *Food and Foodways* 3, 79–98.

Skeat, W.W. 1900. *Malay Magic. Being an introduction to the folklore and popular religion of the Malay Peninsula*. Macmillan and Co., Ltd, London.

Weech, A.A. 1954.. Signposts on the highway of growth. *American Journal of Diseases of Children.* 88, 452–457

Wilson, C.S. 1970. *Food Beliefs and Practises of Malay Fishermen: An ethnographic study of diet on the East Coast of Malaya*. Ph.D. dissertation, Department of Nutritional Sciences, University of California, Berkeley.

Wilson, C.S. 1974. Child following: A technique for learning food and nutrient intakes. *Journal of Tropical Pediatrics and Environmental Child Health* 20, 9–14.

Wilson, C.S. 1975. Rice, fish and coconuts—the bases of Southeast Asian flavours. *Food Technology* 29(6),42–44.

Wilson, C.S. 1980. Nutritional reliance on income in a partially subsistent economy. *Federation Proceedings* 39, 654.

Wilson, C.S. 1985a. Malay medicinal uses of plants. *Journal of Ethnobiology* 5, (2),123–133.

Wilson, C.S. 1985b. Effects of sudden economic change on nutrition in a Malay village. XIII International Congress of Nutrition, Brighton, England.

Wilson, C.S. 1985c. Staples and calories in Southeast Asia: The bulk of consumption. In D.J. Cattle and K.H. Schwerin, (eds.), *Food Energy in Tropical Ecosystems*. Chapter 4. Gordon and Breach, New York.

Wilson, C.S. 1986a. Changing calorie sources in a newly affluent Malay village. Triennial Joint Meeting, American Institute of Nutrition, American Society of Clinical Nutrition, Canadian Society for Nutritional Sciences, Davis, CA.

Wilson, C.S. 1986b. Changing health beliefs and attitudes in a Malay village in transition. Joint Society for Medical Anthropology—British Medical Anthropology Society meeting, Cambridge, England.

Yassin, Z., and R.D. Terry 1990. Dietary patterns of rural elderly females in Malaysia. *Ecology of Food and Nutrition* **24**, 213–221.

Yassin, Z., and R.D. Terry 1991. Anthropometric characteristics of rural elderly females in Malaysia. *Ecology of Food and Nutrition* **26**, 109–117.

——— 13 ———

Polynesian Responses to Modernization: Overweight and Obesity in the South Pacific

JAMES R. BINDON

INTRODUCTION

Due to the time lag built into the process of natural selection, human metabolism is still conditioned by the physical and cultural environment of the last several millennia (Crews and James, 1991; Eaton, Konner and Shostak, 1988; McGarvey et al., 1989). Recent changes in our cultural environment have far out-paced the ability of selection to optimise our gene pool. As populations have gone through the transition from subsistence production to wage labor in a cash economy, increases in body size and mass have frequency been found (Damon, 1974; Walker, 1964; Hiernaux, 1972; Cassel, 1975; Hornabrook, Serjeantson and Stanhope, 1977). The more rapid the transition, the more likely it is that metabolic maladjustments will occur. Some Polynesian populations have experienced the transition primarily since World War II, and many of these populations exhibit extremely high body weights and rates of obesity and overweight (Bindon and Baker, 1985; Hunter, 1962; Prior, 1971; Prior et al., 1974; Pawson and Janes, 1981;

227

Zimmet and Björntorp, 1979). Today Polynesians are living lifestyles all along the continuum from traditional farming and fishing to urban industrial wage-earning. By examining groups at different points along this continuum, tentative inferences about the process of biological adjustment to modernization can be drawn. This paper presents the results of several studies of obesity and overweight among Samoans living in various settings. The pattern of the Samoan response to modernization is then compared to those of other Polynesian populations. Diet and activity are considered as causes of obesity in these groups. Finally, I will propose a model to explain the patterns of obesity found in Polynesian populations.

Modernization in Samoa

Comparisons between Samoan populations living in different environmental situations afford an opportunity to examine the relationship between various life style factors and obesity. Different segments of the Polynesian population of the Samoan Archipelago have undergone quite diverse modernization trajectories since European contact began in earnest in the 1830s. The development history of Samoa is, of course, unique to its historical particulars; however, the general outline is common to most Polynesian societies. I will provide a sketch of the course of development in Samoa as a background for my discussion of the relationship between modernization and obesity among Samoans. The first emissary from the London Missionary Society (LMS), John Williams, actively encouraged the Samoans to desire European products and to ready their island goods for traders. The LMS missionaries taught the Samoans to make presses for the extraction of coconut oil for export. The Samoan Islands became a major center during the middle of the 19th century for supplying coconut oil to Europe. The chief items of import (until about 1870) were cotton prints, shirts and trousers with which the missionaries determined to properly clothe the islanders.

Later in the nineteenth century the Germans entered the picture in the form of the commercial firm Godeffroy & Son, which established an agency in Apia Harbour in 1857. Apia (the modern-day capital of Western Samoa) became a hub of coconut oil, and later copra, collection for many surrounding island groups. Since German designs for the islands were centered on agricultural production, they were naturally drawn to the western part of the archipelago where the majority of the land lies (see Map, Figure 1). The land area of the two large is-

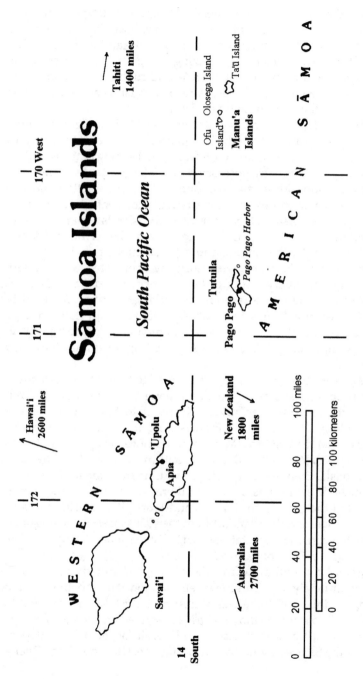

Figure 1. Map of the Samoan Archipelago.

lands in the west is approximately 2,823 km^2 (1,090 square miles) as opposed to the land area of the five eastern islands of 197 km^2 (76 square miles). The Germans bought Samoan land and established agricultural plantations, emphasizing the production of coconuts, and experimenting with coffee, cocoa and rubber. From about 1880 on, U.S. goals were shaped by a desire to establish a naval base in Pago Pago Bay on the eastern island of Tutuila.

Germany, the U.S. and Great Britain contested the right to control the archipelago throughout the last quarter of the nineteenth century. The end result of this competition was a partitioning of the islands in 1899 that gave Germany possession of the large islands in the west, and the U.S. took administrative control of the five smaller islands in the east. German control of the western islands continued only until 1918, when New Zealand took control of the islands as part of its protectorate in the Pacific. The U.S. islands became the Territory of American Samoa under the administrative jurisdiction of the U.S. Navy.

The American Samoans were abruptly confronted with western technology and life style through the advent of World War II. The U.S. Naval Base in Pago Pago harbour became a very active military facility. Briefly during the war, U.S. military troops actually outnumbered Samoans on the island of Tutuila. The Samoan way of life rapidly altered as imported goods and employment opportunities increased explosively.

The process of migration has also served to facilitate the transition away from subsistence production among Samoans. Both the migrants and their sedente relatives are exposed to the economic milieus of Honolulu, Auckland, San Francisco, or the other urban centers where the Samoans settled. MIgration was not a new phenomenon to Samoans as of World War II. Movements from village to village and island to island appear to have been routine from the initial time of settlement of the islands. However, there was no large-scale migration out of the islands until the second World War. During the war, some Samoans left the islands, but in the 1950s many more migrated out, as the economic expectations that had been generated by wartime employment could not realized.

The U.S. Navy withdrew from Pago Pago, and shifted its operations to Hawaii after the war. This meant elimination of most of the jobs that had opened up, and there was almost no industrial employment to lessen the impact of the move. The Navy offered an avenue of escape in the form of free transportation to Hawaii for relatives or dependents of the Samoans who had moved to work for the Navy. Over a thousand Samoans left Tutuila for Hawaii in 1952 alone. Between 1951 and 1956 almost 2,000 Samoans (about 1 in every 10 residents) left from the Territory of American Samoa to take up residence in the U.S. These Samoans established themselves in numerous communities, primarily in Hawaii and California. In spite of their absence from the islands, the Samoans retained their family ties, and hence their participation in *fa'alavelave* (the celebrations that mark various life crises such as births, marriages and title ceremonies) in the form of cash sent back to their families still living in the islands.

While the children in American Samoa were growing up with cola drinks and rock and roll, the American influence was much less invasive in the western half of the archipelago. As noted above, the lands of Western Samoa had been sought by Germany for agricultural production for export. This tradition was continued under the protectorate established by New Zealand at the conclusion of World War I. Two crops account for almost all of the agricultural exports from Western Samoa: coconut and cocoa. This situation remained essentially unchanged when Western Samoa became the first independent Polynesian nation in 1962. Demands for goods began to increase as the Western Samoans saw the increased flow of cash and goods into American Samoa. However, much of that demand can only be satisfied by migration across the seventy miles that separates Western and American Samoa. Currently (1993) Western Samoa is classified by the United Nations as a least developed nation.

While agricultural development has played an important role in Western Samoa, it has had only a minimal effect on American Samoa. In the more westernized setting, copra is the only significant crop export, but exports have declined sharply since World War II. Growth in subsistence production of breadfruit, banana, taro and coconut has seriously lagged behind population growth, and no new crops or agricultural techniques have taken root. As a consequence, American Samoa has had to import much of its food since World War II.

In American Samoa, a major campaign to improve economic and educational opportunities was begun by Governor Rex Lee, who administered the territory from 1961 to 1967. The U.S. congressional grant-in-aid to the territory increased to $9.5 million in 1962 from $2.1 million in 1961, and has continued to grow. In addition, a major tuna cannery began operating in the 1950s, and a second cannery and can manufacturing plant was opened in 1963, providing employment for thousands of Samoans. Products from fishery operations now account for over 90% of all export income. The school system was ex-

panded using educational television, which necessitated the
extension of electrical power to all villages throughout islands. The
electrification project was completed in 1971. A major road construction project has been completed, connecting almost all of the villages
on Tutuila with a good-quality paved road. At the same time, the medical facilities were upgraded, and construction of the Lyndon Baines
Johnson Tropical Medical Center was completed in the early 1970s.

The development histories of Western and American Samoa encompass both ends of the economic spectrum. Western Samoa, chart-
ing an independent course, continues as an economically under-
privileged country while American Samoa stands out as a pocket of
prosperity among the Polynesian countries. As a result of their history, there are groups of Samoans living under widely varying environmental conditions. The contrast between samples from Western and
American Samoa permits an examination of the influences of *in situ*
modernization. By virtue of the separate political and economic histories of the two Samoas, a natural experiment is available for study
whereby a relatively homogeneous group has been subjected to very
different processes of socioeconomic change. Similarly, comparisons
between samples in American Samoa and Hawaii allow an investigation of the influence of migration while at least partially controlling
for socioeconomic modernization.

METHODS

Sampling Procedures

The samples for this presentation were surveyed between 1975 and
1979. They comprised 2,657 Samoans between the ages of 20 and 85. In
Western Samoa, a whole village sample was surveyed in the rural village of Salamumu. In American Samoa, 42 villages were surveyed; the
samples are separated into villages in the outer Manu'a Islands, and
on the main island of Tutuila. In Hawaii, Samoan migrants living in
both urban and suburban settings on the island of Oahu were surveyed. While sampling was neither strictly random nor deliberately
stratified, the sample is generally representative of the populations
from which they are drawn in terms of age composition, employment
and education, although participation was substantially greater for
females than for males in all areas (Bindon and Baker, 1985).

The sample.   The sample from Salamumu, Western Samoa, consists of 142 males and 199 females, representing over 90% of the adult population of the village. Average years of education is fewer than nine, and less than 10% of the adults are employed for wages.

The sample from the Manu'a Islands, American Samoa, represents an intermediate level of modernization. This sample includes 96 males and 169 females representing about 40% of the adults in Manu'a. Average educational level is less than nine years, but about half the men and a quarter of the women are employed.

The sample from the villages on the island of Tutuila represents the most modernized group living in Samoa. This sample comprises 624 men and 842 women denoting 12% of the Tutuilan adults. Educational attainment averages slightly greater than 10 years, and about 60% of the men and 30% of the women are employed.

The Samoan migrants living in Hawaii include 250 males and 335 females. They average about 11 years of schooling, and over two thirds of the men and one third of the women are employed.

Measurements.   Height and weight were taken according to standardized techniques (Weiner and Lourie, 1969). Height was measured with an anthropometer made by GPM on barefoot subjects. Weight was measured on a balance scale with the subject wearing light tropical clothing. Weight has been corrected for clothing by subtracting 1 kg. Triceps skinfolds are reported for the samples in Manu'a, Tutuila and Hawaii. These measurements were taken using a Lange caliper, following Weiner and Lourie (1969). Body Mass Index (BMI) has been calculated as weight in kilograms, divided by height in meters squared. In studies of other Polynesian groups in which height and weight or BMI have been reported in alternate units, they have all been recalculated to correspond to the definition of BMI given above.

Obesity has been defined in a variety of ways in different studies. Most of this study will be concerned with overweight (more weight for a given height than is desirable according to some standard), as opposed to obesity (higher percentage of body fat than deemed desirable by some standard). For this study, the overweight boundaries used by the (U.S.) National Center for Health Statistics (NCHS) in their 1987 monograph on prevalence of overweight in the United States, 1976–1980, will be applied (Najjar and Rowland, 1987). This monograph uses the 85th percentile of BMI for young adults aged 20–29 years as the overweight criterion (27.8 for men, 27.3 for women), and the 95th percentile defines the severe overweight group (31.1 for men and 32.3 for women). These cutoff points correspond approximately to 20 and 40% above desirable weight according to the 1983 Metropolitan Life Insurance Company tables (Metropolitan Life Insurance Company, 1983; 1984).

RESULTS

Table I presents the percentage of each Samoan male from each area that would be considered nonoverweight, overweight, and severely overweight by the NCHS criteria. In Western Samoa, 20% or less of the men under age 40 are overweight, compared to about 60% in Manu'a and Tutuila, and about 70% in Hawaii. Over age 40, about 45% of the men in Western Samoa are overweight as compared to about 55% in Manu'a, 65% on Tutuila and 75% in Hawaii. The total adult overweight percentages for males are about 29% in Western Samoa, 55% in Manu'a, 59% on Tutuila and 67% in Hawaii. The comparable figures for Samoan females from the four areas are presented in Table II. Among Samoan females, about one third of the Western Samoan sample under 30 is overweight, compared to about 55–65% of the young women. Over age 30, about 60% of the Western Samoan women are overweight compared to over 80% of the other groups. The overall overweight percentages for women are 53% in Western Samoa, 73% in Manu'a, 78% in Tutuila and 74% in Hawaii. There are several features to note about the patterns of overweight displayed by the Samoans. First, it should be pointed out that these rates of overweight are extremely high, even among the Western Samoans. The NCHS reported that about 25% of males and 27% of females in the U.S. are overweight (Najjar and Rowland, 1987). While the rate among Western Samoan males is comparable to the U.S. rate, Western Samoan females have almost double the U.S. overweight frequency. The more modern Samoans have overweight frequencies more than double those of U.S. adults. Another striking detail in these tables is the great discrepancy in overweight between the samples from Western Samoa and all the other Samoan groups. There is relatively little difference between the Samoans in Manu'a, Tutuila and Hawaii by comparison with the gap from the Western Samoan samples.

A third notable element is the age patterning of overweight. Among Samoan males, the maximum frequency of overweight occurs in the 50s in Western Samoa, 30s in American Samoa, and 40s in Hawaii. For

TABLE I. Overweight according to BMI among four groups of Samoan males

Group (N)	Average BMI	% Normal	% Overweight	% Severely overweight
Salamumu, Western Samoa		71.4[a]		
20–29 (37)	24.6	83.8	13.5	2.7
30–39 (26)	26.2	80.8	11.5	7.7
40–49 (24)	27.1	58.4	20.8	20.8
50–59 (17)	29.8	52..9	11.8	35.3
60–69 (22)	26.6	54.5	31.8	13.7
Manu'a, American Samoa		44.3[a]		
20–29 (8)	28.4	37.5	62.5	0.0
30–39 (18)	29.9	27.8	38.9	33.3
40–49 (17)	28.7	41.2	35.3	23.5
50–59 (25)	27.4	48.0	32.0	20.0
60–69 (22)	27.9	50.0	27.3	22.7
Tutuila, American Samoa		40.8[a]		
20–29 (125)	27.5	59.2	20.0	20.8
30–39 (133)	31.2	25.6	33.1	41.4
40–49 (117)	30.9	32.5	22.2	45.3
50–59 (107)	31.1	26.2	25.2	48.6
60–69 (69)	29.0	37.7	30.4	31.9
Samoan migrants, Hawaii		33.3[a]		
20–29 (63)	30.5	36.5	28.6	34.9
30–39 (50)	32.1	18.0	30.0	52.0
40–49 (44)	30.8	13.6	38.6	47.7
50–59 (37)	32.2	27.0	27.0	46.0
60–69 (20)	32.3	35.0	20.0	45.0

[a]Percent adults nonoverweight over all age groups.

the females, maximum frequency of overweight occurs during the 30s and 40s for all groups. Among U.S. adults, maximum overweight occurs around age 50 for males and older for females (Najjar and Rowland, 1987).

A fourth point to emphasize is the much higher rate of overweight

TABLE II.   Overweight according to BMI among four groups of Samoan
females

Group (N)	Average BMI	% Normal	% Overweight	% Severely overweight
Salamumu, Western Samoa		47.4[a]		
20–29 (62)	26.4	66.1	22.6	11.3
30–39 (41)	28.3	43.9	36.6	19.5
40–49 (33)	29.8	33.3	30.3	36.4
50–59 (21)	30.3	33.3	38.1	28.6
60–69 (24)	29.9	41.7	20.8	37.5
Manu'a, American Samoa		26.6[a]		
20–29 (23)	29.4	43.5	30.4	26.1
30–39 (19)	34.4	5.3	26.3	68.4
40–49 (40)	33.5	10.0	32.5	57.5
50–59 (56)	31.4	33.9	25.0	41.1
60–69 (16)	30.3	25.0	37.5	37.5
Tutuila, American Samoa		22.3[a]		
20–29 (198)	29.3	42.4	32.8	24.8
30–39 (181)	34.1	10.5	32.6	56.9
40–49 (168)	35.1	8.9	29.2	61.9
50–59 (135)	35.2	14.1	23.0	63.0
60–69 (78)	32.4	25.6	19.2	55.2
Samoan migrants, Hawaii		25.9[a]		
20–29 (111)	31.2	33.3	28.0	38.7
30–39 (59)	34.7	11.9	23.7	64.4
40–49 (63)	35.5	9.5	25.4	65.1
50–59 (34)	33.6	17.6	26.5	55.9
60–69 (17)	34.1	17.6	29.4	52.9

[a]Percent adults nonoverweight over all age groups.

among females. In Western Samoa the females have about twice the
obesity rate, whereas in the other groups the female rate of overweight is about 30% higher than for the males.

Before comparing this pattern to that of other Polynesian groups, I want to briefly characterize the rest of the life cycle among Samoans. Birth weights in Western Samoa are in the middle of the range of world values, while birth weights in American Samoa are among the highest in the world (Bindon and Zansky, 1986a). Infants in both Western and American Samoa gain weight at an extremely rapid rate, especially during the first six months of life (Bindon and Cabrera, 1988; Bindon and Pelletier, 1986; Pelletier and Bindon, 1986). In Western Samoa, children and adolescents have BMIs near the U.S. median, while children in American Samoa and Hawaii average much higher than U.S. standards (Bindon, n.d.; Bindon and Zansky, 1986b). So the pattern of adult overweight and obesity is mimicked throughout the growth period.

How does the pattern of overweight among Samoan adults compare to that found among other Polynesian groups? First we must segregate the different Polynesian studies according to the position along the traditional-modern continuum. While there are many different ways to characterize modernization, one useful measure found to be related to a host of biological measures is the degree of participation of adult males in wage labor. Tables III through V provide population averages for body mass index among groups in which almost all males are engaged in subsistence production (Table III), in which some modernization has taken place, but fewer than half of the males are employed (Table IV), and in which over half of the males are working for wages (Table V).

One way to compare the disparate figures of average body mass index compiled in these three tables is simply to note whether the average exceeds the overweight boundaries of Najjar and Rowland (1987). Among the more traditional groups listed in Table III, none of the averages for males exceeds the BMI overweight boundary of 27.7, whereas five of the seven groups of females have averages of 27.3 or greater, the female overweight criterion. The two groups not having overweight female averages are the Pukapukans and the traditional Marquesans. There are a number of differences between these two groups. The Pukapukans were surveyed in the mid-1960s by Prior and his colleagues (Evans and Prior, 1969). The setting in Pukapuka is that of a coral atoll far off the beaten path in the Northern Cook Islands. By contrast, the Marquesas Islanders were studied in 1979 by a French team including Darlu and his colleagues (Darlu, Couilliot and Drupt, 1984). These islanders live on a high volcanic island, not far from the large Southern Marquesas island of Hiva Oa.

In spite of differences in time of surveys, type of island and proximi-

TABLE III. Average body mass index for selected Polynesian populations in relatively traditional settings (most males engaged in subsistence production)

	Males		Females	
Population (source)	N	BMI	N	BMI
Cook Islands:				
Atiu-Mitiaro (Hunter, 1962)	208	25.3	66	29.0[a]
Pukapuka (Evans and Prior, 1969)	172	25.1	163	26.4
Marquesas Islands:				
Traditional	27	23.4	53	25.1
(Darlu, Couilliot and Drupt, 1984)				
Tokelau Islands:				
(Prior et al., 1974)	255	26.7	319	29.4[a]
Tonga:				
Foa (Prior, 1977)	197	25.6	171	27.3[a]
Western Samoa:				
Rural (Jackson et al., 1981)	356	26.2	382	27.9[a]
Rural (this study)	140	26.2	196	28.3[a]

[a]Above NCHS overweight boundary.

ty to central areas, these two groups share several characteristics, including a heavy reliance on traditional farming and fishing foods at the time of the survey. Moreover, both groups are living in relatively undesirable Polynesian habitats. The coral atolls of Oceania are very limited systems ecologically, susceptible to disruption from major tropical storms (Pollock, 1975), and the Marquesas are considered among the least desirable of high volcanic Polynesian islands due to the lack of suitable arable land (Linton, 1923). Thus, not only do both groups represent a traditional life style, they both exemplify an environment where substantial effort is necessary to maintain subsistence production. The group from the Tokelau Islands also lives in a harsh setting on a series of coral atolls, but they have the highest average BMIs of all the more traditional groups. There is an historical explanation for this deviation from expectation. The Tokelau survey was carried out beginning in 1968, just two years after a major hurricane had

TABLE IV. Average body mass index for selected Polynesian populations in relatively traditional settings ($\leq$ 50% males in subsistence production)

	Males		Females	
Population (source)	N	BMI	N	BMI
Cook Islands:				
Rarotonga (Hunter, 1962)	151	26.9	38	27.8[a]
Rarotonga (Evans and Prior, 1969)	222	25.7	194	30.0[a]
Marquesas Islands:				
Westernized	24	26.6	33	28.1[a]
(Darlu, Couilliot and Drupt, 1984)				
New Zealand:				
Rural Maoris	89	28.7*	71	29.2[a]
(Prior, Rose and Davidson, 1964)				
Tuvalu:				
Funafuti (Zimmet et al., 1977)	189	26.7	207	29.0[a]
American Samoa:				
Manu'a (this study)	95	28.0*	164	31.5[a]

[a]Above NCHS overweight boundary.

devastated the islands. Following the hurricane, the New Zealand government established the Tokelau Island Resettlement Programme to cope with an expanding population in the face of limited resources (Prior et al., 1974). The relatively high BMIs for traditional Polynesians are no doubt the result of the New Zealand involvement with the people of the Tokelaus.

Among the intermediate populations represented in Table IV, all of the females have average BMIs in excess of the overweight standard, whereas only two of the groups of males exceed the criterion. The two groups with overweight male averages are the 1962 study of New Zealand Maoris (Prior, Rose and Davidson, 1964) and the Manu'ans reported in this study. These two groups of Polynesians probably have the highest male employment rate among all of the intermediate societies. One dramatic contrast should be noted between the males and females in Prior's study of the Rarotongans (Evans and Prior,

TABLE V. Average body mass index for selected Polynesian populations in relatively traditional settings (> 50% males employed for wages)

	Males		Females	
Population (source)	N	BMI	N	BMI
New Zealand:				
Tokelau migrants (Baker, 1984)	464	27.8[a]	363	30.1[a]
Tonga:				
Nuku'alofa (Prior, 1977)	179	28.4[a]	201	29.4[a]
Western Samoa:				
Urban (Jackson et al., 1981)	318	28.1[a]	412	30.9[a]
American Samoa:				
Tutuila (this study)	620	29.6[a]	820	32.8[b]
Hawaii:				
Samoans (this study)	246	30.6[a]	324	32.6[b]
Hawaiians (Bassett et al., 1966)	30	28.9[a]	—	—
California:				
Samoans (Pawson, 1986)	103	35.3[b]	105	36.4[b]

[a]Above NCHS overweight boundary.
[b]Above NCHS severely overweight boundary.

TABLE VI. Assignment of occupations to activity levels for Samoans in American Samoa and Hawaii

Activity level	Occupations
Low	Housewife, unemployed (in Hawaii), janitor, salesman, teacher, nurse, police, student, clergy
Medium	Plumber, electrician, cook, cannery worker
High	Construction worker, carpenter, agriculturalist

1969). The males have the lowest average BMI of the intermediate groups, a value that is in line with the BMIs among the studies listed in Table III. However, the females in this same study have one of the higher average BMIs, which would be more in line with the societies in Table V.

When we look at the groups in the modernized settings, the average BMI measurements for all groups, both male and female, exceed the boundary conditions of overweight. The most extreme condition is found among the massively overweight Samoan migrants living in California (Pawson, 1986). The Samoan males in California are the only males with average BMIs exceeding the severely overweight boundary criterion (31.1), whereas the Samoan females from Tutuila, Hawaii and California all have averages in excess of the severely overweight boundary (32.3). The BMIs for the rural Samoans are not out of line with the average measurements of the other traditional Polynesian groups. However, among the intermediate and modernized groups, the Samoans are at or near the top of the distribution of BMIs for both males and females.

As a cautionary note, it should be pointed out that Polynesians have very robust physiques. They are skeletally large and they also tend to have large muscle masses. Thus a BMI of 28 for a Polynesian does not necessarily mean the same thing as a BMI of 28 in the U.S. Black or white populations. That fact notwithstanding, there are clearly many overweight Polynesians. These tables confirm some of the patterns noted among Samoans. First, females have higher BMIs on average than males in all groups except the extremely overweight Samoans living in California. Second, the Polynesian females reach the overweight boundary at a lower exposure to modernization than do the males.

Consideration of causes of obesity usually starts with the diet, and in fact, in Samoa, one of the questions I was most asked by overweight adults was "Do you think I eat too much taro?" However, several dietary studies have been unable to demonstrate a relationship between obesity and dietary intake, either in terms of types of foods or amount of energy, for Polynesians (Bindon, 1982; 1984; Darlu, Couilliot and Drupt, 1984; Hanna, Pelletier and Brown, 1986). As a result, most attention has focused instead on the caloric expenditure or activity side of the energy equation.

In Rarotonga, Prior (1971) reported that the males are habitually hard-working, whereas the females are much less active, hence they display much greater obesity than do the males. Prior (1971) also noted that the wives of men who were employed in Pukapuka were substantially heavier than the other women on the island. Prior suggests (1971; 1977) that activity plays an important role in the development of overweight among Polynesian populations.

Many other workers have also emphasized the importance of changes in activity accompanying modernization as one of the primary causative factors in increasing obesity. Among the Marquesan villages studied by Darlu, Couilliot and Drupt (1984), a negative association between caloric intake and weight was found. However, these workers noted that the highest weights were found in the village with the lowest level of physical activity.

As part of my research in 1976 and 1977 on Samoan adults living in American Samoa and Hawaii, I investigated the relationship between occupational activity and obesity. Table VI illustrates the assignment of occupations to activity categories. The three activity categories (low, medium and high) were based on estimations of energetic expenditures in the different jobs (Leslie, Bindon and Baker, 1984). There was a very strong association between the area of residence of the Samoans (Manu'a, Tutuila, or Hawaii) and the level of activity, but the relationship was different for males and females. The highest levels of activity for males occurred in Manu'a, the most traditional of these three settings, whereas for females the highest level of activity occurred in Hawaii (Table VII).

Among the males, in whom there was appreciable variability in occupational activity levels, there was a highly significant association between activity and obesity (as assessed by the triceps skinfold measurement), with the least active males demonstrating nearly twice the rate of obesity of the more active males (Table VIII). The same relationship did not hold for females, which I attributed to a lack of variability in occupational activity among Samoan females (Bindon, 1981; Table VII). Zimmet and Whitehouse (1981) also attribute increasing rates of obesity among modernising Samoans to decrease in activity, although they provide no measure of activity.

Two other researchers have considered causes of obesity among Samoan adults. Pelletier (1984; 1987) has come up with an interesting hypothesis about caloric balance differences between Sundays and weekdays. Studying diet and activity among men in a rural village and in the capital (Apia) of Western Samoa, he found a pattern in which both groups of men indulged in substantial excess caloric intake on Sundays (a feasting day from early missionary times in Samoa). However, in the village, the men compensated for the excess by

TABLE VII.   Percent of Samoan adults in different occupational activity
categories by area of residence

Activity level	Manu'a	Tutuila	Hawaii
	Males		
Low (%)	33	28	62
Medium (%)	12	27	19
High (%)	55	45	19
Total (%)	100	100	100
(N)	95	619	243
	Females		
Low (%)	95	86	85
Medium (%)	5	13	4
High (%)	0	1	11
Total (%)	100	100	100
(N)	164	815	315

Significance of association (Kendall's tau): $p \leq 0.001$

TABLE VIII.   Percent of Samoan males in different fatness categories as
assessed by triceps skinfold by level of occupational activity

Level of fatness	Triceps Skinfolds (mm)	Level of Activity		
		Low	Medium	High
Lean	≤ 10	15	22	22
Medium	11 – 20	45	54	54
High	> 20	40	24	24
Total		100	100	100

Significance of association (Kendall's tau): $p \leq 0.001$

high weekday activity, and a slight negative energy balance throughout the rest of the week. By contrast, the urban men were more sedentary, and failed to balance their Sunday excesses during the rest of the
week. Schendel (1988) looked at two aspects of daily activity among

Samoan men and women in the same settings used by Pelletier. He found that overall levels of daily energy expenditure were not associated with obesity, but the maximum intensity of activity was, with the Samoans engaging in the highest energy-cost tasks being less obese than those pursuing less intense activity.

DISCUSSION

Several workers have endorsed various versions of the "thrifty gene" hypothesis proposed by Neel (1962) to account for relatively high frequencies of non-insulin dependent (Type II) diabetes mellitus (Baker, 1984; Prior, 1977; Zimmet and Whitehouse, 1981). Neel (1962) proposed that high rates of type II diabetes could be explained by genetic adaptations to limited and fluctuating food supplies. As others have pointed out, the Polynesians satisfy such conditions extremely well. Prior (1977) and Zimmet and Whitehouse (1981) focus on the sporadic availability of foods as a selective mechanism favouring genes for energy storage among Polynesians. The hazardous nature of their voyages of settlement as well as famine occasioned by severe tropical storms are emphasized by these authors. In addition to food limitation during such times, adequate energy storage prior to voyaging would provide a measure of insulation from the cold stress almost certainly experienced at night (Baker, 1984).

While these genes may have served the Polynesians well during the millennia prior to European contact, they appear to have become a detriment to health as life styles have changed to accommodate a cash economy. It is clear, however, both from the Samoan case and from other Polynesian populations, that it is not a simple matter of more modern groups becoming progressively more obese. The interaction of modernity with obesity is sex-specific, and to understand the pattern, the separate sex roles of Polynesian men and women in the context of modernization must be discussed. To begin with, what are the traditional economic roles of men and women? In Rarotonga and in Samoa, as well as many other Polynesian societies, there are clear-cut sexual divisions of labour. While the overall pattern is similar, I will discuss the Samoan case in detail, since it is the one with which I am most familiar.

Agricultural jobs are done predominantly by males. Men clear the bush where the taro gardens are planted. It is also men's work to carry the cuttings from harvested taro that are used to plant the new garden. Men will go to the gardens to bring taro, bananas, breadfruit and coconuts. Men and boys scrape the breadfruit and taro, and peel the green bananas. Most importantly, they grate the meat from ripe coconuts, and then squeeze the gratings to make coconut cream. Building the rock oven (*umu*) and cooking the food is also the task of the untitled men. Men engage in fishing, both within the reef and out to sea. The small dugout canoes (*paopao*) as well as the larger ocean-going bonito-canoes (*va'aalo*) require energetic rowing. If fishing is to be done within the reef, extensive swimming and diving is frequently necessary.

The traditional role of Samoan women includes gathering fish and shellfish from the reef. Women help in the weeding and harvesting of the gardens, but the success of the garden is said to depend on the hard work of the men. Women also help by gathering firewood, and collecting banana or breadfruit leaves to cover the rock oven. They are responsible for child-care and house cleaning, although in Samoa the older children play an important part in doing the household tasks.

Thus, the traditional division of labour dictates that men travel farther and work physically harder women. We saw that in the relatively traditional Polynesian groups, none of the males had average BMIs above the overweight boundary, while five out of the seven groups of females exceeded the overweight criterion (Table III). In rural villages in Western Samoa over 50% of the adult females were overweight (Table II), whereas in the very traditional and limited setting of Pukapuka, Prior (1971) reported that about one fourth of the women were overweight. At the same time, only about half as many Samoan men and a third as many Pukapukan men, as compared to their respective groups of women, were overweight.

Modernization also has gender-related concomitants. Men were the first to be incorporated into the wage-earning force in Samoa, and so they were the first segment of the household to be taken out of the family pool. The jobs available to men early in the process of development tend to be labour-intensive. So while they are producing cash instead of food, their level of activity is little changed. This phase of development would be exemplified by most of the intermediate societies in Table IV, where only two of the six groups of males surpassed the overweight boundary.

On the other hand, the early phases of development are conducive to a reduction in activity levels among women. All six of the groups in the intermediate table (Table IV) had average BMIs for females that were greater than the overweight criterion. In Samoa, when male labor is taken out of the household labor pool, changes in food gathering and preparation are necessary. Some of the first European dietary items incorporated into the Samoan diet were tinned meat and fish—taking the place of the protein foods that were previously gathered by the women (Bindon, 1982). In addition, food preparation shifted from the rock oven that the men make to kerosene stoves—more appropriate for women's use. That also freed women from having to gather firewood and the leaves used to wrap food and to cover the rock oven daily. These changes are reinforced by Samoan food ideology (Bindon, 1988). Samoan garden staples are traditionally prepared and cooked by men, whereas imported foods are appropriate for women to prepare. This distinction is related to the orientation of the Samoan village (*see* Shore, 1982:48–50) with the bush (*'i uta*) and its starchy products (*mea a'ano*) being in the realm of men, while light protein foods and imported goods (*mea lelei*, literally good things) come from the sea (*'i tai*), and are appropriate for females to prepare. There is much slippage of these divisions in practice, but it provides a rationale in traditional Samoan terms in favor of shifting from the traditional starches to imported ones since more female labor was available as the men started working outside the household.

As development progresses further, education and employment opportunities open up for the Polynesians, and they move from labor-intensive to knowledge-intensive jobs (see Table VII). As this happens, the men reduce their activity levels and substantial rates of overweight are found, such as those exemplified by the high average BMIs among the modernised groups in Table V, including the Samoans on Tutuila, in Samoa and Hawaii. At the same time, after the initial changes of development, little alteration of female activity patterns can be anticipated until they enter the wage pool in large numbers. Even when female employment accelerates, the women tend to take low-activity jobs, so there is no appreciable decline in obesity levels with additional modernization among Polynesian women. On the other hand, as more men take advantage of education, more of them end up in low-activity jobs, so there tends to be an increase in rates of overweight with modernization among men.

In summary, there are good reasons in the history of the Polynesians for them to have a genetic predisposition for obesity. Such a genetic tendency was probably strongly selected for during voyaging and settlement of the islands, and thereafter following storm damage to crops. However, as Polynesians move away from subsistence production and toward wage labour and purchased foods, the metabolic bias toward fat accumulation has become a detriment. As illustrated by both the Samoans and other Polynesian groups examined in this study, modernization of life style has varying effects depending upon the cultural context. Because the traditional division of labour in many Polynesian societies has the men performing much heavier work than the women, and because males get drawn into labour-intensive wage jobs early in development, females are at a greater risk of developing obesity earlier in the process than are the Polynesian men.

Other studies have demonstrated that modernising Polynesians suffer from increasing levels of chronic diseases including hypertension, coronary heart disease, and diabetes among others (Bindon, Crews and Dressler, 1991; Bindon and Crews, 1993; Crews, 1988; Janes and Pawson, 1986; McGarvey and Schendel, 1986; McGarvey and Baker, 1979; Prior and Tasman-Jones, 1981). From this presentation, it should be obvious that in the study of these problems the importance of the cultural context cannot be overlooked.

NOTES

James Bindon is a professor of Anthropology and Chairman of the Department at the University of Alabama. He has been studying Samoan diet, obesity and health for over 15 years. He recently has begun studies of obesity and obesity-related disease among the Mississippi Choctaw. Current interests include prevention and control of diabetes among Samoans and Choctaw.

REFERENCES

Baker, P.T. 1984. Migrations, genetics, and the degenerative diseases of South Pacific Islanders. In A.J. Boyce (ed.), *Migration and Mobility*. Taylor & Francis, Ltd., London. pp. 209–239.

Bassett, D.R., G. Rosenblatt, R.C. Moellering, Jr., and A.S. Hartwell 1966. Cardiovascular disease, diabetes mellitus and an anthropometric evaluation of Polynesian males on the island of Niihau—1963. *Circulation* **43**, 1088–1097.

Bindon, J.R. 1981. *Genetic and Environmental Influences on the Morphology of Samoan Adults*. Ph.D. Dissertation. Department of Anthropology, Pennsylvania State University.

Bindon, J.R. 1982. Breadfruit, banana, beef, and beer: Modernisation of the Samoan diet. *Ecology of Food and Nutrition* **12**, 49–60.

Bindon, J.R. 1984. An evaluation of the diet of three groups of Samoan adults: Modernisation and dietary adequacy. *Ecology of Food and Nutrition* **14**, 105–115.

Bindon, J.R. 1988. Taro or rice, plantation or market: Dietary choice in American Samoa. *Food and Foodways* **3**, 59–78.

Bindon, J.R. (n.d.). Body build and composition of Samoan children: Modernisation and migration influences. Unpublished observations.

Bindon, J.R., and P.T. Baker 1985. Modernisation, migration and obesity among Samoan adults. *Annals of Human Biology,* **12**, 67–76.

Bindon, J.R., and C. Cabrera 1988. Infant feeding patterns and growth of infants in American Samoa during the first year of life. *Human Biology* **60**, 80–92.

Bindon, J.R., and D.E. Crews 1993. Changes in some health status characteristics of American Samoan men: a 12 year follow up study. *American Journal of Human Biology* **5**, 31–38.

Bindon, J.R., D.E. Crews, and W.W. Dressler 1991. Life style, modernization and adaptation among Samoans. *Collegium Anthropologicum* **15**, 101–110.

Bindon, J.R., and D.L. Pelletier 1986. Patterns of growth in weight among infants in a rural Western Samoan village. *Ecology of Food and Nutrition* **18**, 135–143.

Bindon, J.R., and S.M. Zansky 1986a. Growth and morphology. In P.T. Baker, J.M. Hanna and T.S. Baker (eds.), *The Changing Samoans: Behaviour and health in transition.* Oxford University Press, New York.

Bindon, J.R., and S.M. Zansky 1986b. Patterns of growth in height and weight among three groups of Samoan pre-adolescents. *Annals of Human Biology* **13**, 171–178.

Cassel, J.C. 1975. Ponape-Palau blood pressure comparison. In J.M. Stanhope (ed.) *Migration and Health in New Zealand and the Pacific.* Epidemiology Unit, Wellington, N.Z.

Crews, D.E. 1988. Body weight, blood pressure and the risk of total and cardiovascular mortality in an obese population. *Human Biology* **60**, 417–433.

Crews, D.E., and G.D. James 1991. Human evolution and the genetic epidemiology of chronic degenerative diseases. In G.A. Lasker and N. Mascie-Taylor (eds.), *Application of Biological Anthropology to Human Affairs.* Cambridge University Press, London. pp. 185–206.

Damon, A. 1974. Human ecology in the Solomon Islands: Biomedical observations among four tribal societies. *Human Ecology* **2**, 191–215.

Darlu, P., M.G. Couilliot and F. Drupt 1984. Ecological and cultural differences in the relationships between diet, obesity and serum lipid concentrations in a Polynesian population. *Ecology of Food and Nutrition* **14**, 169–183.

Eaton, S.B., M.J. Konner and M. Shostak 1988. Stoneagers in the fastlane: Chronic diseases in evolutionary perspective. *American Journal of Medicine* **84**, 739–749.

Evans, J.G., and I.A.M. Prior 1969. Indices of obesity derived from height and weight in two Polynesian populations. *British Journal of Preventive and Social Medicine* **23**, 56–59.

Hanna, J.M., D.L. Pelletier, and V.J. Brown 1986. The diet and nutrition of contemporary Samoans. In P.T. Baker, J.M. Hanna and T.S. Baker (eds.), *The Changing Samoans: Behaviour and Health in Transition*. Oxford University Press, New York.

Hiernaux, J. 1972. A comparison of growth and physique in rural, urban and industrial groups of similar ethnic origin: A few case studies from the Congo and Chad. In D.J.M. Vorster (ed.). *Human Biology of Environmental Change*. London International Biological Programme.

Hornabrook, R.W., S. Serjeantson and J.M. Stanhope 1977. The relationship between socioeconomic status and health in two Papua New Guinean populations. *Human Biology* **5**, 369–382.

Hunter, J.D. 1962. Diet, body build, blood pressure and serum cholesterol levels in coconut eating Polynesians. *Federation Proceedings* **21**, 36–43.

Jackson, L., R. Taylor, S. Faaiuso, S.P. Ainuu, S. Whitehouse and P. Zimmet 1981. Hyperuricaemia and gout in Western Samoans. *Journal of Chronic Diseases* **34**, 65–75.

Janes, C.R., and I.G. Pawson 1986. Migration and biocultural adaptation: Samoans in California. *Social Science and Medicine* **22**, 821–834.

Leslie, P.W., J.R. Bindon and P.T. Baker 1984. Caloric requirements of human populations: A model. *Human Ecology* **12**, 137–162.

Linton, R. 1923. *The Material Culture of the Marquesas Islands*. Bernice P. Bishop Museum Memoirs, Honolulu. Vol. 8, No. 5.

McGarvey, S.T., and P.T. Baker 1979. The effects of modernization and migration on Samoan blood pressure. *Human Biology* **51**, 461–475.

McGarvey, S.T., J.R. Bindon, D.E. Crews and D.E. Schendel 1989. Modernization and adiposity: Causes and consequences. In: M.A. Little and J.D. Haas (eds.), *Human Population Biology: A Transdisciplinary Science*. Oxford University Press, London. pp. 263–279.

McGarvey, S.T., and D.E. Schendel 1986. Blood pressure of Samoans. In P.T. Baker, J.M. Hanna, and T.S. Baker (eds.), *The Changing Samoans: Behavior and health in transition*. Oxford University Press, New York. pp. 351–393.

Metropolitan Life Insurance Company 1983. 1983 Metropolitan height and weight tables. *Statistical Bulletin, Metropolitan Life Insurance Co.* **64**, 2–9.

Metropolitan Life Insurance Company 1984. Measurement of overweight. *Statistical Bulletin, Metropolitan Life Insurance Co.* **65**, 20–23.

Najjar, M.F., and M. Rowland 1987. *Anthropometric Reference Data and Preva-*

250   James R. Bindon

lence of Overweight: United States. 1976–1980. National Center for Health
Statistics, Vital and Health Statistics, Series 11, No. 238. DHHS Pub. No.
(phs) 87–1688. U.S. Government Printing Office, Washington, D.C.

Neel, J.V. 1962. Diabetes mellitus: A "thrifty" genotype rendered detrimental
by "progress"? *American Journal of Human Genetics* **14**, 353–362.

Pawson, I.G. 1986. The morphological characteristics of Samoan adults, In
P.T. Baker, J.M. Hanna and T.S. Baker (eds.), *The Changing Samoans: Behaviour and Health in Transition*. Oxford University Press, New York.

Pawson, I.G., and C. Janes 1981. Massive obesity in a migrant Samoan population. *American Journal of Public Health* **71**, 508–513.

Pelletier, D.L. 1984. *Diet, Activity and Cardiovascular Disease Risk Factors in
Western Samoan Men*. Ph.D. Thesis, Department of Anthropology, Pennsylvania State University.

Pelletier, D.L. 1987. The relationship of energy intake and expenditure to
body fatness in Western Samoan men. *Ecology of Food and Nutrition* **19**,
185–199.

Pelletier, D.L., and J.R. Bindon 1986. Patterns of growth in weight and length
among American Samoan infants. *Ecology of Food and Nutrition* **18**,
145–157.

Pollock, N.J. 1975. The risks of dietary change: A Pacific atoll example. In M.
Arnott (ed.), *Gastronomy: The anthropology of food and food habits*. Mouton,
The Hague.

Prior, I.A.M. 1971. The origins of civilisation. *Nutrition Today* (July-August) **6**,
2–11.

Prior, I.A.M. 1977. *Nutritional Problems in Pacific Islanders*. Nutritional Society
of New Zealand, Auckland, NZ.

Prior, I.A.M., B.S. Rose and F. Davidson 1964. Metabolic maladies in New
Zealand Maoris. *British Medical Journal* **1**, 1065–1069.

Prior, I.A.M., J.M. Stanhope, J.G. Evans and C.E. Salmond 1974. The Tokelau
Island Migrant Study. *International Journal of Epidemiology* **3**, 225–232.

Prior, I.A.M., and C. Tasman-Jones 1981. New Zealand Maori and Pacific
Polynesians. In H.C. Trowell and D.P. Burkitt (eds.), *Western Diseases:
Their emergence and prevention*. Harvard University Press, Cambridge,
MA.

Schendel, D.E. 1988. Daily activity, energy intake and body composition
among Western Samoans. *American Journal of Physical Anthropology* **75**,
267.

Shore, B. 1982. *Sala'ilua: A Samoan Mystery*. Columbia University Press, New
York.

Walker, A.R.P. 1964. Overweight and hypertension in emerging populations.
American Heart Journal **68**, 581–585.

Weiner, J.S., and J.A. Lourie 1969. *Human Biology*. F.A. Davis Co., Philadelphia.

Zimmet, P., A. Seluka, J. Collins, P. Currie, J. Wicking and W. DeBoer 1977.

Diabetes mellitus in an urbanised isolated Polynesian population. *Diabetes* **26**, 1101–1108.

Zimmet, P., and S. Whitehouse 1981. Pacific Islands of Nauru, Tuvalu and Western Samoa. In H.C. Trowell and D.P. Burkitt (eds.), *Western Diseases: Their emergence and prevention.* Harvard University Press, Cambridge, MA.

Zimmet, P., and P. Björntorp 1979. Adipose tissue cellularity in obese non-diabetic men in an urbanized Pacific Island (Polynesian) population. *American Journal of Clinical Nutrition* **32**, 1788–1791.

——14——

Activity Level
and Obesity among
Samoans

LAWRENCE P. GREKSA

Many societies are currently undergoing significant social, economic and biological changes due to exposure to a modern way of life. For simplicity, this process will be referred to as modernization. The purpose of this paper is to examine the impact of modernization on the activity levels of one group of Polynesians, Samoans, and to evaluate the impact of these activity level changes on the body size and body composition of Samoans.

The Samoan islands were first discovered by Europeans in 1722 but, for a variety of historical and cultural reasons, American Samoa was not significantly affected by contact with western nations until a U.S. government program of economic and technologic aid was instituted in the early 1960s. Some of the biological and social consequences of these changes have recently been summarized (Baker, Hanna and Baker, 1986). The present paper is concerned with one specific consequence of modernization in American Samoa, a substantial increase in body fatness.

The magnitude of obesity in modern American Samoans is emphasized in Figures 1 through 3, in which body size and body composi-

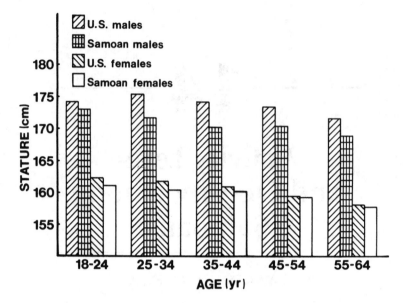

Figure 1. Stature in Samoan and U.S. adults.

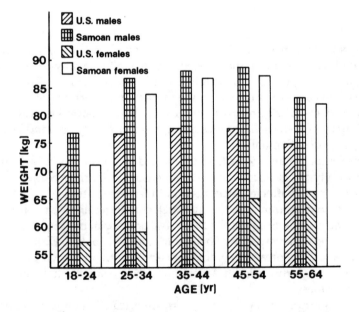

Figure 2. Body weight in Samoan and U.S. adults.

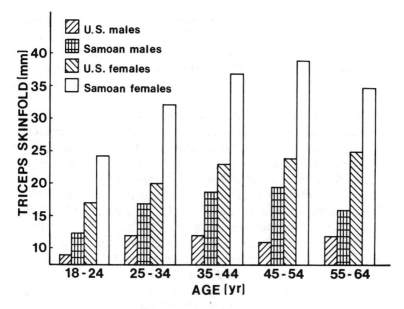

Figure 3. Triceps skinfold measures in Samoan and U.S. adults.

tion in a combined sample of American Samoans residing in American Samoa and Hawaii (1088 males and 1120 females) are compared with National Center for Health Statistics standards for U.S. adults (Stoudt, Damon and Roberts, 1965; Stoudt, Damon and McFarland, 1970; *see* also Chapter 13). As can be seen in Figure 1, median stature is similar between these populations, with American Samoans being somewhat shorter than U.S. adults. However, American Samoan adults are considerably heavier than U.S. adults (Figure 2) and, as demonstrated in the comparison of the median triceps skinfold, this difference in weight is largely due to differences in fatness (Figure 3). It is clear from an examination of these figures that modern American Samoans tend to be very fat. These comparisons are all the more striking when it is remembered that the U.S. population is itself noted for a high prevalence of obesity (Bray, 1977).

The role of modernization in the development of high levels of obesity in Samoans has been examined by comparing individuals living in Western Samoa, different regions of American Samoa, and Hawaii. These comparisons roughly reflect an acculturation gradient, with Samoans residing in Western Samoa being the least acculturated and Samoans residing in Hawaii being the most acculturated. These studies have found a generally positive relationship between level of modernization and degree of body fatness in both Samoan children and adults (Bindon and Baker, 1985; Bindon and Zansky, 1986a, 1986b; McGarvey, 1991; Pawson, 1986; Pawson and Janes, 1981). (*see* also Chapter 13).

The factors affecting energy balance are complex, but increase in body weight must ultimately be due either to increased energy intake, decreased energy output, or a combination of both. As is the case for most modernizing societies, American Samoa has undergone changes which have affected both components of energy balance. (Bindon, 1982, 1984, 1986; Greksa, Pelletier and Gage, 1986; Hanna, Pelletier and Brown, 1986; McGarvey et al., 1989; Pearson, 1990; Pelletier, 1987, 1988). For example, Bindon (1982) found that traditional foods make up only 68% of the diet in the most traditional areas of American Samoa. Also, Pirie (1970) estimated that the primary form of employment for Samoan males in 1960 was bush-fallow agriculture, but 14 years later only 3% of all economically active males in American Samoa were full-time agriculturalists (Levin and Pirie, 1974). Thus, both nutritional and activity patterns have undergone substantial modifications in American Samoa during the last 20 to 30 years and both are undoubtedly responsible to some extent for the substantial increases in body fatness which have occurred over the same period. In the remainder of this paper the importance of changes in one of these components, or activity level, on the body composition of adult American Samoans is evaluated by comparing the time and energy costs of traditional Samoan subsistence with those for modern wage labour. Little ethnographic information is available on the activity patterns of women and therefore the following discussion is limited to males. Where possible, energy costs for specific tasks are provided, standardized for a 65 kg man.

Since the time of the first European explorers, most observers have commented on the ease with which nutrient resources are acquired in Samoa (Stair, 1897; Turner, 1884). Traditional subsistence was based primarily on bush-fallow agriculture and secondarily on the exploitation of marine resources (Holmes, 1958; Kraemer, 1902; Watters, 1958). The division of labor was by sex and social status (Holmes, 1974; Mead, 1969). Females were concerned with household tasks and the harvesting of lagoon and reef resources while males were responsible for all other food production and preparation activities (Lockwood, 1971). All males, except perhaps those of very high social status, participated to some extent in subsistence activities. However, the more strenuous work was performed by untitled men under the supervision of titled men, or *matai* (Keesing, 1934). Since most untitled men were less than 30 years old (Holmes, 1958), this was equivalent to a division of labour by age.

A wide variety of plants was cultivated by Samoans but the bulk of the diet was provided by a few fruit and root crops. The primary staples were breadfruit, taro and bananas while coconuts, giant taro and yams were secondary staples (Holmes, 1974; Watters, 1958). Breadfruit, as in other Polynesian societies, was the preferred food and provided a substantial proportion of the diet during the approximate six months when it was available. Quantitative data on the composition of the Samoan diet are available for Manu'a, a group of three small American Samoan islands. The inhabitants of these islands are the most traditional in American Samoa. In a dietary survey conducted during the breadfruit season, Bindon (1982) found that breadfruit, bananas and coconuts provided 51% of the daily caloric intake in Manu'a. In a later study, Gage (1982) measured nutrient intake in one of the most conservative villages in Manu'a and found that an average of 66% of the daily caloric intake was provided by breadfruit and bananas during the breadfruit season.

Although fruit crops provided a substantial proportion of the Samoan diet for at least one half of the year, little time or energy was involved in their cultivation or collection, other than the initial planting (Gage, 1982; Holmes, 1974). For example, breadfruit trees were seldom systematically planted and only banana trees were weeded at all, and then only occasionally (Coulter, 1941; Gage 1982). The minimal requirements of these crops can best be emphasized by noting that the average *aiga* of about 8 individuals in rural American Samoa invests a total of only 30 minutes and 773 kJ (185 kcal) per day in the production and harvesting of breadfruit and bananas (Gage, 1986). These are the same crops which can provide up to two thirds of the caloric content of the diet during the breadfruit season.

The important root crops in the Samoan diet were taro, giant taro and yams. Taro was the primary staple during those periods when breadfruit was not available. Bindon (1982) found that taro provided 3.5% of the daily caloric intake in Manu'a during breadfruit season while Gage found that it provided 16% of the caloric content of the diet when breadfruit were not in season. Even though root crops were less important to the diet than fruit crops, their energy and time requirements for growing were three to four times those of the fruit crops (Gage, 1986). The root crops were grown on plantations located 3 to 8 km (0.62 to 5 miles) behind the village on the mountain side, often on slopes of 45 to 60 degrees (Coulter, 1941). The trip to and from the plantation was probably the most strenuous habitual task associated with traditional agriculture, with an energy cost of about 29.3 kJ/min (7.0 kcal/min) on the trip to the plantation and about 16.7 kJ/min (4.0 kcal/min) on the return trip.

The most strenuous single task associated with root crop production was the clearing of a new plantation. After the removal of the larger trees, brush was cleared, collected and burned. Even with steel tools the energy cost of this work is about 41.8 kJ/min (10.0 kcal/min), heavy work by most criteria. Although strenuous, this task was infrequent since a plantation was abandoned after only 2 to 4 years (Farrell and Ward, 1962; Watters, 1958). Taro, which were planted in holes created with digging sticks (oso), occupied approximately 70% of each plantation (Watters, 1958) and were weeded only once or twice during their 6 to 10 month maturation (Lockwood, 1971). Successive planting of the crowns of harvested taro (tiapula) was the practice. The weighted average energy cost of all tasks associated with plantation agriculture, including travel time, was about 27.2 kJ/min (7.1 kcal/min) (Greksa, Pelletier and Gage, 1986).

Gage (1986) reviewed the available data on the time requirements of Samoan agriculture (Fairbairn, 1973; Farrell and Ward, 1962; Gage, 1982; Lockwood, 1971) and concluded that only 6 to 12 hours per week of agricultural work would have been required of productive males in traditional Samoa. Expressed differently, an aiga's requirements for agricultural products could be met by 2 to 3 hours of work each week per aiga member. Thus, an aiga of 20 individuals would only need to provide a total of 40 to 60 hours of agricultural labor each week.

The other component of the Samoan economic system was the exploitation of marine resources, which provided the bulk of the daily protein in traditional Samoa. In general, fishing was performed by males while females harvested reef and lagoon resources (Holmes, 1974). Modern time-motion studies in Western Samoa indicate that 8 to 12 hours per week or less per aiga is spent in fishing activities (Farrell and Ward, 1962; Lockwood, 1971). No data are available on the energy cost of marine exploitation but few of the available strategies appear to have been strenuous.

In summary, the work associated with traditional Samoan subsistence was occasionally strenuous but, on the whole, was neither time-nor energy-costly. There is not a great deal of information available on nonsubsistence activities in traditional Samoa, but the data that are available suggest that few, if any, of these activities were more than moderately strenuous on an habitual basis. Thus, the activities associated with subsistence work, particularly plantation agriculture, were probably more strenuous than most other activities and therefore provide a very conservative estimate of activity levels of traditional Samoa.

The energy requirements of occupations in modern American Samoa will be discussed next, based primarily on a 1974 census conducted by the East-West Center (Levin and Pirie, 1974). In 1974, only 74% of all males above the age of 20 years were economically active. The proportion of economically active men varied with age: 68% of all men in the 20–29 year age group were employed, while about 87% of 30–39 year olds, 83% of the 40–49 year olds, 74% of the 50–59 year olds and 37% of the men greater than 60 years old were economically active. As noted earlier, only 3% of these men were full-time agriculturalists. Therefore, the remainder of this discussion will focus on wage laborers, the majority of whom (56% of all employed males) were employees of the Government of American Samoa. Forty-two per cent of these men had sedentary occupations while 58% were manual laborers.

The average energy requirements of the occupations available in modern American Samoa were determined from the literature (Durnin and Passmore, 1967; Katch and McArdle, 1983) and standardized for a 65 kg man. The average energy cost of the sedentary occupations (that is, professional occupations, clerical, sales) in modern American Samoa varies from 7.1 to 10.4 kJ/min (1.7 to 2.5 kcal/min). The average energy requirements of the available manual labor occupations (that is, service personnel, mechanics, construction workers) varies from 14.6 to 16.7 kJ/min (3.5 to 4.0 kcal/min). The work week is, of course, 40 hours in duration, but no information is available on the amount of time actually spent working. However, it is certainly reasonable to assume that a minimum of 6 to 12 hours per week, or an amount equivalent to that expended in traditional Samoa, is spent actively working.

Very few strenuous nonoccupational activities exist in modern American Samoa. For example, automotive transportation is used extensively, even for trips of a few hundred yards. The only strenuous sport in which many individuals participate is rugby and this is a seasonal sport primarily restricted to younger men. Thus, it is likely that occupational activity patterns are reasonably representative of over-all activity patterns for sedentary workers and may be a conservative estimate for manual laborers.

By their nature, the types of reconstructions attempted in this paper are speculative and thus only permit the drawing of tentative conclusions. Nevertheless, the available data suggest that the time and energy requirements of traditional Samoan subsistence were only moderate and certainly less than often envisaged for a traditional agricultural population. The average energy cost of plantation agriculture, the most strenuous of the subsistence activities, was about 27.2 kJ/min (7.1 kcal/min). Even if it is assumed that all subsistence activities were performed at this level of energy expenditure, a maximum of only 6 to 12 hours of agricultural labor and perhaps 5 to 10 hours of marine exploitation per week were required of males. In addition, due to the division of labor in traditional Samoa, younger males performed the most strenuous work so that older males worked at even lower levels of energy expenditure. In other words, although traditional Samoan males were certainly not inactive and occasionally performed highly strenuous work, the activity levels of young males were, on average, only in the low moderate range according to standard criteria (Karvonen, 1974) while older men were even less active. On the other hand, all of the wage labor occupations in modern American Samoa are classified as light work, or of lesser intensity than much of the work in traditional Samoa. In addition, almost one fourth of all modern American Samoan adult males are not economically active. Therefore, even given the relatively low level of work in traditional Samoa, there stills appears to have been a decrease in average occupational energy expenditure with modernization, although not necessarily a large decrease, especially for manual laborers.

Given that there appears to have been a decrease, albeit a moderate one, in average occupational energy expenditure with modernization in Samoa, it would be interesting to estimate the effect of such changes on energy balance and, in particular, to estimate the role that such changes have played in the development of the high levels of obesity found among modern American Samoans. An estimate of this effect can be obtained using the data presented in Figure 4. This figure compares average body weight in various subsamples of Samoans (Bars C to E) with the Metropolitan Life Insurance median ideal weight for large framed men of the same average height as American Samoan males (Bar A). Bar B is the average weight of 20–30 year old

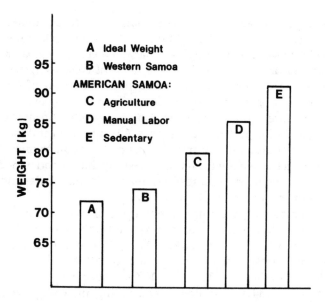

Figure 4. Body weight in Samoan populations by locale and activity patterns.

Western Samoan males, primarily village agriculturalists (Baker and Hanna, 1981). The last three bars represent, respectively, the age- and stature-adjusted weights of American Samoan agriculturalists, manual laborers and sedentary workers. The American Samoan agriculturalists are primarily from Manu'a, the most traditional part of American Samoa.

As noted earlier, Western Samoans tend to be the least acculturated Samoans. Thus, the sample of Western Samoan village agriculturalists most closely resembles the activity patterns of traditional Samoans. American Samoan wage laborers (manual laborers and sedentary employees) are among the least traditional Samoans and, as a result, differ from Western Samoan agriculturalists in many lifestyle characteristics, including nutritional and activity patterns. Comparison between these groups thus provides an estimate of the total average impact of modernization, via changes in both energy intake and energy expenditure, on body weight in Samoans. Next, comparisons between American Samoan wage laborers (manual laborers and sedentary workers) and American Samoan agriculturalists estimate the average independent effect of changes in occupational activity patterns as a result of modernization on body weight, since these men have otherwise similar lifestyles. Finally, American Samoan agriculturalists perform activities similar to those of Western Samoan agriculturalists. However, even the most traditional parts of American Samoa have been affected by modernization to some extent so that these men differ from the Western Samoans in other lifestyle characteristics, including nutritional patterns. A comparison of Western and American Samoan agriculturalists thus provides an estimate of the average effect on weight of changes in energy intake and nonoccupational activity patterns as a result of modernization, independent of changes in occupational activity level.

The average body weights of the samples of Western Samoan agriculturalists, and American Samoan agriculturalists, manual laborers and sedentary workers are 74.3 kg, 80.2 kg, 85.4 kg and 91.6 kg, respectively. The corresponding Metropolitan Relative Weights for these samples are 103%, 111%, 119% and 127%, respectively. The necessary comparisons can be simplified by calculating an average weight for the two categories of wage laborers. Thus, a weighted mean weight for these men, based on their participation rates in the work force (42% sedentary workers, 58% manual laborers), is 88.0 kg. It should be noted that the average weight of the Western Samoan agriculturalists is, as might be expected, similar to the Metropolitan ideal weight for men of that stature.

Using these data, one can infer a total average positive effect of modernization on the weight of Samoan males, due to changes in both components of energy balance, of about 14 kg (range: 11–17 kg), based on a comparison between Western Samoan agriculturalists and American Samoan wage laborers. Comparisons between American Samoan agriculturalists, on the one hand, and American Samoan wage laborers, on the other hand, suggest an independent effect due to change in activity patterns of, on average, about 8 kg (range: 5–11 kg). Finally, American and Western Samoan agriculturalists differ in average weight by about 6 kg.

These data thus suggest that modernization-induced changes in both components of energy balance have played important roles in the development of the high levels of obesity found among modern American Samoans. The comparisons described above suggest that modernization has resulted in a total average increase in weight in adult Samoan males of about 14 kg, with over half of this increase, or about 8 kg, on average, being due to changes in occupational activity patterns. These data thus suggest that changes in occupational activity patterns have played a more important role in the development of obesity in Samoans than was suggested by comparisons of the average energy requirements of traditional and modern work in Samoa. These comparisons indicated a decrease in average energy requirements of occupational tasks with modernization but ones of only moderate magnitude, especially in manual laborers. The simplest explanation for this apparent discrepancy is that even small differences in average energy expenditure could have a major impact on body weight over a lifetime. An alternative explanation, and possibly a complementary one, involves consideration of components of occupational activity patterns other than average energy expenditure. In particular, although average energy expenditure does not appear to have decreased greatly between traditional and modern Samoa, there was a decrease in the frequency of episodes of heavy intensity work (Schendel, 1988). Such episodes may not have been sufficiently frequent in traditional Samoa to have had a major effect on total energy expenditure, but they may have facilitated the proper functioning of the biochemical mechanisms which control food intake regulation or perhaps energy metabolism, especially given the possibility of genetic predisposition for obesity in Polynesian populations (Baker, 1984; Prior, 1977; McGarvey, 1991). Thus, even though the actual decrease in daily energy expenditure with modernization may not have been large, its effect on energy balance, both directly through energy expenditure and indirectly through an interaction with energy intake, may have been as important as increases in energy intake in the development of obesity in modern American Samoans.

NOTES

Lawrence Greska is an Associate Professor of Anthropology at Case Western Reserve University, Cleveland, Ohio. His research focuses on the nature and effectiveness of human biological responses to a variety of stresses, including social stresses such as modernization, and environmental stresses such as hypobaric hypoxia.

REFERENCES

Baker, P.T. 1984. Migrations, genetics, and the degenerative diseases of South Pacific islanders. In A.J. Boyce (ed.), *Migration and Mobility*. Taylor and Francis, New York. pp. 209–239.

Baker, P.T. and J.M. Hanna. 1981. Modernization and the biological fitness of Samoans: A progress report on a research program. In C. Fleming and I. Prior (eds.), *Migration, Adaptation and Health in the Pacific*, Epidemiology Unit, Wellington Hospital, Wellington, New Zealand., pp. 14–26.

Baker, P.T., J.M. Hanna and T.S. Baker (eds.), 1986. *The Changing Samoans: Behavior and health in transition*. Oxford University Press, New York.

Bindon, J.R. 1982. Breadfruit, banana, beef and beer: Modernization of the Samoan diet. *Ecology of Food and Nutrition* 12: 49–60.

Bindon, J.R. 1984. An evaluation of the diet of three groups of Samoan adults: Modernization and dietary adequacy. *Ecology of Foods and Nutrition* 14, 105–115.

Bindon, J.R. 1986. Dietary patterns of children in American Samoa: Multivariate analyses of food groups and household associations. *Ecology of Food and Nutrition* 18, 331–338.

Bindon, J.R., and P.T. Baker, 1985. Modernization, migration and obesity among Samoan adults. *Annals of Human Biology* 12, 67–75.

Bindon, J.R., and S.M. Zansky, 1986a. Growth patterns of height and weight among three groups of Samoan preadolescents. *Annals of Human Biology* 13, 171–178.

Bindon, J.R., and S.M. Zansky. 1986b. Growth and body composition. In P.T. Baker, J.M. Hanna and T.S. Baker (eds.), *The Changing Samoans: Behavior and health in transition*, Oxford University Press, New York. pp. 222–253.

Bray, G.A. 1977. Obesity in America: An overview. In George Bray (ed.), *Obesity in America*, National Institutes of Health, Washington. pp. 1–19.

Coulter, J.W. 1941. Land Utilization in American Samoa. *Bernice Bishop Museum Bulletin* 170. Bernice Bishop Museum, Honolulu.

Durnin, J.V.G.A., and R. Passmore, 1967. *Energy, Work and Leisure*. Heinman Educational Books, London.

Fairbairn, I.J. 1973. *The National Income of Western Samoa*. Oxford University Press, Melbourne.

Farrell, B.H., and R.G. Ward, 1962. The village and its agriculture. In J.W. Fox and K.B. Cumberland (eds.), *Western Samoa: Land, life, and agriculture in tropical Polynesia*, Whitcombe & Tombs, Ltd., Christchurch, New Zealand. pp. 177–238.

Gage, T.B. 1982. *Ecological Theories of Diet and Food Production: A case study of Samoan subsistence agriculture*. Ph.D. dissertation, The Pennsylvania State University, University Park.

Gage, T.B. 1986. Environment and exploitation. In P.T. Baker, J.M. Hanna and T.S. Baker (eds.), *The Changing Samoans: Behavior and health in transition*, Oxford University Press, New York. pp. 19–38.

Greksa, L.P., D.L. Pelletier, and T.B. Gage 1986, Work in contemporary and traditional Samoa. In: P.T. Baker, J.M. Hanna and T.S. Baker (eds.), *The Changing Samoans: Behaviour and health in transition*, Oxford University Press, New York. pp. 297–326.

Hanna, J.M., D.L. Pelletier and V.J. Brown, 1986. The diet and nutrition of contemporary Samoans. In P.T. Baker, J.M. Hanna and T.S. Baker (eds.), *The Changing Samoans: Behavior and health in transition*, Oxford University Press, New York. pp. 275–296.

Holmes, L.D. 1958. *Ta'u: Stability and change in the Samoan Village*. Polynesian Society Reprints No. 7. Wellington, New Zealand.

Holmes, L.D. 1974. *Samoan Village*. Holt, Rinehart & Winston, New York.

Karvonen, M.J., 1974. Work and activity classifications. In L.A. Larson (ed.), *Fitness, Health and Work Capacity*. MacMillan, New York. pp. 38–54.

Katch, F.I. and W. D. McArdle, 1983. *Nutrition, Weight and Exercise*. 2d ed. Lea and Febiger, Philadelphia.

Keesing, F.M. 1934. Samoa: Islands of conflict. *Foreign Policy Reports* 9, 293–304.

Kraemer, A. 1902. *Die Samoan-inseln*. vol. 1, 2, 3. E. Schweizerbart, Stuttgart.

Levin, M.J., and P.N.D. Pirie, 1974. *Report on the 1974 Census of American Samoa*. East West Population Institute, Honolulu.

Lockwood, B.A. 1971. *Samoan Village Economy*. Oxford Univ. Press, Melbourne.

Mead, M. 1969. *Social Organization of Manu'a*. 2d ed. Bernice P. Bishop Museum, Honolulu.

McGarvey, S.T. 1991. Obesity in Samoans and a perspective on its etiology in Polynesians. *American Journal of Clinical Nutrition* 53, 1586S–1594S.

McGarvey, S.T., J.R. Bindon, D.E. Crews and D.E. Schendel 1989. Modernization and adiposity: Causes and consequences. In M.A. Little and J.D. Haas (eds.), *Human Population Biology: A transdisciplinary science*. Oxford University Press, New York. pp. 263–279.

Pawson, I.G. 1986. The morphological characteristics of Samoan adults. In P.T. Baker, J.M. Hanna and T.S. Baker (eds.), *The Changing Samoans: Behavior and health in transition*, Oxford University Press, New York. pp. 254–274.

Pawson, I.G., and C.G. Janes, 1981. Massive obesity in a migrant Samoan population. *American Journal of Public Health* 71, 508–513.

Pearson, J.D. 1990. Estimation of energy expenditure in Western Samoa, American Samoa and Honolulu by recall interviews and direct observation. *American Journal of Human Biology* 2, 313–326.

Pelletier, D.L. 1987. The relationship of energy intake and expenditure to body fatness in Western Samoan men. *Ecology of Food and Nutrition* 19, 185–199.

Pelletier, D.L. 1988. The effects of occupation, leisure activities, and body composition on aerobic fitness in Western Samoan males. *Human Biology* 60, 889–899.

Pirie, P. 1970. Samoa: Two approaches to population and resource problems. In: W. Zellinsky, L. Kosinski and R.M. Prothero (eds.), *Geography and a Crowding World*. Oxford University Press, New York. pp. 493–508.

Prior, I.A. M. 1977. Nutrition problems in Pacific Islanders. *The 1976 Muriel Bell Memorial Lecture*. Nutrition Society of New Zealand, Wellington.

Schendel, D. 1988. Daily activity, energy intake and body composition among Western Samoans. *American Journal of Physical Anthropology* 75, 267 (abstract).

Stair, J.B. 1897. *Old Samoa, or Flotsam and Jetsam from the Pacific Ocean*. Religious Tract Society, London.

Stoudt, H., A. Damon and J. Roberts, 1965. Weight, height and selected body dimensions of adults, United States, 1960–1962. *Vital and Health Statistics*, Series 11, No. 8. U.S. Government Printing Office, Washington.

Stoudt, H., A. Damon and R.A. McFarland, 1970. Skinfolds, body girths, biacromial diameter and selected anthropometric indices of adults, United States, 1960–1962, *Vital and Health Statistics*, Series 11, No. 35. U.S. Government Printing Office, Washington.

Turner, G. 1884. *Samoa a Hundred Years Ago and Long Before*. Macmillan, London.

Watters, R.F. 1958. Cultivation in old Samoa. *Economic Geography* 34, 338–354.

——15——

Obesity and Fatness as seen by the Azande in Central Africa

ARMIN PRINZ

INTRODUCTION

The Azande are a farming and hunting population living at the Nile-Congo watershed in the corner between the boundaries of Sudan, Central African Republic and Zaire (*See* Map, Figure 1). They resisted European conquest as late as the beginning of this century. They have an exogamic clan organisation, with the exception of the chiefs and noblemen, who are members of the endogamic Avungara clan. Since about 1920 European influence, especially the work of Christian missionaries, has changed the tribal situation completely. Not only have traditional beliefs in witchcraft and sorcery, which had played an important role in stabilizing the society (Evans-Pritchard, 1937), been opposed, the whole social structure also has been nearly completely destroyed. One serious problem lies in the fact that the young people, educated in mission schools, are unwilling to take part in the necessary farm work. Influenced by their European training and education, they are drawn towards "modern" jobs and a "civilised" way of life. Many of them believe that such opportunities are only to be found in the cities, and thus, a great number of

Armin Prinz

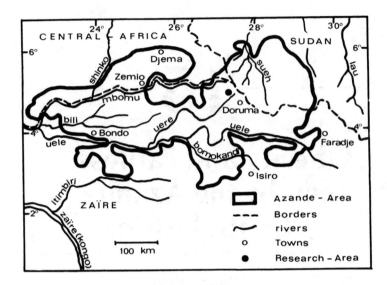

Figure 1. Map of south central Africa showing the location of the Azande people.

young people leave the tribal areas in order to look for work (usually unsuccessfully) away from home. In this way, they only strengthen the ranks of the uprooted and the unemployed urban proletariat and fall easy victims to alcoholism and crime. Yet, even those young people who remain in the tribal area after leaving school are frequently unwilling to take up "lowly" farm work to an adequate degree and prefer to be supported by their older relatives, who, however, are unable to produce sufficient food for everybody (Prinz, 1986).For this investigation I used an open-ended questionnaire. The answers were recorded on a tape recorder and translated later by native speakers into French. Altogether 43 men and 39 women were interviewed on their opinions on obesity.

NUTRITIONAL PROBLEMS

The Azande suffer from a considerable degree of infertility, which started after European conquest at the beginning of this century. Around 1955 the tribal population numbered about 700,000 persons, of which 450,000 inhabited Zaire, 200,000 the Sudan and 50,000 the

Central African Republic. According to my research, the population has been decreasing by approximately 2% per year, while female sterility amounts to 45%. The ratio of women capable of childbearing, which should be 100:140 to keep the population figures consistent, is here only 100:70 (Prinz, 1986).

Reasons for this development are given as widespread diseases such as venereal diseases, leprosy and sleeping sickness, increasing social disintegration, abortion, and rural exodus, as well as nutritional problems (Abbott, 1950; Retel-Laurentin, 1974; Farrell, 1954; have given these reasons.). Shortly before his death, Sir Edward Evans-Pritchard, the most distinguished ethnographer of the Azande, in a personal letter to the author, in 1972, called for urgent investigation into this problem, "...because, as you know, the interference with the traditional family life and the continued poverty of the manioc diet, make it hard to pinpoint the reasons for the extreme wane in population" (Evans-Pritchard, 1972).

The most serious nutritional problem of the Azande results from the increasing popularity of manioc. Although this starchy root was imported to Africa by the Portuguese beginning in the 16th century (Jones, 1959), it was introduced by the Europeans to the Azande as late as the 1920s. This has brought about a drastic deterioration in the nutrient content of Azande food, due to its lack of proteins and vitamins of the B-complex. Simple cultivation methods and the permanent availability of manioc have all but supplanted millet, the former diet staple of the Azande, which is rich in proteins and vitamins but requires intensive cultivation. In colonial times, manioc cultivation was purposely promoted by the authorities with a view to using the free labour capacity of the population in cotton plantations (Reining, 1966). The difficult nutritional situation is further exacerbated by the high prussic acid concentration in manioc, which could only be balanced by additional high sulphur-amino acid intake, since the organic sulphur contributes to rapid detoxification in the body via thiocyanate, which is easily excreted (Prinz, 1988).

The Azande have a high incidence of goitre, partially due to the lack of iodine in the food and partially to presence of thiocyanate, the sulphur salt of prussic acid, which is produced via manioc consumption. Up to 80% of the population, according to my own investigations of a sample of nearly 1,000 patients, are afflicted by goitre, which also significantly reduces fertility. Particularly, individuals suffering from congenital cretinism caused by a lack of iodine are considered to be sterile. As can be gathered from historical sources,

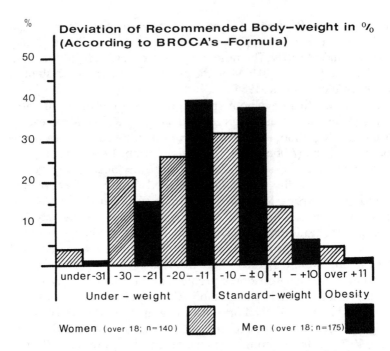

%

Deviation of Recommended Body–weight in %
(According to BROCA's –Formula)

| under-31 | -30 – -21 | -20 – -11 | -10 – ±0 | +1 – +10 | over +11 |

Under – weight   Standard–weight   Obesity

Women (over 18; n=140)   Men (over 18; n=175)

Figure 2. Deviation of recommended body weight of Azande adults in percent according to the formula of Broca[a].

[a]P.P.B. Broca was a French surgeon (ca. 1824–1880) and anthropologist, who introduced the formula centimeters/1 meter reduced by 10% for men, 15% for women, as the ideal weight. Thus a man with a body height of 180 cm (70.9 inches) would have an ideal weight of 72 kg (158.4 lbs.) and a woman 160 cm (63 inches) would have an ideal weight of 51 kg (112.2 lbs.).

goitres were practically unknown to the Azande only 60 years ago (Lagae and Vanden Plas, 1922). The development of this disease has been triggered not only by increased manioc consumption but also by a decrease of the traditional home-production of ash-salt, which prevents goitre, and the increased use of noniodised salt sold at the markets (Prinz, 1988).

The nutritional situation is furthermore exacerbated by an increase of alcoholism. This leads not only to negligence of the necessary farm work, but even the few high-quality cereals available are being used almost entirely for the production of beer and spirits, there being less available for general consumption (Prinz, 1986).

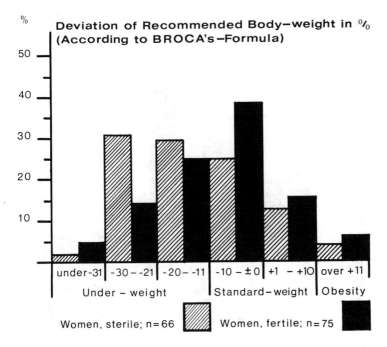

Figure 3. Deviation of recommended body weight of nonfertile and fertile Azande women in percent according to the formula of Broca[a].
[a]See Footnote a, Figure 2, for explanation of Broca's formula.

In accordance with the purpose of the present study, I will deal exclusively with the body weight of the Azande without referring more closely to qualitative aspects of their nutritional condition (see Figures 2 and 3). This study is based on data collected in the course of my own field work in the years 1984 and 1986 (Prinz, 1988).

The prevailing conditions are generally those of slight underweight and practically no obesity (see Figure 2). An interesting fact is that men are predominantly of average weight, while women tend more strongly to be either underweight or overweight. Yet the only two individuals more than 20% overweight (they are not presented separately in the diagram) were men, namely two influential and wealthy (by Azande standards) Avungara chiefs.

Comparing infertile with fertile women, one notices a significantly better nutritional condition in the latter (Figure 3). This also confirms

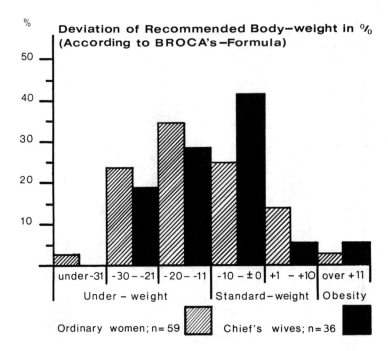

Figure 4. Deviation of recommended body weight of ordinary Azande women versus chiefs' wives according to the formula of Broca[a].
[a]See Footnote a, Figure 2, for explanation of Broca's formula.

the findings of fertility studies elsewhere in which anorexia is linked to an insufficiency of ovarian functions (Frisch, 1985). (It is noted that Frisch's hypothesis regarding the role of body fat in onset and mainte-nance of menstrual cycles has been questioned by others (Scott and Johnston, 1982).

The weight comparisons undertaken also point towards social dif-ferences. Chiefs' wives display considerably better health than women not married to chiefs (Figure 4). These weight comparisons show significant differences between the nutritional condition of vari-ous population groups. Although these differences are noticeable nei-ther to strangers nor to the Azande themselves, they do have an unequivocal bearing on the Azande ideas concerning obesity and the position that well-fed individuals enjoy amongst this ethnic commu-nity.

SOME ETHNOGRAPHIC REMARKS ON OBESITY

All enquiries relating to obesity proved a source of immense amusement to the persons approached. They could not believe that such a question might be of interest to a European ethnographer; especially so, as this person was quite obviously above average weight himself as compared to Central African standards, and because it was known from the author's previous stays with the Azande that he used his time then also for the purpose of reducing his own weight.

Consequently, it was somewhat difficult to obtain unbiased statements. To begin with, problems were involved in explaining what exactly constitutes obesity (overweight), as these people are generally undernourished and sometimes even individuals of average-weight are regarded as obese. Thus, it was necessary to explain obesity with the help of examples; and here, one could use two widely known prototypes: Chief Ukwatutu, an obese but greatly respected man who had died in 1979, on the one hand; and the hospital doctor of this area, a man who, though obese, was generally hated and did not come from this area but from the Kassi (from the Kassai province of Zaire). Whether the views on status and role of obese individuals in the community were couched in positive or negative terms seemed to depend also on the fact that the respondents were thinking of one or the other of these men as a model.

There was a similar pattern concerning women. For the quiet Azande women the doctor's wife, extremely obese and generally disliked, an always loudly voicerous Bantu woman, was contrasted strongly with the obese widow of a highly esteemed Azande merchant and ivory smuggler, a well-perfumed woman with gleaming skin who lived on a fine farm.

For a selection of typical answers to the questioning by men on fat men, men on fat women, women on fat women, and women on fat men *see* the Appendix.

EVALUATION

What is remarkable about these results is that men held a preponderance of negative views about fat men, while women held positive views about fat men and fat women. It seems evident that the reason for the men's negative view lies in a feeling of envy of the supposed wealth and obvious attractiveness of fat men for women.

The contradictory answers by average-weight persons to my open-

TABLE I. Azande men's opinions on obesity (n=43) (standard-weight, multiple answers)

Fat men		Fat women	
Shorter life	42	Indifferent[a]	37
Unhealthy	39	Lazy	36
Weak, bodily	35	Fertile	35
Wealthy	29	Shorter life	34
Ugly	27	Handsome	30
Weak, sexually	27	Strong bodily	26
Healthy	15	Sterile	19
Small penis	9	Good mother	15
No witch	5	Weak, bodily	14

[a]As partner.

ended interview questions made it difficult to evaluate their positions.

Thirty-nine of the 43 men queried believed that obesity in men was unhealthy, yet 11 of them stated that fat men were healthier than thin ones. Forty-three men (all those questioned) said that fat women were more fertile than thin ones, while 8 of them later stated the opposite.

These discrepancies arose from the conflicting positions taken vis-a-vis the reference prototypes mentioned above and also from the uncertainty by the persons questioned as to the criteria by which someone could be termed obese. The traits and characteristics that were most often mentioned by the Azande men in connection with obese persons were: shorter life for fat men and indifference or laziness for fat women. Women saw fat women as more fertile while they saw fat men as wealthy (see Tables I and II).

Men are indifferent about obese persons as sexual partners, in the sense of "I don't care how someone looks, what counts for me is personal attraction" (*see* the Appendix for comments by men on fat men). On the other hand, for women the idea of wealth and sexual prowess in their partner is stressed, putting the idea of personal affection only in third position.

Physical weakness is a trait considered typical of obese persons, but only by men questioned, and applied more frequently to men than to women. Sexual prowess is attributed to obese men solely by the women questioned, while men consider them sexually weak. Another classical demonstration of sexual envy can be identified in the frequently and strongly stated view of the men, that fat men possessed only a small penis.

Obesity is considered unhealthy for men by both men and women, although only the men attributed a shorter life expectancy to obese persons. The high value placed on fertility in this population, so afflicted by sterility, is expressed in a view maintained by both sexes, namely that obese women are more fertile than thin ones. This attitude almost automatically prevents obese women from being classified as unhealthy; to have many children is a mark of perfect health.

The laziness attributed to obese women by both women and men should not be regarded as an absolute negative classification. The term lazy is applied only to people who can afford financially, and who are widely respected, to employ helpers to do the everyday field and farm work.

However, the most interesting result of these interviews, from the ethnographer's point of view, lies in the fact that obese persons are not at all, or only very infrequently, regarded as witches. Only thin, emaciated individuals are considered dangerous in this sense, a point that seems not to have been noted, or at least commented on by Evans-Pritchard, as there is no reference to this in his comprehensive

TABLE II. Azande women's opinions on obesity (n=39) (standard-weight, multiple answers)

Fat women		Fat men	
Fertile	34	Wealthy	35
Lazy	29	Strong, sexually	31
No witch	26	Indifferent[a]	28
Wealthy	25	No witch	23
Healthy	22	Handsome	21
Strong, bodily	20	Unhealthy	14
Ugly	17	Strong, bodily	9
Strong sexually	11	Ugly	8
Handsome	8	Healthy	5

[a]As partner.

standard work on Azande witchcraft (Evans-Pritchard, 1937). The enormous potency of witchcraft, which is believed to be located in an organ in the upper part of the belly, is regarded as all-consuming, so that the people who possess such an organ have no extra energy left on put on weight.

To sum up, it can be said generally that obese persons enjoy a much higher social status with the Azande than in western societies. Poor nutrition and economic difficulties bring about this concept of obesity as a sign of success. What also contributes considerably to this positive view of obesity is the observation made by the Azande (correct in the sense of dietetics as well) that well-fed women are more fertile than badly nourished ones. This view is especially important, as this population is afflicted by an enormously high rate of sterility.

APPENDIX

Responses to questions regarding views of fat people

A selection of some typical answers:

MEN ON FAT MEN

"Fat men are weak. Therefore, they have a shorter life as well. But a better life, too; they are wealthy, have good food and several wives."

"Fat men are ugly but wealthy. Therefore they still have beautiful women. But these women aren't good women, they live with the fat men because they are wealthy, and cheat on them with young men to whom they give presents."

"They don't live long. It's not healthy to be fat, they have to make efforts to do even the simplest little things; even when they defecate they often break out in a sweat."

"Being fat is a sign of health in a sick man. Sick men are thin; you lose weight when you are ill."

"Fat men aren't handsome but good and friendly. They take care of their families and help their relatives if they are in trouble. They are not witches either, for *mangu* (witchcraft) consumes the body."

"I don't want to be fat. Fat men have only a small penis and can only rarely have intercourse with their wives. These women then sleep with other men and have children by them."

MEN ON FAT WOMEN

"The Azande love fat women. They've got to be strong; they must make it comfortable for their men during the nights, they've got to protect them from the cold, lie between them and the cold wall, cushion their heads in their arms. And fat women are good women, they aren't witches and mean no danger. They don't fly on trees to strike down other people with their flames (of witchcraft)."

"Fat women are lazy. They move slowly, are always sitting down and letting their husbands wait for their meals. There is never any water for washing in the house. But they make eyes at other men."

"My mother was a fat women. Her upper arm was as thick as my thigh; she always cooked good meals. For me and my brothers and sisters she was a good woman."

"People always say that fat women are lazy. But they've got to take care of a big household. They've got to determine who's going to do what work, where the new granary will be built, what field must be tilled. They are there to tell us what to do."

"A fat woman may or may not be a good women. I don't think it's a very healthy thing to be that fat. They have no strength, and they must make a lot of effort to do any kind of work. They sweat a lot and again lose a lot of strength with their sweat. Fat people have trouble breathing when they get older."

"Fat women are beautiful. I'd like to be with a fat women. Not too fat, but strong. Thus, I'd have strong children as well."

"I don't care whether a woman is fat or not. If I like her I will court her; the only thing that counts is that she's a good woman. What is important in a woman is her character."

"I'm interested in the sex I have with a woman, not in whether she's fat or not."

WOMEN ON FAT WOMEN

"They have a lot of children because they're healthy. Fat women are strong, and they love intercourse. A man needs a lot of strength if he's got a fat woman, but then again, she will take care of him."

"Fat women are lazy, but they're wealthy, too, they've got all they need, food, clothes and people working for them on the fields."

"You don't have to be afraid of fat women, they are not witches. But they do have magic powers, yet they won't harm you if you leave them in peace."

"Fat women eat a lot of vitamins: some of them are strong, some are weak. I'd rather stay thin, but it's up to God to decide whether we grow fat or not."

"A fat woman needs a man with a big penis, she can't have children by a man with a small one. They are good mothers and give their children a lot to eat, so they in turn become fat as well. Many fat women have children."

"Fat women have more children, thin women more miscarriages."

WOMEN ON FAT MEN

"Fat men are wealthy. And they can have a lot of women. Not only because they're wealthy but also because they have a lot of sexual prowess."

"I like fat men. They're respected. As the wife of a fat man you're respected as well. Fat men also look better, you like to feel them sleeping with you."

"If you like a man, he can be fat or thin, that doesn't matter."

"Fat men are ugly but wealthy. They can have a lot of women because many women think fine clothes are more important than love. I wouldn't want a fat man."

"It's a good thing to be the wife of a fat man. He's no witch and will protect his wife from other witches. You're well protected in a fat man's farm."

"I'd like to have a fat man; they're well off, strong and healthy. And I like them, they've got the better character. Also, they're esteemed, and even the chief will ask for their advice in important matters."

"Weight is no indicator of capability and fitness, sexual prowess is congenital and is not dependent on weight."

As mentioned above in the text, I am somewhat stout, too, and try to use my time in the field in order to lose weight. When I had proudly lost some 33 pounds (15 kg) due to a diet of manioc and termites and was already considering myself extremely attractive, an Azande woman of my acquaintance one day came up to me, full of regret, feeling very sorry for me, and said:

"My poor one, are you ill to lose such a lot of weight? You were so good-looking when you came three months ago. And now one can see the bones in your face, your ribs stick out, and your trousers are too big for you. I will bring you some good food every day, chicken and

rice, bananas and peanuts, so that you will again become healthy and strong."
At this moment my weight was still 178 pounds (80.9 kg) at a height of 5 feet 9 inches! (175 cm)

NOTES

Armin Prinz is a Lecturer in the Department of Medical Anthropology of the Institute for the History of Medicine of the University of Vienna, Vienna, Austria, and has a doctorate in medicine and philosophy.

REFERENCES

Abbot, P.H. 1950. A survey of signs of nutritional ill-health among the Azande of the southern Sudan. *Transactions Royal Society of Tropical Medicine and Hygiene* **43**, 477–492.

Evans-Pritchard, E.E. 1937. *Witchcraft, Oracle and Magic among the Azande.* Clarendon Press, Oxford.

Evans-Pritchard, E.E. 1972. Personal letter to the author. 15th March 1972. Personal Communication.

Farrell, McD.B.H. 1954. Death of children among the Azande. *Sudan Notes and Records* **35**(1), 7–19.

Frisch, R.E. 1985. Fatness, menarche, and female fertility. *Perspectives in Biology and Medicine* **28**(4), 611–633.

Jones, W.O. 1959. *Manioc in Africa.* Stanford University Press, Stanford, CA.

Lagae, C.R., and V.H. Vanden Plas 1922. *La langue des Azande.* Vol. II, *Dictionaire Francais-Zande.* "Goitre." Gand. Editions Vertias.

Prinz, A. 1986. Medizinanthropologische uberlegungen zum bevolkerungsruckgang bei den Azande Zentralafrikas. *Curare* **9**, 257–268.

Prinz, A. 1988. Le manioc en Afrique. Historie, toxicologie, ethnographie. *Al Biruniya. Review marture pharmacie* **4**, 45–65.

Reining, C.C. 1966. *The Zande Scheme.* Northwestern University Press, Evanston, IL.

Retel-Laurentin A. 1974. *Infecondié en Afrique noire.* Masson et Cie, Paris.

Scott, E.C., and F.E. Johnston 1982. Critical fat, menarche and the maintenance of menstrual cycles. A critical review. *Journal of Adolescent Health Care* **2**, 249–260.

—16—

Evaluation of Fatness in Traditional Japanese Society

NAOMICHI ISHIGE

Since the 1970s, the Japanese have generally regarded fatness as being unhealthy, and a plump figure has now become undesirable. But this was not always the case, for just as in Europe, until the nineteenth century, as well as even now in other parts of Asia, so too in Japan a "proper" degree of fatness was well-regarded.

Of course, even in the Japanese society of earlier centuries excessive fatness was regarded with derision, except that of the Sumo wrestler (*see* Chapter 2). People regarded it as a type of sickness. A story of an overweight aristocrat who was prescribed a strict diet by his doctor in *"Konjaku-monogatari-shu"* (Tales of Once-upon-a-time") and a portrait of a woman disabled by her excessive fatness in *"Yamai-no-soshi"* (A Story Book of Disease and Sickness), both from the 12th century, well reflect some degree of social awareness. However, the excessively fat person was a rarity in historical Japan, owing probably to the poor nutritional levels of most people. Further, in this respect, it should be noted that the consumption of the meat of terrestrial mammals was taboo, according to Buddhist tenets, that there was no tradition of eating dairy products, and that the use of vegetable oils was rare in traditional Japanese cuisine.

However, the evaluation of body figures has not been unchanging throughout the centuries. In Table I I have indicated broadly the transition in Japanese concepts from a traditional to a modern evaluation of body shapes.

I sought to combine an analysis of portraits in "*emaki*" and "*ukiyoe*," together with a perusal of Japanese literature after the 10th century A.D. "*Emaki*" are scroll paintings, which were popular between the 10th and the 17th centuries, and took the form of serial scenes, each with its own commentary, painted on a single scroll to tell a story. More than several dozen people of identifiable occupations from various social classes are commonly depicted in these works. Their number sometimes exceeds one hundred, and they offer reliable information on the then stereotypic physique of each social class. In my analysis, approximately fifty of these works were utilized. "*Ukiyoe*," a woodblock print of the Edo period (which lasted from the 17th to the 19th century) provides another useful resource. The most popular theme was a portrait accompanied with an explanatory title, although it comprised other features such as landscape, too. Research into body shape at that time, based on the evidence of "*ukiyoe*," has already been done (Araki, 1985).

Compared with these paintings and prints, traditional literature offers little information as to contemporary body shape, since authors were more preoccupied with the correct portrayal of their characters' psychological aspects than with the question of mere physique.

The analysis, concerning which I presented a monograph in Japanese explaining its detailed procedure (Ishige, 1989), reveals some general points regarding the evaluation of human body shapes in Japan (Table II) . For both males and females the desirable figure was plump and rotund. This was regarded as symbolizing health, beauty, satiation, wealth, membership in the upper classes, and generosity. In contrast, a skinny body was regarded as undesirable, since it symbolized unhealthiness, ugliness, hunger, poverty, membership in the lower classes and a narrow mind.

According to traditional concepts, the soul of males resided in the abdomen, and thus a big belly accommodated a big soul. On the other hand, a big belly on a woman was not well-regarded, since it conveyed the impression of pregnancy, as well as being unaesthetic. (Here I might digress to note that *seppuku*, or *harakiri*, as it is more commonly but erroneously termed, was regarded as the most honourable

TABLE I. Traditional versus current Japanese concepts of human body shape

Figure type	Traditional evaluation		Current evaluation
Extremely corpulent	Undesirable figure -----unhealthy	→	Undesirable figure ----unhealthy
Plump	Desirable figure---------healthy	→	Undesirable figure ----unhealthy
Normal	Ordinary figure---------healthy	→	Desirable figure -------healthy
Skinny	Undesirable figure -----unhealthy	→	Ordinary figure---------healthy

TABLE II. Traditional general Japanese concept of imputed personality characteristics and body shape

Figure	Imputed personal characteristics						
Plump	desirable	healthy	beauty	satiation	wealth	upper class	generosity
	↔	↔	↔	↔	↔	↔	↔
Skinny	undesirable	unhealthy	ugliness	hunger	poverty	lower class	narrow mind

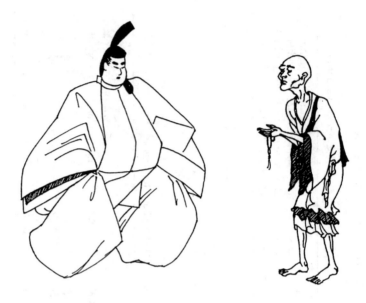

Figure 1. A plump noble and a skinny monk.

form of suicide, since by slitting the abdomen one exposed the pure soul (Chiba, 1971)).

However, as in some instances, in contrast to those general concepts mentioned above, a skinny body was desirable, as in the case of monks, shamans and ascetics (Figure l). A plump monk, for example, was thought of as being a priest of high rank, and would be a symbol of the high but degenerate authority which symbolizes the secular. As a result, it would have been thought that his personal religiousity was weak. In contrast, a skinny ascetic person symbolized holiness and saintliness, and was regarded as a person of "high voltage" religiosity (Figure 1; Table III).

Generally, in traditional Japanese society, a plump female was re- garded as beautiful, but from the latter half of the 18th century, in the cities, a slender woman became the symbol of beauty.

Such was the beauty depicted in *ukiyoe* paintings. The actual pro- portion of body length to face length at those times was 5:1, but that depicted in those paintings was 7 or 8:1 (Araki, 1985: 47). The typical *ukiyoe* beauty had small breasts and a "willow" waist. Thus the beauty of the *ukiyoe* was only an idealized form that was rarely, if ever, found

TABLE III. Characteristics traditionally associated with body shapes among priests in Japan

Figure	Associated characteristics		
Plump	secularity	authority	degeneracy
	$\updownarrow$	$\updownarrow$	$\updownarrow$
Skinny	holiness	saintless	asceticism

among ordinary people. Judging from the faces of the *ukiyoe* beauties, and as verified by physical anthropological research, the women depicted were modelled on the wives of aristocrats (Suzuki, 1983: 205). From a modern perspective such *ukiyoe* beauties are too slender, too contrived, and too sexually neutral. And such a figure is now regarded as being extremely unhealthy.

In considering the basis on which such idealized concepts of beauty were founded, the role of the *kimono* costume requires brief discussion, since the form of the *kimono* changed from the 18th century.

In contrast to the idealized beauty of bodily proportions symbolized in the statues of Ancient Greece, for example, that of traditional Japan was based on a body style resulting when wearing the *kimono*. So, in Japan, unlike Europe, it was not the costume that revealed the beautiful bodily proportion, but, rather, that a well–proportioned body provided the props for displaying perfectly a gorgeous *kimono*. Whereas in Europe the costume served the body, in Japan *vice versa*, the body served the costume.

From the 17th century to the early part of the 18th, a major change occurred in Japanese female costume. In the medieval period the lower part of the body was fully enveloped in either voluminous pantaloons or a large, single enveloping piece of cloth. But from the 17th century that gave way to a one piece *kimono* covering both the upper and lower torso, and closed by a belt, called an *obi* (Figure 2).

At first the *obi* was narrow and was tied in front. But by the early 18th century the *obi* had become an art form, and it increased in width more than 20 cm, when folded. Thus women came to wear the *kimono* simply as a background on which to display their increasingly ornate *obi*. To display the *obi* more beautifully it also came to be tied at the back, thus covering the posterior.

To provide a perfect platform for displaying an *obi* without ugly

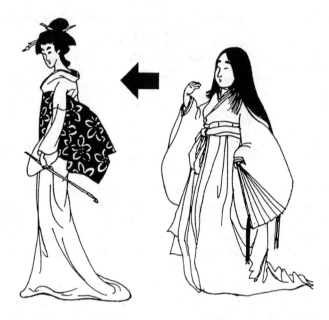

Figure 2. Lady's costume in Medieval period (right) and one-piece *kimono* in the Edo period.

bulges, a flat breast and flat posterior were those attributes of bodily shape deemed most desirable. This type of figure is known as *yanagi-goshi*, or "willow waist," and symbolized elegance, beauty, enjoyment, and the urban environment. On the contrary, a "pigeon breast" and a protruding rump symbolized rurality and barbarousness, and were considered undesirable.

Nevertheless, such ideal beauty, although aesthetically appealing, was not regarded as making for a good wife. It was thought of as being consumptive, not good for child–bearing, and of giving the image of a "tubercular type" of person (Table IV). Regardless of those negative impressions, however, that image of ideal beauty persisted until the 20th century.

In the case of males, the *obi* was narrower, and was tied under the navel. Thus a protruding belly (like mine) was regarded as the ideal type for wearing the *kimono* (Figure 3).

During the American Occupation of Japan (1945–53) the evaluation of female bodily shape changed drastically, as people switched to

TABLE IV. Characteristics traditionally associated with body shapes of women in Japan after the 18th century

Figure	Associated characteristics					
Plump	pigeon breast & protruding rump	↔ barbarousness	↔ ugliness	↔ toil	↔ rural	↔ healthy
Slender	willow waist	↔ elegance	↔ beauty	↔ enjoyment	↔ urban	↔ unhealthy

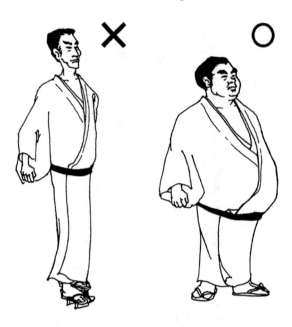

Figure 3. The ideal body figure for wearing the male *kimono*.

wearing mostly western costume. The "glamour girl" type, with big breasts and well–rounded hips, became idealized.

The ideal bodily shape since then has been strongly influenced by the dictates of western fashion. During the 1960s, long-limbed physique became the ideal one for miniskirt fashions, even in Japan. From the 1970s onwards, a strong American influence in favour of a healthy lifestyle gave a final blow to the traditional affirmative consensus towards the plump male physique which had long symbolized wealthy status. It is now regarded as being unhealthy.

The Roher's index which determines a standard weight from correlation between weight and height was applied to data collected in the Tokyo area in 1984 by the Metropolitan Government. It revealed that 18% of the population, regardless of sex, was classified as overweight. People, however, showed greater concern for their excess weight than the statistical evidence suggested. According to self-evaluation data which were collected at the same time, 24% of male and 34% of female respondents were conscious of their weight (Tokyo-to Seikatsubunka-Kyoku, 1984: 21–23). These higher figures, especially among women, seem to imply not only increasing awareness of health among people generally, but also a contemporary public consensus which regards plump physique as undesirable from an aesthetic point of view.

NOTES

Dr. Naomichi Ishige is Professor and Director of the Second Research Department, National Museum of Ethnology, Osaka, Japan. He has a Bachelor's degree in Archeology from Kyoto University and a doctorate in agriculture from Tokyo Agricultural University. His research specialities are cultural anthropology and food culture of Asia. He has published about 20 books in Japanese on Asian food culture, and has done field work in New Guinea, Southeast Asia, China, Korea, and East and North Africa.

REFERENCES

Araki, Y. 1985. Ukioe-nimiru shintaikan-nituite (On a view of the body observed in "*Ukiyoe*"), *Aobagakuen Tankidaigaku Kiyoo* 10, Tokyo.

Chiba, T. 1971. Seppukuko-shou (Psychological analysis on Hara-kiri or self-disembowelment), *Kikan-jinnruigaku* 2(2), Tokyo.

Ishige, N. 1989. Yanagigoshi to decchiri (Willow waist and broad hips), *Kikan-jinnruigaku* 20(3). Tokyo.

Suzuki, H. 1983. *Hone-karamita nihonjin-no ruutu* (Osteological Characteristics of Japanese People and their Origins.) Iwanami-shoten, Tokyo.

Tokyoto-Seikatbuna Yoku 1984. Tominno-kenkonikannsuru-seronchosa (A poll on health awareness of the Metropolitan citizens), Tokyo-to, Tokyo.

17

Social Aspects of
Obesity and Fatness:
A Critique

STANLEY J. ULIJASZEK

Obesity has been described as a culture-bound syndrome (Ritenbaugh, 1982), and this is a theme that recurs throughout this volume. Usage of the terms obesity and fatness is important, since, taken collectively, the authors present, among other things, a cross-cultural overview of perceptions of obesity, fatness and large body size, and desirable body image, health and healthiness, and the impact of modernization on all of these. Obesity, fatness and large body size are terms which vary in the degree to which they describe a desirable or undesirable, healthy or unhealthy state, while health and perceptions of healthiness can vary across cultures and time. And while placing the analysis of change in these factors in the context of modernization, this process varies from place to place and is not uniform in its biological and social effects.

It is instructive to look at the usage of the terms obesity and fatness in a society that underwent modernization in the 19th century, England. The Oxford English Dictionary definition of obesity is "eating to fatness," while fatness has a number of descriptions, including "well supplied with what is needful or desirable" (1563), "plenty, su-per-abundance" (1570), "self complacent" (1588). Only more recent definitions give both positive and negative definitions: "in well-fed condition," as against "corpulent, and dense" (Little, Fowler and Coulson, 1987). Thus, the language of body size and shape is also culture bound, and subject to change; Pollock rightly cites Turner (1984), who states that "obesity is the effect of language and ideas on our bodies." In England, the positive sense with which body fatness was perceived in the past has been displaced by a negative one. This is a theme common to a number of papers in this volume, notably those by van Otterloo, for the Netherlands, Wilson, for Malaysians, and Bindon and Greksa, for Samoa. Thus, as populations modernise, perceptions of body fatness may change.

Authors of various chapters define obesity in different ways, while others use the terms fatness, or large body size, as less negatively oriented terms. However, most of these definitions overlap. Perhaps the best definitions of obesity are those offered by Scrimshaw and Dietz, in their evaluation of the potential advantages and disadvantages of obesity; a social definition is one of fatness beyond the socially accepted norms for a given society, while a medical definition relates to individuals who weigh more than the upper acceptable limit for their height and frame. Although their medical definition relies on actuarial information in the form of United States life assurance statistics, there are many other definitions which rely on other reference data, including body mass index for adults (Garrow, 1988) and children (Rolland-Cachera et al., 1982). However defined, health risks associated with obesity are quite clear: although high blood pressure, raised concentration of plasma low-density cholesterol and a low concentration of high-density cholesterol fractions are all important risk factors for heart disease, weight gain makes these factors worse, and weight loss makes them better, in both men and women (Garrow, 1993). However, these relationships may differ across populations, since if the thrifty genotype hypothesis of Neel (1962) holds true, it is possible there may also be population genetic components to cholesterol metabolism. It has been proposed that apolipoprotein gene alleles that segregate with the inheritance of coronary heart disease may allow prediction from an early age of those individuals predisposed to premature atherosclerosis (Galton, 1987).

The social definition of obesity also varies across societies and time, since although fatness is symbolically linked to psychological dimensions such as self-worth and sexuality, the nature of that symbolic association is not constant (Brown and Konner, 1987). This is made clear by various authors in this volume: Ossipow talks of Swiss vegetarians who are disgusted by omnivores who are fat because they present a "dirty" body which has been poisoned by meat, while in Holland, van Otterloo describes differences in ideal body image between working class and middle class mothers. Pollock describes the positive value with which body fatness is regarded in many traditional societies, and more specifically, de Garine writes that among the Massa of Northern Cameroon and Chad, large body size and weight is associated with strength and prosperity, power and majesty, although obesity and ideal body shape are viewed differently by different people. Brink reports that the Annang of Nigeria value "a woman of substance," while Prinz finds that views about obesity among the Azande of Zaire, Sudan and Central African Republic differ by gender: although obese women were considered in a positive light by both men and women, obese males were viewed negatively by other men, but positively by women. Village-dwelling Malays, reports Wilson, find "plump to be pretty, thin to be ugly." That perception of obesity can change across time is made clear in the chapters by Teti and Ishige, respectively. In Calabria, South Italy, fatness was a model to be attained for the undernourished poor of urban centers during the late 19th century and first half of the 20th century, while in contrast the thin person was perceived as a worrying figure, both threatening and dangerous, to the better nourished. In Japan, plump females were considered desirable by males prior to the second half of the 18th century, while after this time, a slender figure became the symbol of beauty, at least in the cities.

Traditional positive perceptions of obesity and fatness are easy to understand: such societies experienced food shortages and uncertainty of food supply, and individuals with larger, fatter body size represent variously success, better reproductive performance, higher social status, and better survivability in times of shortages. Scrimshaw and Dietz point out the advantages of body fatness in buffering adversity and promoting reproductive success; indeed, the energy store represented by body fat in a normal woman is about equivalent to the energy cost of a pregnancy. Cultural elaboration of the desirability of fatness in the form of ritual fattening practices is described by several authors. Notably, de Garine points to the symbolic importance of this practice among Massa males for the community as a whole, in coping with a highly seasonal often marginal subsistence environment. In Nauru, food supplies are irregular, and Pollock gives a dual focus for the traditional fattening of young females both of which are related to reproductive performance; they nurtured the strength of the young woman at the time when she was becoming an adult, and supported her role in the creation of new life in a community that felt demographically challenged. Elsewhere, Brink describes ritual fattening of Annang women in Nigeria, and how it is perceived to enhance fertility. The Azande of Central Africa are demographically challenged, and Prinz demonstrates that obesity is associated with greater fertility in this group. He reports high levels of infertility related to undernutrition, in a population that is declining in number. For the Azande, obesity is also associated with higher social status. A theme alluded to in many of these chapters is the cultural elaboration of positively attributed fatness; this is considered in some detail by Hattori, who reports on social perception of fatness among Sumo wrestlers in Japan.

The change to more negative perceptions of obesity in industrialised and modernising societies is less easy to understand. Chapters by Bindon, Greksa, Pollock, Wilson, Ishige and Teti discuss obesity in the context of modernization, either directly or indirectly. Comparisons across cultures are made difficult by differences in the process and rate of modernization across societies. In the developed world, the term modernization encompasses all the developments which followed in the wake of industrialisation and mechanisation, and include the loosening of boundaries between social classes, increased social mobility, as well as the growth of wide-spread education, the evolution of procedures of industrial negotiation, and the development of social welfare systems at the national and regional level. These things have happened in most western nations, as their populations underwent the transition from a predominantly agricultural mode of subsistence, to one of wage-earning within an industrialised cash-based economy. The experiences of the newer nation states becoming independent in the twentieth century are quite different from those of western nations which underwent their industrial revolutions in the 18th century. In this context, modernization has been defined as the interaction of less complex energetic, technological and socioeconomic systems characterized by regional production and consumption with contemporary economic systems of industrial technology influences by the national and international market, social and political factors (McGarvey, 1989). Thus, the changes in body size, shape, health and disease risk must be considered in relation to changes in lifestyle and perception associated with the particular set of social and economic changes in any group, community or population.

Pollock describes the cultural importance of food in Nauru society, and the way that puberty ceremonies and fattening processes diminish in importance with new forms of social differentiation, which included cash income and education. However, food as a mark of prestige persisted through a period of introduction of new foods that were energy dense and high in simple carbohydrates. With epidemiological evidence of very high levels of non–insulin dependent diabetes mellitus (NIDDM), the process of modernization seems to have created a contradiction for the Nauruans, who maintain an identity in which food sharing and consumption are very important, but are faced with "the slur of obesity," which they are told, makes them unhealthy. It would be interesting to know if the potential stress associated with this contradiction has health implications. Bindon describes obesity and overweight as biological adjustments to modernization among Samoan populations, showing women to have become more obese than males in the course of this process. Bindon suggests that this gender difference can be largely attributed to gender differences in changing work patterns, women initially becoming less active, but men retaining higher levels of activity despite changes in occupation. Greksa tests Bindon's assertion by examining the impact of modernization on physical activity levels in Samoan men and women. He finds that the increase in body weight across time must be due to both increased dietary energy intake and reduced output. In Malaysia, Wilson finds that between 1968/9 and 1984, changes in food resources of villagers toward greater availability of commercial foodstuffs, increased income, and reduced physical activity led to an increase in the number of overweight individuals, and greater concern about obesity, as a consequence of exposure to western views on this matter.

The chapters by Bindon, Pollock, and Wilson refer to Neel's (1962) "thrifty genotype" hypothesis when explaining relationships between obesity and NIDDM in Pacific Island and Malay populations respectively. Although this is plausible, an alternative explanation in the form of the so-called "thrifty phenotype" hypothesis has been put forward by Hales and Barker (1992). In this, a relationship is proposed between impaired development of the pancreas in the undernourished fetus and the development of NIDDM. The postulated mechanism is illustrated in Figure 1. Briefly, the authors' speculation is that maternal malnutrition and/or other maternal placental ab-

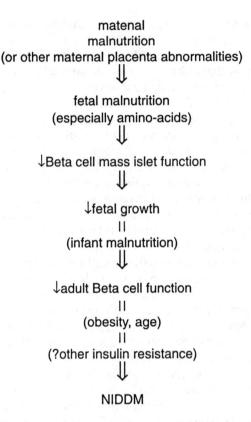

matenal
malnutrition
(or other maternal placenta abnormalities)
⇩

fetal malnutrition
(especially amino-acids)
⇩

↓Beta cell mass islet function
⇩

↓fetal growth
‖
(infant malnutrition)
⇩

↓adult Beta cell function
‖
(obesity, age)
‖
(?other insulin resistance)
⇩

NIDDM

Figure 1. "Thrifty phenotype" hypothesis: non-insulin-dependent diabetes mellitus (Hales & Barker, 1992).

normalities lead to fetal malnutrition. The consequences of a generalised undernutrition include reduced fetal growth, and a postulated reduced beta cell-mass and islet function of the pancreas. Deficiencies of protein and amino acids are believed to be of particular importance in creating these defects of structure and function. The authors suggest that impaired beta-cell function persists into adulthood, predisposing the individual to non-insulin dependent diabetes mellitus. This disease then expresses itself in association with environmental risk factors, obesity and physical inactivity in particular, as well as increasing age, and possibly other processes leading to insulin resistance. In the context of the populations described in this volume, all but one have undergone modernization in recent times, and the possibility that the "thrifty phenotype" may explain the rise in NIDDM incidence cannot be discounted. Longitudinal studies of NIDDM incidence across the next generation will help resolve the issue. However, Pollock reports that obesity was already prevalent at the time of European contact, when diabetes was supposed absent, while the prevalence of diabetes began to increase some way in the course of modernization, suggesting that the "thrifty phenotype" is unlikely to occur in this population.

Modernization has taken place in the industrialised nations, and is underway in most populations of the developing world. However, the former second-world countries of the Eastern bloc are in a rather ambiguous position in relation to theory about modernization, obesity, and disease. The course of modernization in countries like Czechoslovakia and Poland has been very different from elsewhere in the world, and the articles by Parizkova and Charzewska give valuable data about the prevalence of obesity in these countries. Charzewska rightly criticizes existing medical definitions of obesity as being "so vague as to be arbitrary." However, some measure of overweight or fatness is needed for any cross-cultural comparison of this condition, as viewed from a medical perspective. Interestingly, Charzewska attributes different trends in the relationship between social class and obesity to the different definitions of obesity used in the different studies she reports. However, it is also possible that the 1976–9 population, with higher levels of obesity in the higher socioeconomic groupings than in the lower ones, exhibited a pattern which may have reflected positive cultural and social attributes associated with fatness. The social distribution of obesity in Poland prior to the economic transition of the early 1980s is similar to that found in countries prior to, or early in the process of modernization. It would be interesting to know what the social perceptions of obesity were in the 1970s, and whether they have changed since the early 1980s.

The relationship between medically defined obesity and morbidity risk is addressed by most authors. Although association between body fatness, body composition, fat patterning and risk of coronary heart disease and NIDDM have been clearly demonstrated (Garrow, 1993), these relationships vary across populations, and are made complicated by environmental factors associated with different levels of modernisation. Leonetti and colleagues offer an intriguing theory suggesting that stress may be an important intervening factor. They propose that a neuroendocrine link between stress and day-to-day levels of adrenaline may play an intermediate role in fat distribution, and the morbidity risk associated with it, based on a study of American born sons of immigrants from Japan. It can be speculated that in addition to the stress associated with modernization-driven change, changes in the social perception of obesity may also be stressful, and carry a health risk. Leonetti et al.'s work could be extended to consider other modernising populations who face a contradiction between their traditional perceptions of obesity and the "modern" medically-oriented view of obesity as an unhealthy condition.

The relationships between social and biological definitions and perceptions of obesity and fatness in a number of culturally distinct populations show clear patterns: 1) obesity and fatness are usually desirable in the context of general food shortage or uncertainty; 2) this desirability is elaborated in fattening rituals which may have both biological and psychological importance for the whole community in their coping with low food availability; and 3) social desirability of fatness and obesity is usually reversed in the course of modernization, when large body size and fatness become available to all, and the health effects of obesity become apparent. There are exceptions to these generalisations, and a number of these are given in this volume. Furthermore, gender differences in the perception and prevalence of obesity exist and are clearly demonstrated by various authors.

NOTES

Dr. Stanley J. Ulijaszek is a physical anthropologist in the Department of Biological Anthropology of Cambridge University, Cambridge, England, whose research interests include cultural as well as environmental effects of diet change on human adaptation, biological and social. Much of his research has been on traditional populations of Papua, New Guinea. He is author, together with Dr. Simon Strickland, of a recent book exploring the roles of nutrition and the ecology on human evolution and adaptation, Nutritional Anthropology. Prospects and Perspectives.

REFERENCES

Brown, P.J. and M. Konner 1987. An anthropological perspective on obesity. In Human Obesity, R.J. Wurtman and J.J. Wurtman (eds.). New York: New York Academy of Sciences. pp. 29–46.

Galton, D.J. 1987. The genetics of atherosclerosis. *Proceedings of the Nutrition Society*, **46**, 337–43.

Garrow, J.S. 1988. *Obesity and Related Diseases*. Churchill Livingstone, Edinburgh.

Garrow, J.S. 1993. Obesity. In *Human Nutrition and Dietetics*, J.S. Garrow and W.P.T. Jame, (eds.). Churchill Livingstone, Edinburgh. pp. 465–79.

Hales, C.N. and D.J. Barker 1992. Type 2 (non-insulin-dependent) diabetes mellitus: The thrifty phenotype hypothesis. *Diabetologia*, **35**, 595–601.

Little, W., H.W. Fowler, and J. Coulson 1987. *The Shorter Oxford English Dictionary, on Historical Principles*. Clarendon Press, Oxford.

McGarvey, S.T. 1989. Five-year longitudinal changes in fatness and blood pressure in American Samoa. *American Journal of Anthropology*, **78**, 269–70.

Ritenbaugh, C. 1982. Obesity as a culture bound syndrome. *Culture, Medicine and Psychiatry*, **6**, 347–61.

Rolland-Cachera, M.F., M. Sempé, M. Guilloud-Bataille, E. Patois, F. Péquignot-Guggenbuhl, and V. Fautrad 1982. Adiposity indices in children. *American Journal of Clinical Nutrition*, **36**, 178–84.

Turner, B.S. 1984. *The Body and Society. Explorations in Social Theory*. Basil Blackwell, Oxford.

——18——

Social Aspects of Obesity and Fatness: Conclusion

CAROLE M. COUNIHAN

This volume offers a welcome perspective on fatness and obesity across cultures. It presents rich and varied data about how human beings relate to large bodies in many different social settings. The volume is particularly useful for readers interested in addressing four important questions. First, the volume offers data to enable us to think about the relationship between "modernization"—social and economic development—and obesity. Several papers—those by Pollock, Teti, Wilson, Bindon, and Greksa—suggest that as traditional agricultural populations begin to eat more processed foods and be engaged in wage as opposed to subsistence labor, they develop proclivities for obesity. The papers offer reflections on how this fattening will affect the health, aesthetic standards, and fertility of these populations.

Several of the papers offer material to enable readers to think directly about the long-term cross-cultural relationship between body weight, gender, fertility, and beauty ideals. De Garine's fascinating paper on the *guru* describes a case where men are fattened to achieve beauty and desirability prior to marriage, whereas Brink's, Prinz's,

301

302 Carole M. Counihan

and Pollock's articles focus on the fattening of women. Readers can use these data to ponder the adaptive effects of using resources to fatten men vs. women and the prestige that accrues to the fat body in cultures where reproduction is highly valued and potentially problematic due to periodic undernutrition.

Many of the papers provide data for examining gender relations in the context of body size and aesthetics. Ishige's and Hattori's papers examine Japanese body ideals and provide a context for understanding the value on the huge body of Sumo wrestlers in a culture where the usual ideal for body beauty is slim and slight. Bindon's article also considers the significance of gender in the trend towards obesity among modernizing Samoans. Ossipow's paper on vegetarianism is suggestive of gender significance in its recognition that many vegetarians are female. Readers interested in the "tyranny of thinness" oppressing women in western culture will find the papers by Charzewska, van Otterloo, and Parízková interesting in offering further data on cultures where thinness is highly valued and fatness disdained.

Several papers offer insights into the health effects of obesity that provide a helpful context for evaluating social attitudes towards fat. Scrimshaw and Dietz's article is a useful review of the literature on the advantages and disadvantages of human obesity. Leonetti *et al.* give a sharply focused treatment of some of the neuroendocrinological consequences of obesity. Taken in conjunction with Parízková's and Charzewska's biosocial perspectives, these papers offer readers a broad understanding of how physical and cultural forces interact in determining the health and psychological consequences of being fat.

For western readers, there is an innate fascination in reading a collection of papers that surveys the meaning and experience of obesity in an array of cultures. For in western society, obesity is unequivocally negative: in terms of aesthetics, morality, and health. It is enlightening to learn that in some cultures fat is beautiful for both women and men, that fat is valued for conveying fertility or denoting wealth, that fat results from leisure or an easier life, and that fat does not always represent evil, ugliness and sloth. In providing alternative meanings of obesity, the volume takes us a step closer towards a more effective critical understanding of our own beliefs about fat. Is fat really as bad as we make it out to be? Why do we load it with so much negative weight? What do western attitudes about obesity tell us about our culture? This volume makes a valuable contribution to understanding ourselves as well as to the literature on obesity.

NOTES

Carole M. Counihan is an Associate Professor in the Department of Sociology/Anthropology of Millersville University, Millersville, Penssylvania. Her PhD is from the University of Massachusetts, Amherst, and her research interests include gender, food and culture, world hunger and social change.

INDEX